MEDICAL AND CARE COMPUNETICS 2

Studies in Health Technology and Informatics

This book series was started in 1990 to promote research conducted under the auspices of the EC programmes Advanced Informatics in Medicine (AIM) and Biomedical and Health Research (BHR), bioengineering branch. A driving aspect of international health informatics is that telecommunication technology, rehabilitative technology, intelligent home technology and many other components are moving together and form one integrated world of information and communication media.

The complete series has been accepted in Medline. In the future, the SHTI series will be available online.

Volume 114

Recently published in this series

Vol. 113. J.S. Suri, C. Yuan, D.L. Wilson, S. Laxminarayan (Eds.), Plaque Imaging: Pixel to Molecular Level
Vol. 112. T. Solomonides, R. McClatchey, V. Breton, Y. Legré, S. Nørager (Eds.), From Grid to Healthgrid
Vol. 111. J.D. Westwood, R.S. Haluck, H.M. Hoffman, G.T. Mogel, R. Phillips, R.A. Robb, K.G. Vosburgh (Eds.), Medicine Meets Virtual Reality 13
Vol. 110. F.H. Roger France, E. De Clercq, G. De Moor and J. van der Lei (Eds.), Health Continuum and Data Exchange in Belgium and in the Netherlands – Proceedings of Medical Informatics Congress (MIC 2004) & 5th Belgian e-Health Conference
Vol. 109. E.J.S. Hovenga and J. Mantas (Eds.), Global Health Informatics Education
Vol. 108. A. Lymberis and D. de Rossi (Eds.), Wearable eHealth Systems for Personalised Health Management – State of the Art and Future Challenges
Vol. 107. M. Fieschi, E. Coiera and Y.-C.J. Li (Eds.), MEDINFO 2004 – Proceedings of the 11th World Congress on Medical Informatics
Vol. 106. G. Demiris (Ed.), e-Health: Current Status and Future Trends
Vol. 105. M. Duplaga, K. Zieliński and D. Ingram (Eds.), Transformation of Healthcare with Information Technologies
Vol. 104. R. Latifi (Ed.), Establishing Telemedicine in Developing Countries: From Inception to Implementation
Vol. 103. L. Bos, S. Laxminarayan and A. Marsh (Eds.), Medical and Care Compunetics 1
Vol. 102. D.M. Pisanelli (Ed.), Ontologies in Medicine

ISSN 0926-9630

Medical and Care Compunetics 2

Edited by

Lodewijk Bos

ICMCC President, The Netherlands

Swamy Laxminarayan

Institute of Rural Health & Biomedical Research Institute, Idaho State University, USA

and

Andy Marsh

VMW Solutions, UK

IOS Press

Amsterdam • Berlin • Oxford • Tokyo • Washington, DC

ISBN 1-58603-520-7
Library of Congress Control Number: 2005926528

Publisher
IOS Press
Nieuwe Hemweg 6B
1013 BG Amsterdam
Netherlands
fax: +31 20 620 3419
e-mail: order@iospress.nl

Distributor in the UK and Ireland
IOS Press/Lavis Marketing
73 Lime Walk
Headington
Oxford OX3 7AD
England
fax: +44 1865 750079

Distributor in the USA and Canada
IOS Press, Inc.
4502 Rachael Manor Drive
Fairfax, VA 22032
USA
fax: +1 703 323 3668
e-mail: iosbooks@iospress.com

PRINTED IN THE NETHERLANDS

dti

International Federation for Medical and Biological Engineering

IFMBE

IEEE

Information Society
Technologies

Society on Social Implications of Technology

Board Lists

Virtual Hospital Chair
Dr Georgi Graschew
Charité – University Medicine Berlin, Germany

HIV and ICT chair
Murdo Bijl
Health Connections International, The Netherlands

Event Advisory Board
as of April 1, 2005

Contents

Symposium on Imaging

Symposium on Telehomecare

Symposium on Information/Knowledge Management

Medical and Care Compunetics 2
L. Bos et al. (Eds.)
IOS Press, 2005

ICMCC
The Information Paradigm

Lodewijk BOS, Swamy LAXMINARAYAN and Andy MARSH
Members of the Board, ICMCC Council

1. Introduction

Business-to-business (B2B) and Business-to-Customer (B2C) approaches have been considered to be sound practices in the application of ICT (Information and Communication Technology) in commerce and industry.

In the medical and care arena, these concepts have not yet been common practice. But with the enormous explosion of heterogeneous information modalities in health care, the need for applying such concepts is essential. However despite the limited research done so far in evaluating the possible effects, it is to be expected, that these practices will bring forth significant benefits to both the medical and care professionals and the consumer/patients.

2. ICMCC 2004, the History

In September 2004 the International Council on Medical and Care Compunetics (ICMCC) was founded to create the infrastructure necessary for the B2B and B2C concepts in the medical and care domains. The creation of the council was a logical consequence of the first ICMCC Event held in The Hague, in June 2004 [1].

New and innovative in its format, the 2004 Event was an off-shoot of ideas that were put together in April 2003 to emphasize the computing and networking synergies in medicine and (health) care. The term *Compunetics* was coined to represent the union of the latter. Contrary to the traditional *sessions-oriented* conferences, ICMCC 2004 represented a meeting created around a cluster of special workshops in closely interrelated areas of compunetics. The Call for Workshops resulted in 18 workshops of either half a day or a full day. People from all over the world including Europe, USA, South America, and Israel participated in the workshops. Conference participants came from 26 different countries, as far away as Taiwan and Australia.

It became apparent during the preparation of the 2004 Event and more so at the event itself, that a platform for information in all its functionalities is desperately needed. As was to be expected with such a broad range of areas being addressed, the moments of discovery of similarity in the use of ICT between the various fields were revealing. At these instances the "syndrome" of the reinvention of the wheel became apparent.

3. ICMCC, the Council

The concepts that initiated the 2004 Event became the starting points of the newly founded Council, a central place where as many aspects of medical and care ICT and networking (compunetics) could come together in many different ways. Out of that concept, the following goals emerged:

3.1. Goals

The central objective of ICMCC is to create a global technology based knowledge infrastructure that serves as:

1. a global knowledge (transfer) centre
2. a centre of expertise
3. an information dissemination platform
4. a center of excellence
5. an incubator, and
6. an innovation exhibition

3.2. Global Knowledge Centre

Organizations like Healthwise in the US (www.healthwise.org) with its millions of users per year show the necessity as well as the benefit of delivering appropriate information to patients/consumers. According to its CEO, Don Kemper, "Consumers …. helped save between $7,5 million and $21,5 million by avoiding unnecessary ER and doctor office visits" [2].

The availability of information works on both the B2B and the B2C level, as the structure will aim at both the professionals (caregivers) and the consumer. Professionals will be able to find relevant information (medical, technical, scientific) in a fast and efficient way. Industry (and more specifically SME's) will have access to technical information from a central portal. Patients/consumers will be able to obtain information related to their illness or handicaps such that they will be more knowledgeable about possible treatments and treatment alternatives. The shifting paradigm of health from reparative to preventive will enhance the necessity of consumer related information, that, when efficiently obtained, can be of great economical benefit.

In a world where the need for care is growing rapidly and where it is impossible to expect a growth in the number of caregivers, information is becoming more and more crucial. Not only because an informed patient is an economic benefit, as said before, but also because awareness amongst professionals about developments in their own and related fields can save enormous amounts of money. An example is the field of telehomecare in Europe. A growing number of projects can be found both regionally and nationally. Since most of these projects do not know of each other's existence, almost all of them follow, up to a large extent, similar protocols. Centrally available information might help to save considerable amounts of funding, because the previously mentioned reinvention of the wheel can be minimized.

The knowledge centre will be realized as a system of systems.

3.3. Centre of Expertise

ICMCC will build a global network of professionals in medicine and care. Clinicians, pharmacologists, managers, care practitioners, patients, policy makers, IT specialists, all will be represented on national and international levels within the ICMCC organization, thus providing the world with an important network structure that can be used for advisory and counseling purposes.

3.4. Dissemination Platform

Fundamental to the structure of ICMCC is the dissemination of information. There is a need for a central platform for many organizations and initiatives. Many of the largest umbrella organizations in the world lack a platform where all the various aspects of medicine and care in relation to ICT can be integrated.

Awareness will be one of the key words within the description of the ICMCC mission. Patient awareness seems an obvious goal, but also amongst professionals one can see the need. Many clinicians still see ICT (computers) as a thread to their existence and not, as it should be in our view, as a tool towards efficiency, in time as well as in costs, but also in treatment [3].

In Germany the insurance foundation for miners (Bundesknappschaft) started a trial in 1999 in which they linked ("vernetzen"), with the help of ICT, both general practitioners and clinicians and delivered a "Gesundheitsbuch" (health book) to patients. The reason why they started this trial in the Bottrop area was because 20 percent of the insured caused 80 percent of the expenditures. In the third year (2001) the savings in costs were 7%, and the average number of days spent in hospital decreased from 12 to 8,9 [4].

In addition to its role as a dissemination platform, ICMCC will independently serve as a meeting and discussion platform for any and all parties involved in medical and care compunetics.

3.5. Centers of Excellence

As stated in its goals, ICMCC will help to stimulate research in a number of areas as well as bring the experts together. Across the world a limited number of highly specialized centers will be created in cooperation with industry and universities.

3.6. Incubator

As much as ICMCC can stimulate research, the Council can also be instrumental in bringing together research and industry (especially the SME's). Here as well we want to act as a link between the various, national incubator facilities.

3.7. Innovation Exhibition

ICMCC will also serve as a window to the world of ICT related innovations in the medical and care fields in the way of an exhibition where both research and industry can jointly show there latest results.

4. The ICMCC Event 2005

ICMCC was started as a means to show the synergies in medical and care compunetics. While writing this article, a discussion has been going on between some of the chairs of the ICMCC Event 2005 as to which paper/workshop should be part of which symposium.

This discussion demonstrates the effectiveness of the ICMCC concept. The proposals were delivered by the authors themselves to a specific symposium, e.g. the symposium on e-health. But looking at the various inputs it became clear that a classification was not that easy to make. For example, some papers deal for a large part with standardization more than with e-health, others could as well be scheduled within the symposium on information management.

Some of the symposia clearly illustrate the role of ICMCC as an international discussion platform, especially the presentations on e-health and the virtual hospitals. The latter is one of the first in Western Europe on this issue. Taking these two symposia as an example, essential for both discussions is the change in the perception of concepts that is actually taking place. What is the difference between e-health, tele-health and tele-medicine? Is there any difference? Should the concept of the virtual hospital really be called that way? Does it have any relationship with a "building"? And what will be the benefit for the patient in these concepts? To what extent will the type of patient, influence the definition of a concept? It might very well be that the outcome of the discussion on virtual hospitals might result in varying definitions depending on whether one is talking about a soldier, a rural citizen or an urban citizen, or maybe even a handicapped or elderly person.

We have been very proud that so many outstanding key-individuals in the medical and care fields have joined the ICMCC initiative. During our first meeting at the 2004 event, there was a lively discussion on whether the Event should focus on specific subjects. The Event board had the wisdom to decide that it would be far too early to do so. They agreed with ICMCC's founder that crystallizing at this stage would deliver a massive rock that would lack all the flexibility that was at the base of the initiative. Out of that "freedom" the Council was founded. This year's Event as well as the rapidly growing international recognition shows how wise that decision has been.

References

[1] Bos, L, Laxminarayan, S., Marsh, A., Medical and Care Compunetics 1, IOS Press, 2004.
[2] Kemper, DW; Mettler, M., Information Therapy, Healthwise, 2002, p.133.
[3] See: Kopec, D. et al, Errors in Medical Practice: Identification, Classification and Steps towards Reduction, in: Medical and Care Compunetics 1, IOSPress 2004, pp. 126ff.
[4] Müller, H, Gewinnen durch Kooperation, Aerzte Zeitung, 13.11.2002.

Medical and Care Compunetics 2
L. Bos et al. (Eds.)
IOS Press, 2005

Understanding the Social Implications of ICT in Medicine and Health: The Role of Professional Societies

Brian M. O'CONNELL[a] and Swamy LAXMINARAYAN[b]
[a]*President, IEEE Society on Social Implications of Technology Department of Computer Science, Central Connecticut State University New Britain, CT USA 06050*
email: OconnellB@mail.ccsu.edu
[b]*Biomedical Information Engineering, Idaho State University Pocatello, Idaho 83209*
email: s.n.laxminarayan@ieee.org

Abstract. In past times, engineers and other ICT professionals could normally function exclusively within an environment of purely technical dimensions. This sphere could be easily delineated from those involving policy, political or social questions. Consequently, these professions could well be characterized as generally isolated from mainstream society, engendering a condition that Zussman (1985) has described as a "technical rationality that is the engineer's stock-in-trade requir[ing] the calculation of means for the realization of given ends. But it requir[ing] no broad insight into those ends or their consequences". This condition has often led to a perceived technical mindset that according to Florman (1976), draws upon "the comfort that comes with the total absorption in a mechanical environment. The world becomes reduced and manageable, controlled and unchaotic".

In a relatively short period of time, ICT has been radically transformed in both its capabilities and reach. Specifically, within the context of this event, the permeation of digital technologies into nearly every aspect of bioengineering and healthcare delivery have broken down the borders between technological pursuits and the larger dynamics of society. This has in turn has produced, according to Williams (2000) a discipline that has "evolved into an open-ended Profession of Everything in a world where technology shades into science, into art, and into management, with no strong institutions to define an overarching mission". Within ICT, H.C. von Baeyer (2003) affirms this status in noting "the frustration of engineers who have at their disposal a variety of methods for measuring the amount of information in a message, but to none deal with its meaning".

The cybernetics pioneer, Norbert Wiener (1964) presaged the current climate when he wrote that "as engineering technique becomes more and more able to achieve human purposes, it must become more and more accustomed to formulate human purposes". This observation is particularly relevant to the global challenges presented within the context of e-Health. as characterized by the Commission of the European Communities (2000):

The development of medical technologies in the coming decades will make an ever greater impact on health services. Important innovations include the use of computers and robotics, the application of communications and information technology, new diagnostic techniques, genetic engineering, cloning, the production of new classes of pharmaceuticals, and the work now beginning on growing replacement tissues and organs. These developments can contribute significantly to improved health status.

The massive nature of the challenge is evidenced by a recent report of the Commission (2004) which notes that:

- Increased networking, exchange of experiences and data, and benchmarking, is also
- necessary at the European level in the health sector. Drivers for this include the need for
- improvements in efficiency, and the increased mobility of patients and health professionals
- under an emerging internal market in services. The situation requires the integration of
- clinical, organizational, and economic information across health care facilities, so as to
- facilitate virtual enterprises at the level of jurisdictions and beyond.

As predicted by Wiener and Williams, the far-reaching implications of these advances cannot be confined to infrastructure alone, and are certain to impact contemporary societal norms. It is notable that at the onset of its initiative, the Commission report (2000) refers to the "significant ethical issues raised" raised in the process of developing new technologies. Viable responses to these challenges will not result from unilateral or detached applications of expertise. Instead they will require innovative approaches that reflect the present convergence of the technical and the social. Of foremost concern will be the establishment of a working dialogue among those in technological, legal, social and philosophical fields. Although such interactions have occurred in the past, the present need is arguably unique in history as it requires a dynamic and permanent partnership that is typified by more than superficial familiarity with other, often unfamiliar disciplines.

Diversity in Biology and Medicine: The diversity in biology and medicine has grown beyond belief especially with the introduction of advancing technologies. With diversity comes controversies, raising a whole gamut of ethical, legal, social, and/or policy issues. Typical examples include genetic engineering and biotechnology. Health care is a very sensitive area that requires individual protection against the invariable consequences of the social issues. As scientists and engineers, we have ambitious plans for ourselves. For example, as Francis Collins of the National Human Genome Research, has predicted (TIME, 2003), "I think it is safe to say we will have individualized, preventive medical care based on our own predicted risk of disease as assessed by looking at our DNA. By then each of us will have had our genomes sequenced because it will cost less than $100 to do that. And this information will be part of our medical record. Because we will still get sick, we will still need drugs, but these will be tailored to our individual needs. They will be based on a new breed of designer drugs with very high efficacy and very low toxicity, many of them predicted by computer models." These plans are already in action in ways that have triggered a whole series of social, ethical and policy issues associated with genetic and genomic knowledge and technology. No single institution can address on its own the various issues that are in interplay. Professional societies have a commitment to serve as an information base and provide the synergies required to bring together the interdisciplinary stakeholders to become involved in the debates.

SSIT as a Model

While formal institutional paradigms for this new mode of interaction are understandably sparse, the thirty-three year history of the Society on Social Implication of Technology (SSIT) of the Institute of Electrical and Electronic Engineers (IEEE) provides a useful model to explore interdisciplinary efforts. The SSIT consists of approximately 2000 members worldwide. The scope of the Society's interests includes such issues as engineering ethics and professional responsibility; the use of technical expertise in public policy decision making; environmental, health and safety implications of technology and social issues related to energy, information technology and telecommunications. Throughout its existence, the SSIT has attracted a diverse membership consisting of engineers in academe and industry, computer scientists, educational specialists, attorneys, academic ethicists, philosophers, librarians, historians and other scholars and practitioners working in the humanities, the sciences and technology. The unique nature of SSIT is evidenced in the collaborative efforts of its members. Experience and knowledge are shared across disciplinary boundaries, making it possible to construct comprehensive pictures of socio-technical issues as well as strategies toward resolution of conflicts.

Conclusions

This presentation will consider the model of SSIT and those of other global professional societies in an effort to investigate the elements of successful collaboration within the context of ICT issues. It will further examine the dynamics that lead to open and fruitful dialogues across the disciplines.

References

[1] Baeyer, C. von, Information: The New Language of Science (Cambridge: Harvard University Press, 2003).
[2] Commission of the European Communities, Communication from the Commission to the Council, the European Parliament, the Economic and Social Committee and the Committee of the Regions on the Health Strategy of the European Community, Brussels.16.5.2000, available at: http://europa.eu.int/eur-lex/en/com/pdf/2000/en_500PC0285.pdf.
[3] Commission of the European Communities, Communication from the Commission to the Council, the European Parliament, the Economic and Social Committee and the Committee of the Regions on e-Health – making healthcare better for European citizens: An action plan for a European e-Health Area, Brussels, 30.4.2004, available at: http://europa.eu.int/information_society/doc/qualif/health/COM_2004_0356_F_EN_ACTE.pdf.
[4] Florman, S., The Existential Pleasures of Engineering (New York: St. Martin's Press, 1976).
[5] Wiener, N., God and Golem, Inc. (Cambridge: MIT Press, 1964).
[6] Williams, R., Retooling: A Historian Confronts Technological Change (Cambridge: MIT Press, 2002).
[7] Zussman, R. Mechanics of the Middle Class: Work and Politics Among American Engineers, (Berkeley: University of California Press, 1985).

Symposium HIV and ICT, Breaking Down the Barriers

Medical and Care Compunetics 2
L. Bos et al. (Eds.)
IOS Press, 2005

iPath – a Telemedicine Platform to Support Health Providers in Low Resource Settings

K. BRAUCHLI[a], D. O'MAHONY[b], L. BANACH[c] and M. OBERHOLZER[a]
[a]*Department of Pathology, University Hospital Basel, Switzerland*
[b]*Family Practitioner, Port St Johns, South Afric*
[c]*Telemedicine Unit, University of Transkei, South Africa*

Absract. In many developing countries there is an acute shortage of medical specialists. The specialists and services that are available are usually concentrated in cities and health workers in rural health care, who serve most of the population, are isolated from specialist support [1]. Besides, the few remaining specialist are often isolated from colleagues. With the recent development in information and communication technologies, new option for telemedicine and generally for sharing knowledge at a distance are becoming increasingly accessible to health workers also in developing countries. Since 2001 the Department of Pathology in Basel, Switzerland is operating an Internet based telemedicine platform to assist health workers in developing countries. Over 1800 consultation have been performed since. This paper will give an introduction to iPath – the telemedicine platform developed for this project – and analyse two case studies: a teledermatology project from South Africa and a telepathology project from Solomon Islands.

Keywords. Telemedicine, telepathology, internet, developing countries, knowledge sharing

1. Introduction

Health providers like doctors and hospitals in developing countries often suffer from limited or non-existing access to specialists [1–4]. For example, the National Referral Hospital (NRH) in Honiara, the only major hospital on Solomon Islands serves a population of approximately 450'000 people and there is not a single pathologists or dermatologist. In 2001, a simple histology laboratory was set up in Honiara. Microscopic slides are prepared in the lab and subsequently photographed with a digital camera and submitted via email to an Internet-based telemedicine platform located at the University of Basel, Switzerland. Several pathologists in Europe review these images and within 8.5 hours (median) a diagnosis is made available to the surgeon in Honiara [4].

Following the successful example of telepathology in Honiara, other projects started using that telemedicine platform and now there are approximately 70 consultations from developing countries every month. While pathology had been the first applications, there are now several teledermatology projects in Africa using this platform and also one large project for neonatology consultations in Ukraine.

In all these examples, telemedicine is not used directly by the patient but primarily by doctors and nurses who need the additional input from specialists to improve the services that they are delivering.

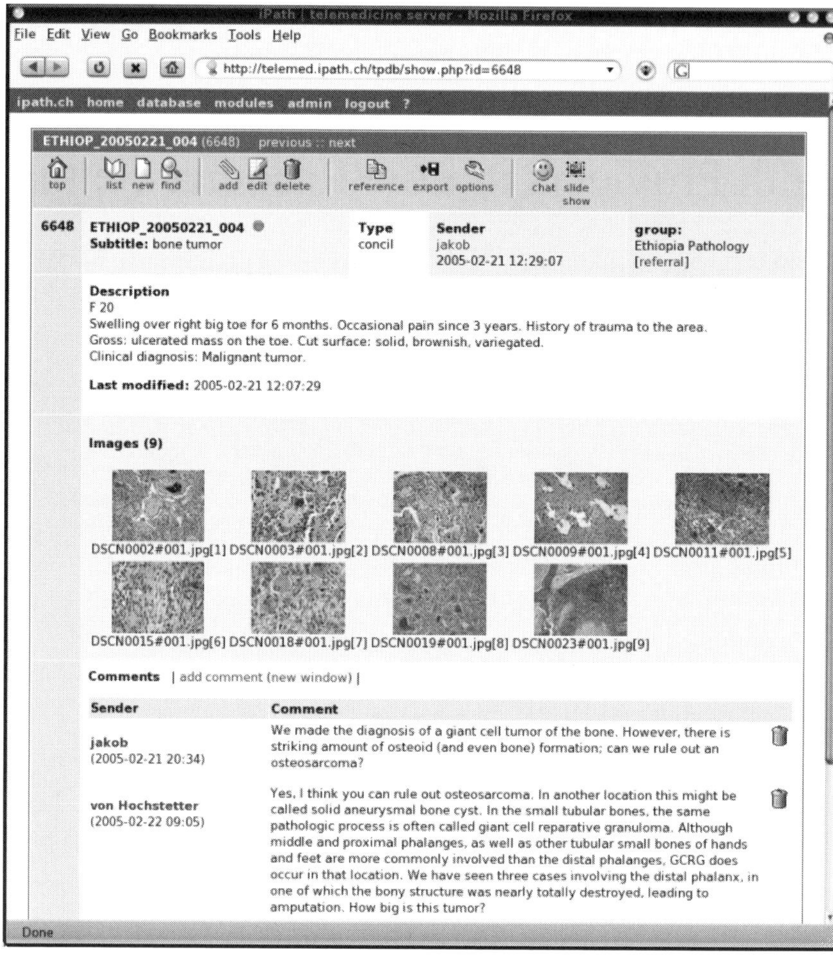

Figure 1. A typical case in iPath. This is an example of a telepathology consultation from Ethiopia. At the top there is the general case information (sender, submission date) followed by a clinical description and an image gallery. Below, specialists can state their comments and diagnosis.

2. iPath – a Hybrid Web and email Based Telemedicine Platform

Since 2001, the Department of Pathology of the University Hospital Basel has been developing the iPath software (http://ipath.ch), an open source framework for building web and email based telemedicine application [5,6]. iPath provides the functionality to store medical cases with attached images and other documents into closed user groups (c.f. Fig. 1). Within these groups, users can review cases, and write comments and diagnosis. Additionally, users can subscribe for notifications so that they get an automatic email if e.g. a new comment was added to one of their cases or if a new case is entered into a group.

Technically, iPath is a web application written in PHP. From the functionality it is somewhere between a content management system (CMS) and a group-ware tool. All users are organised into several discussion groups. Every discussion group has at least one moderator who can assign other users to the group and who can delete erroneous

Table 1. Usage statistics of iPath (24.12.2004).

	Users	Cases	Images	daily logins (2004)	submission by email
total	1213	5016	33247*	38	32.12%
developing countries	84**	1798	14006		74.17%

* average file size 93KB. Besides images there were another 5864 files (pdf, powerpoint etc)
** only 47% of users specified country of origin.

data. Thus, the system does not need to be administrated centrally as every group is administrating itself [5].

A very useful function of iPath, especially for areas with limited resources is the automatic email import. Users must once specify a group into which they would like to store cases sent by email. Then they can send a case to iPath as an ordinary email from any email client, typing the case title as the subject of the email, the clinical description as main text and simply attaching images. iPath will automatically import such cases into the group specified. Table 1 illustrates that out of 1798 cases submitted from developing countries, 74% were submitted by email (compared to 32% of all case submissions world wide).

The iPath software has been released as an open source project that can be used for regional networks and by other projects. Currently, the main usage of iPath is the telepathology network at the University of Basel with over 1000 users world wide (c.f. Section 2.1). However, we are aware of iPath being used for regional telemedicine networks in South Africa, Nepal, North West US, West Africa, Switzerland and in Germany. However, as the code is freely available, there might be more applications that we are not aware of.

2.1. Telemedicine Platform at University of Basel

Since 2001, the Department of Pathology of the University Hospital Basel, Switzerland, is operating an open telemedicine platform based on iPath – http://telepath.patho.unibas.ch [4–6]. In the beginning the platform was mainly used for telepathology projects in Switzerland and for collaboration with some pathologists in developing countries. Meanwhile, the platform has over 1300 users and more than 5000 cases have been discussed so far (c.f. Table 1). Besides the pathology projects at our department, the platform is used for a wide range of application – from telepathology on Solomon Islands [4] to neonatology discussion in Ukraine (59 users) to teledermatology consultations in Africa (over 50 consultations).

Table 1 shows the basic usage statistics of this platform. By the end of 2004 there were 1213 users of which 84 had specified coming from a developing country (only 47% of all users specified a country of origin, so probably there are more form developing countries). Since the start of the project in September 2001 a total of 5016 cases with totally 33247 images have been sent to the server – on average 6.7 images per cases. The average image size was 93KB. If we look at developing countries only, there were 1798 cases submitted with a total of 14006 images – on average 7.7 images per case. For the year 2004 there was an average of 67 consultations from developing countries submitted every month. Figure 2 illustrates the origin of all these consultations. The largest contribution was from a telepathology project at the Sihanouk Center of Hope in Phnom Penh, Cambodia, which submitted over 700 cases.

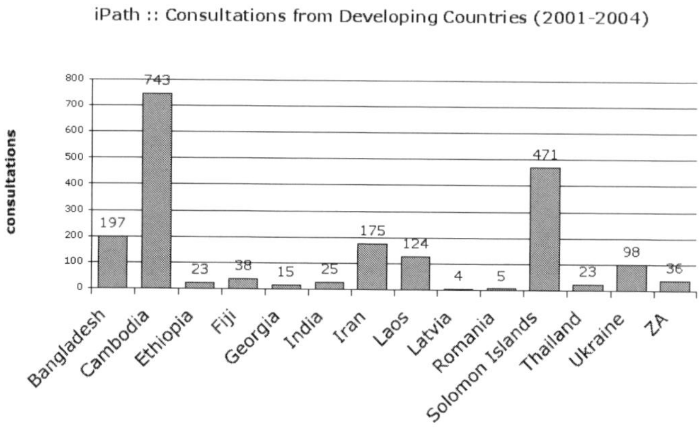

Figure 2. Consultations submitted from developing countries since the start of the iPath server in Basel in September 2001. Two major parts of the submissions are from the telepathology projects in Cambodia (743) and Solmon Islands (471).

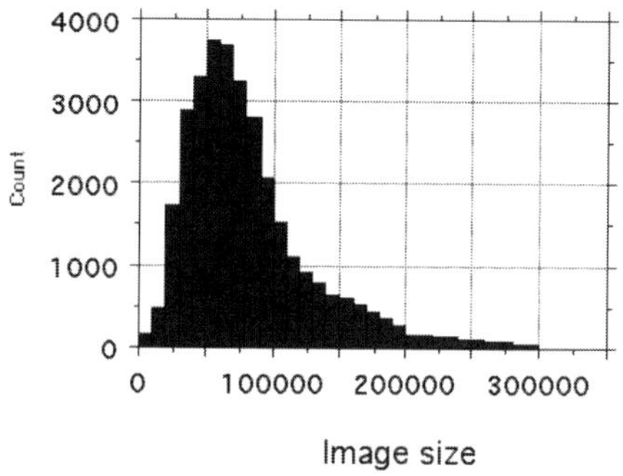

Figure 3. Distribution of image size for consultations submitted to the Basel telepathology server. From September 2001 to December 2004 a total amount of 33'247 images with an average file size of 93KB have been submitted. (c.f. Table 1).

3. Case Studies

iPath is used for a wide range of telemedicine applications. To illustrate the practical application and outcome in low resource settings we will study two examples.

3.1. Teledermatology in Port St. Johns, South Africa

Port St. Johns is a small provincial town on the east coast of South Africa. It is located in the former Transkei which used to to be an "independent" homeland during the apartheid. Now, the region is one of the poorest in South Africa. In the rural Port St Johns district, the population numbers about 75 000, the majority of which lives below the poverty line. Primary health care is provided mainly by nurses at state funded clinics, supported by general practitioners in the public and private sectors. In the last decade, the number of doctors in the district has varied between two and six. The referral hospital at Umtata is 100 Km distant but since 1998, has no had a specialist dermatologist permanently. At times the closest dermatology specialists was in East London, 350km from Port St. Johns. Hence, family practitioners have to diagnose and treat practically all dermatology problems (~15% of all consultations). To improve access for patients to dermatological care and to improve family practitioner clinical skills, a teledermatology project was initiated in April 1999 [7]. The project started with email based store-and-forward teledermatology, and since 2002 it is using iPath. In the first year the server in Basel was used but since 2003 the Telemedicine Unit [7,8] of the University of Transkei (UNITRA) in Umtata is running a regional telemedicine network based on the iPath software (http://telemed.utr.ac.za) which is now being used by the teledermatology project in Port St. Johns.

For the telemedical consultations images are captured with a digital camera (first an Olympus C-1400XL and later an Fuji 2 mega-pixel). Images were resized using Adobe Photoshop or GIMP[1]. In the beginning images were submitted by plain email with attached pictures. However, text and pictures easily got separated and misfiled. Thus patient information and images were compiled into an html page which worked well but was a very time consuming process. Finally, using iPath, clinical information and images are sent by plain email to the iPath server, where they are automatically inserted into a database and presented to the dermatology specialist in form of a concise web page. Besides the ease of use, the automatic email notifications system of iPath has also helped to reduce turnaround times. From an average response time of over 30 days, it is now at 6.5 days since consultation are done using the iPath platform at UNITRA.

Since 1999, 110 patients from Port St. Johns have been diagnosed using teledermatology. 76 patients where female and 34 male with an average age of 32 years. In 105 cases a telemedical diagnosis was possible and in 104 cases this assistance was judged helpful by the general practitioner (GP). For 57 cases, the telemedical diagnosis enabled an improvement of the treatment (unpublished data, an evaluation of the project is in preparation). The major outcome however is not only the direct improvement for the patient but also the fact that teledermatology helped the GP to improve his skills in diagnosing and treating dermatology problems appropriately, or, citing the GP: "The number of cases dropped off over the years. This is definitely due to my improved skill in diagnosis due to learning."

3.2. Telepathology on Solomon Islands

The National Referral Hospital (NRH) in Honiara is the only major hospital in Solomon Islands, an independent state with approximately 450'000 inhabitants, tucked away in the south west of the pacific ocean. The NRH is the only referral hospital for the 8 provincial hospitals. The country has about 40 doctors but not a single pathologist and consequently tissue samples for histological examination have to be sent by airmail to the nearest pathology service in Brisbane, Australia and it is not unlikely that the doctors at the NRH have to wait 3–6 weeks before the histological diagnosis is returned from Brisbane. Besides, the state of Solomon Islands consists of over 900 islands, spread out over hundreds of kilometers. Patients from remote islands have to travel by boat for days to reach the hospital on the main island. For many patients it is difficult to return home to wait until a diagnostic result has arrived at the NRH and as a consequence, treatment decisions often have to be made without a histological diagnosis.

A small histology laboratory was established at the National Referral Hospital (NRH) in Honiara, Solomon Islands, in September 2001, allowing the preparation of

---

[1]Open Source image manipulation program – http://www.gimp.org.

Table 2. Telepathology consultations from National Referral Hospital in Honiara, Solomon Islands. Phase I are the consultations before the introduction of the virtual institute (cf. text) which is the time from January 2002 to October 2002. Phase II describes the situation from November 2002 to December 2003 after the introduction of the virtual institute. The second line indicates the median time between submission of the case by email and the first response from a pathologist. (Figure from Brauchli et al. 2004).

	Phase I	***Phase II***	***total***
Number of consultations	73	260	333
First response after (median)	28h	8.5h	12h
Consultation possible	93.2%	94.2%	94%
Additional images requested	24.7%	10%	13.2%

H&E stained sections. Gross specimen are prepared by the surgeon, processed in the laboratory and the slides are usually ready two or three days later. From the microscopic sections prepared in this laboratory, digital photographs are taken using a Nikon CoolPix 990 Camera mounted on a Nikon OptiPhot 2 microscope. These pictures are usually scaled to approximately 600x400 pixels (typically 20KB – 70KB) then sent via email to the telepathology server at University of Basel [4].

During a two year period from January 2002 and December 2003 a total of 333 pathology consultations where submitted from NRH to the telepathology server in Basel. These consultations were submitted by email with a short clinical description and with images as attachments (average 8.8 images per consultation). In 50% of all consultations a first report from a pathologist was issued in 12h or less (cf. Table 2).

A major improvement in the project was the introduction of a virtual institute [4,6]. A virtual institute is a group of experts with a duty plan. Every week one specialist is "on call" and the iPath system automatically notifies the "expert on call" about any new cases and also about new comments from other experts. Besides, the expert on call was asked to mark a diagnosis as final if in his or her opinion, a diagnostically conclusive response was possible based on the submitted material. This organisation helped to reduce the turn around time for diagnosis from 28h in the beginning (phase I in Table 2) to 8.5h after the introduction of the virtual institute (phase II).

4. Discussion

When iPath was developed it was not primarily intended for telemedicine in low resource settings, however, it turned out that an easy to use telemedicine solution which does not have high demand on bandwidth can be a very helpful tool in developing countries. The platform has been very well used by health professionals working in developing countries to consult with specialists from other parts of the world to overcome the professional isolation often present in remote hospitals and to improve their skill and services they can deliver to their patients.

Looking at the usage of iPath over the past 3 years we can observe a number of different types of applications. Firstly there are remote consultations where typically a doctor at a remote hospital consults with a group of distant specialists. Secondly there is a growing number of general discussion groups (not only on iPath) where specialists working in isolation are sharing knowledge and experience with distant colleagues. Besides, iPath is more and more used for decentralised studies, where a number of partners are jointly collecting data on a special topic (research, quality control, etc). Data can be text, images and also custom forms for capturing structured data. The advantage of an Internet based solution is that every partner can at any time review the whole collection and compile statistics.

As iPath is developed as an open source project and distributed under the General Public License (GPL[2]) its use is not restricted to the telemedicine server of the University of Basel. The open source license allows other projects to use iPath and adapt it to their needs. As telemedicine is primarily used by specialists in centrally located institutions, it bears the risk of inducing a digital divide within a developing country if the periphery of the health system is not involved in the development of the network [9]. Besides there are often cultural differences and language barriers that are difficult to address in large international projects. The open source nature of iPath allows such adaptations and it is easily possible to reproduce working regional solutions as free and open source software can be adapted and distributed.

References

[1] Fraser, H.S. and S.J. McGrath, *Information technology and telemedicine in sub-saharan Africa.* Bmj, 2000. **321**(7259): p. 465–6.

[2] Johnston, K., et al., *The cost-effectiveness of technology transfer using telemedicine.* Health Policy Plan, 2004. **19**(5): p. 302–9.

[3] Schmid-Grendelmeier, P., P. Doe, and N. Pakenham-Walsh, *Teledermatology in sub-Saharan Africa.* Curr Probl Dermatol, 2003. **32**: p. 233–46.

[4] Brauchli, K., et al., Telepathology on the Solomon Islands–two years' experience with a hybrid Web- and email-based telepathology system. J Telemed Telecare, 2004. **10 Suppl 1**: p. 14–7.

[5] Brauchli, K., et al., *Telemicroscopy by the Internet revisited.* J Pathol, 2002. **196**(2): p. 238–43.

[6] Brauchli, K., et al., Diagnostic telepathology: long-term experience of a single institution. Virchows Arch, 2004. **444**(5): p. 403–9.

[7] O'Mahony, D., et al., *Teledermatology in a Rural Family Practice.* S A Fam Pract, 2002. **25**(6): p. 4–8.

[8] Stepien, A., et al., *Histo- and cytopathologic remote diagnosis (telepathology). Preliminary report.* Ann Univ Mariae Curie Sklodowska [Med], 1999. **54**: p. 313–8.

[9] Geissbuhler, A., et al., Telemedicine in Western Africa: lessons learned from a pilot project in Mali, perspectives and recommendations. AMIA Annu Symp Proc, 2003: p. 249–53.

[2]Free Software Foundation – http://www.fsf.org.

Medical and Care Compunetics 2
L. Bos et al. (Eds.)
IOS Press, 2005

Telemedicine for HIV/AIDS Care in Low Resource Settings

Maria ZOLFO[1], Line ARNOULD, Veerle HUYST and Lut LYNEN
Institute of Tropical Medicine, Department Clinical Sciences, Antwerp, Belgium

Abstract. Telemedicine is a way to support health care delivery in remote areas. With our telemedicine project the Institute of Tropical Medicine, Antwerp, Belgium, intended to facilitate the introduction of antiretroviral therapy (ART) for patients affected by Human Immunodeficiency Virus (HIV) and Acquired Immune Deficiency Syndrome (AIDS) in developing countries, providing training, distance support and education to healthcare providers working in those settings.

Keywords. Telemedicine, HIV/AIDS, internet, low resource settings, developing countries

Introduction

Worldwide there are more than 40 million people infected with Human Immunodeficiency Virus (HIV), and 90% of them are living in low resource settings [1]. In many countries, but particularly in Africa, HIV and Acquired Immune Deficiency Syndrome (AIDS) are now the most important health problems. Besides continuous efforts for prevention, the introduction of antiretroviral therapy (ART) has become a humanitarian and economic necessity and possibility.

Today ART is increasingly available in resource limited settings thanks to global initiatives like the World Health Organization's "3x5" strategy [2] and global efforts like Global Fund against AIDS, Tuberculosis and Malaria [3]. The speed at which clinicians and paramedics are going to be trained in the South will be determinant for the rapid scaling up access to ART. Therefore there is an urgent need to develop good quality training programs on ART and clinical management of HIV/AIDS patients and to guarantee mentoring systems for the upgrading and continuous medical education of those colleagues working in isolated areas.

Telemedicine is a way to assist delivery of care in remote areas [4–7]. Facing the necessity to support physicians in treating patients with newly introduced ART, the Institute of Tropical Medicine, Antwerp (ITMA) set up a computer aided training programme for healthcare providers, working in developing countries.

Expert advices from HIV/AIDS specialists on ART and management of Opportunistic Infections (OIs) have been offered to colleagues working in different countries.

The telemedicine advice has been organized initially through an e-mail network on a list server but later, in response to the need of continuous medical education on HIV

---

[1]Corresponding Author: Maria Zolfo, Institute of Tropical Medicine, Nationalestraat 155, 2000 Antwerp, Belgium; E-mail: mzolfo@itg.be.

and ART, through a discussion forum on a telemedicine web site (http://telemedicine.itg.be).

Short Course on Antiretroviral Therapy (SCART)

Responding to the recent progresses made in the care of HIV/AIDS patients using ART also in countries with limited resources, ITMA organises a 3 weeks training on HIV clinical care for medical doctors, specifically targeting the use of ART.

The third edition of this course will take place in the summer 2005. The participants are trained in order to be able to:

- choose, and explain to the HIV positive patient, the appropriate antiretroviral (ARV) regimen taking into account:
  - the goal of the therapy (treatment, prevention of transmission of the HIV; post exposure prophylaxis and prevention of mother to child transmission)
  - the optimal timing for initiation of treatment (including assessment of the stage of the HIV infection and present clinical condition of the patient)
  - the general characteristics of the patient
  - the availability of resources in a specific setting.
- Plan a monitoring strategy for a patient on ARV including:
  - clinical follow up
  - adherence monitoring
  - laboratory follow up
  - identification and management of immune reconstitution inflammatory syndrome (IRIS) and side effects.
- Identify and predict ARV treatment failure (clinical, immunological and virological), to be able to assure the management of it, including the prescription of the appropriate alternative ARV therapy taking into account the available resources.
- Evaluate the quality of care for patients with chronic health problems like AIDS patients and relate quality aspects to the organisation of a clinic taking into account the different resources needed for AIDS care.
- Explain the possible impact ARV can have on mortality and the role of clinical care within the whole spectrum of interventions addressing the health and social care challenges related to the HIV epidemic.

Teaching consists of "state of the art" lectures, seminars, discussions and practical sessions with site visits to HIV/STI clinics. ITMA staff gives most of the lessons but internationally known experts from other academic institutions and field experts are invited to complement specific areas of expertise.

The Telemedicine Project

The telemedicine project has been conceived in 2003 by the department of Clinical Sciences at ITMA. The basic aim of the project is to facilitate the introduction of high-

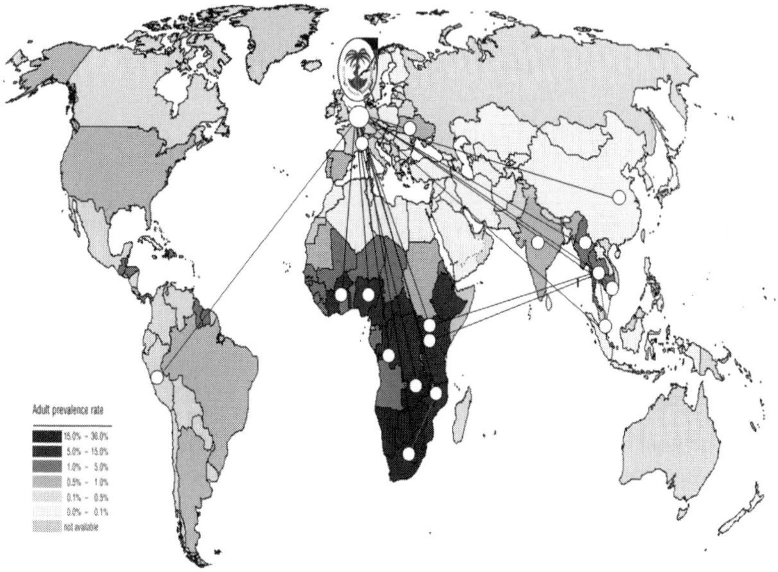

Figure 1. ITMA telemedicine active sites.

quality ART care for HIV/AIDS patients living in resource limited settings, by providing on-line technical support in the field of ART and management of OIs to clinicians working in the South. Some of those clinicians have followed the SCART.

Advices have been given through e-mail messages from a list server and afterwards through a discussion forum on a telemedicine web site, which has been officially launched during the SCART 2004. Patient's history, physical examination, pictures, laboratory findings and questions to be answered have been sent from more than 17 different countries. [Figure 1]

Between April 2003 (date of first referral) and March 2005, the department has answered to 342 requests: 93% (318) of questions patient oriented and 7% (24) of general questions (organization of health services for AIDS care, TB DOTS, vaccination programs, buddy groups, guidelines delivery). 49% of the questions patient oriented were related to ARVs (drug-drug interaction, adverse effects, drug combinations, …) and 44% to OIs diagnosis and treatment [Table 1, 2]. 81% (257) of the requests were presented under the form of clinical cases and the rest was presented as open questions.

Telemedicine Web Site

In the summer 2004, during the second edition of the SCART training, the telemedicine web site has been officially launched (http://telemedicine.itg.be).

As of end March 2005, after 7 months of web site activity more than 150 health care professionals, from 40 different countries, and mainly poor resource settings, subscribed to the discussion forum. The 88 cases and questions described on the discussion forum, resulted in 380 interactions between colleagues with a total number of 12 300 accesses on the web site, discussion forum and educational web pages combined.

Table 1. Telemedicine referrals in the first 2 years of existence: 342 cases and questions.

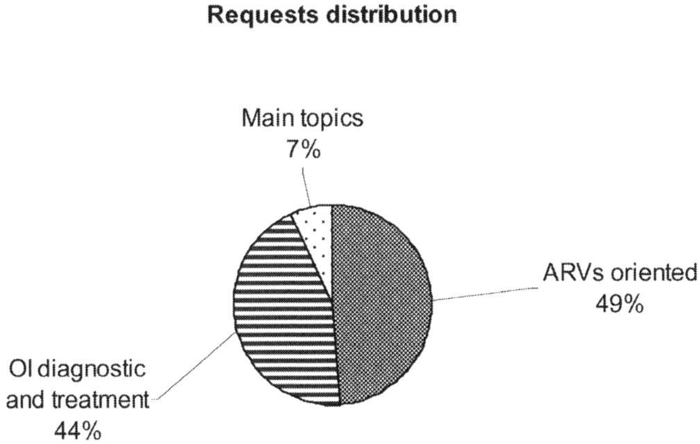

Table 2. Questions on ARVs.

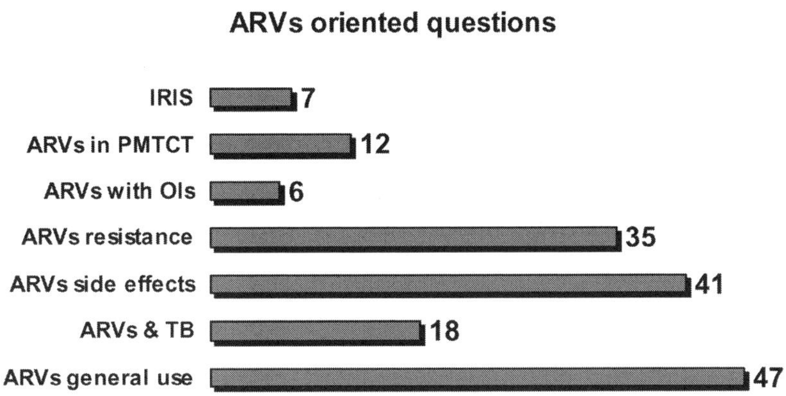

All postings are archived in an electronic database, with a personal list of postings from each user. An internal e-mail account is available for direct contact between the members, facilitating the exchange of recent literature and policy documents. All postings are visible to the discussion forum members, who can contribute to them and search for the old ones through a search function. A system of warning messages is available giving early notice on the personal e-mail account when a new posting is available on the discussion forum.

Interesting cases and recurring questions are elaborated as case rounds or frequently asked questions (FAQs), which are consultable through the search function for continuous education on the web site. Also user-friendly guidelines, links, and policy documents with particular focus on low resource setting are available for consultation. The aim of interactive programs as web quizzes, FAQs, case rounds and the databases of cases is intended as tool of distance learning. An international accreditation system is under evaluation.

Conclusion

E-mails have been used for years by ITMA as a low cost telemedicine support for colleagues working in low resource countries. This is the first pilot computer aided training project centred on HIV and AIDS care delivered by our center, with the intent to guide doctors in the scaling up ARVs process and HIV/AIDS patients care.

After a short course on antiretroviral therapy, a web site discussion forum (http://telemedicine.itg.be) is offered to colleagues working in low resource settings as a tool to support medical decision making and management of difficult HIV/AIDS cases, in the daily clinical practice. Clinical images and bibliographic material are used to accompany questions and answers. Guidelines, links, case discussions, quizzes and FAQs are available for continuous education on the web site.

Although the use of ART remains limited in low resource settings, there are global initiatives making those drugs available to hundred thousands HIV infected persons. The speed at which clinicians and paramedics are going to be trained in the South will be determinant for the speed of the scaling up access to ARVs.

By giving the opportunity to trained clinicians to access continuous support and education through a discussion forum and policy documents on the web site, we intend to lower the threshold to launch ARVs projects in low resource settings.

References

[1] UNAIDS 2004. Report on the global AIDS epidemic. WHO Library, 2004.

[2] WHO. Treating 3 million people in the developing world by 2005. http://www.who.int/3by5/publications/documents/en/3by5StrategyMakingItHappen.pdf.

[3] The Global Found to fight AIDS, Tuberculosis and Malaria, 2004. http://www.theglobalfound.org.

[4] L.E. Graham, M. Zimmerman, D.J. Vassallo, V. Patterson, P. Swinfen, R. Swinfen, R. Wootton, Telemedicine – the way ahead for medicine in the developing world, *Trop Doct* **33** (2003), 36 38.

[5] R. Swinfen, P. Swinfen, Low-cost telemedicine in the developing world, *J Telemed Telecare* **8** (2002), 63 65.

[6] M. Kuntalp, O. Akar, A simple and low-cost Internet-based teleconsultation system that could effectively solve the health care access problems in underserved areas of developing countries, *Comput Methods Programs Biomed* **75** (2004), 117 126.

[7] Brauchli K, Jagilly R, Oberli H, Kunze KD, Phillips G, Hurwitz N, Oberholzer M, Telepathology on the Solomon Islands–two years' experience with a hybrid Web- and email-based telepathology system. *J Telemed Telecare* **10** Suppl 1 (2004), 4 7.

Medical and Care Compunetics 2
L. Bos et al. (Eds.)
IOS Press, 2005

A Home Integral Telecare System for HIV/AIDS Patients

Cesar CACERES [a], Enrique J. GOMEZ [a], Felipe GARCIA [b], Paloma CHAUSA [a], Jorge GUZMAN [a], Francisco DEL POZO [a] and Jose Maria GATELL [b]
[a] *Bioengineering and Telemedicine Unit. Universidad Politecnica de Madrid, Spain*
[b] *Infectious Diseases Unit. Clinic Hospital, Barcelona, Spain*

Abstract. VIHrtual Hospital is a telemedicine web system for improving home integral care of chronic HIV patients through the Internet. Using the videoconference, chat or messaging tools included in the system, patients can visit their healthcare providers (physician, psychologist, nurse, psychiatrist, pharmacist, and social worker), having these access to the Electronic Patient Record. The system also provides a telepharmacy service that controls treatment adherence and side effects, sending the medication to the patient's home by courier. A virtual community has been created, facilitating communication between patients and improving the collaboration between professionals, creating a care plan for each patient. As a complement, there is a virtual library where users can find validated HIV/AIDS information helping to enhance prevention. This system has been developed using low cost technologies in order to extend the number of patients involved in its trial. Thus, VIHrtual Hospital is now on trial in the Hospital Clinic (Barcelona, Spain) involving a hundred patients and twenty healthcare professionals during two years.

Although we are still waiting for the final results of the trial, we can already say that the use of telemedicine systems developed ad hoc for a chronic disease, like HIV/AIDS, improve the quality of care of the patients and their care team. The system described is a good example of the possibilities that technologies are offering to create new chronic patient care models based on telemedicine.

1. Introduction

Since the appearance of the Highly Active AntiRetroviral Treatments (HAART), people living with HIV are lengthening their lives, delaying the manifestation of the virus in its final state of AIDS [1,2]. The goal now is to improve their quality of life [3], deteriorated by multiple clinical [4], psychosocial [5–7] and organizational [8] factors.

In this article we will describe a new approach to improve this quality of care, through a telemedicine system that will provide both patients and healthcare professionals with tools for an integral HIV/AIDS care. In this domain, integral care means that there is a multidisciplinary care team of health professionals, integrated by medical doctors, nurses, psychologists, psychiatrists, pharmacists, and social workers, that jointly with the patient will care him/her. This challenge has been faced by the creation of the "VIHrtual Hospital" project. Its main goal is the definition, development, clinical routine installation and evaluation of a telemedicine service that complements standard care with a telecare follow-up for attending stable HIV infected patients, in a chronic phase of their disease, and study if that improves the quality of assistance and the expense per patient comparing to the conventional control (without telemedicine service) that patients usually have.

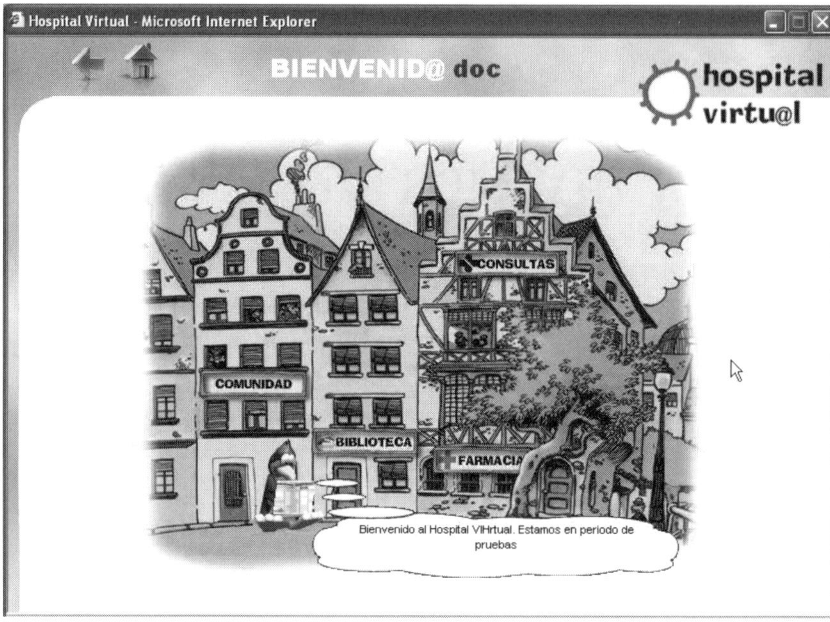

Figure 1. Main Menu of the VIHrtual Hospital System.

2. System Services Description

To describe this VIHrtual Hospital system we will go through the main services it provides. These services can be accessed from the main menu of the system shown in Fig. 1.

2.1. Virtual Consultation

Virtual consultations are proposed as a complement of the conventional visits of the patient to any health professional of the care team. This can be achieved through: a videoconference, always started by the professional; a chat session; and exchanging messages, through the database without using e-mail client programs for anonymity purposes.

An Electronic Health Record is available during these visits for both professionals and patients, as shown in Fig. 2. It can be emphasized that we have included psychological and social data to integrate the patient's records seeing their care as a whole. An agenda is also available so that, at the end of the visit, patient and professional can agree and make the next appointment.

2.2. Telepharmacy

The follow-up of the treatment is done by the doctors and pharmacists and, obviously, the patient. They commonly agree the ideal treatment taking into account multiple factors. This therapy usually consists of three or four drugs that, after a visit, the doctor prescribes to the patient. Up to now the patient goes with those prescriptions to the

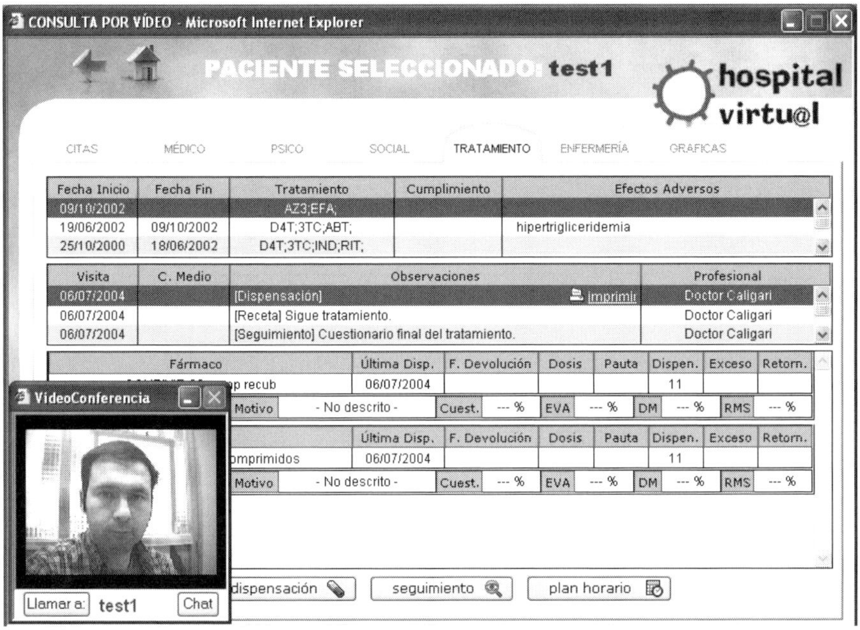

Figure 2. Videoconference Session with a Patient.

hospital pharmacy, where the pharmacist delivers the drugs (in Spain antirretroviral drugs are not sold in the usual "street" pharmacies, but only delivered in hospital pharmacies).

Now, with the telemedicine system, the doctor could have visited his/her patient online, so the prescription is sent to the hospital pharmacy automatically by the system. In this case the pharmacist will be informed that the patient needs more medication and therefore consults the compliance data that the patient should have introduced already. With these data the pharmacist can make a significant follow-up of the compliance, adverse effects, interactions with other drugs, etc. Before sending the medication to the patient's home by courier, the pharmacist usually wants to visit the patient and check if is having any problem with the treatment. This is also done virtually, with the videoconference facility of the VIHrtual Hospital system. This new process is shown in the diagram of the Fig. 3. The patients can also in this section visualise the evolution of their own treatments on charts and consult basic information on the available antiretroviral drugs.

2.3. Virtual Community

This virtual community doesn't pretend to substitute the HIV/AIDS communities that already exist in the Internet. It is meant to create spaces to exchange information about the disease, about the project, share their opinions, comment articles, news, etc. Patients have their own discussion forum where the healthcare professionals are not allowed, and these professionals have as well their own section where they can discuss particular clinical cases.

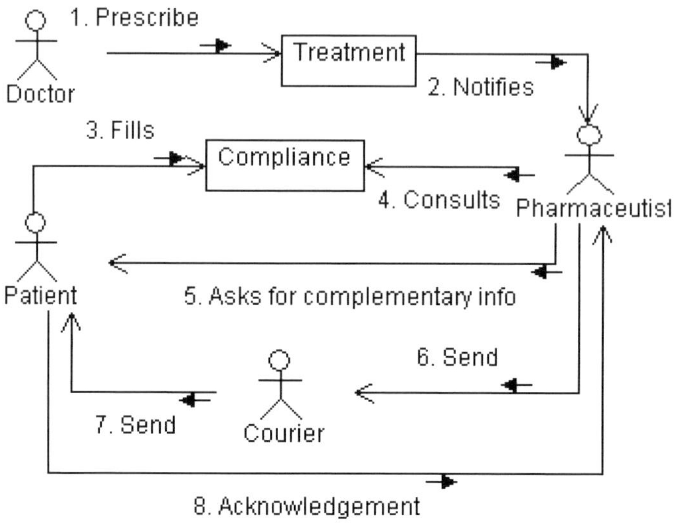

Figure 3. Telepharmacy Workflow Process.

2.4. Virtual Library

There are huge amounts of information about HIV/AIDS in the Internet. But this, that could seem an advantage, turns out to be a disadvantage because you need to distinguish valid information from that which is not [9]. Therefore the aim of this virtual library is to store validated basic information about the HIV/AIDS disease, as links to other web pages, for both patients and professionals.

2.5. User Administration

A complete separate tool has been developed outside the web system, so only the administrator will have access to it. When adding new professionals in the trial, their data and timetable will be entered. This tool also administers patient's inclusions in the trial. Every time that a new patient is added to the trial, the system accesses to the existing HIV database of the hospital and copies all the patient data (but the personal identification data) into the trial database.

3. System Architecture and Security Issues

To accomplish all these goals, the following architecture has been implemented (see Fig. 4) and integrated into the Hospital Information System network of the Clínic Hospital of Barcelona.

The server is placed in the demilitarized zone (DMZ) that the Clínic Hospital has behind a firewall. Professionals connect to this server from their own computers through the hospital intranet. Patients access the system from their homes with ADSL using a secure connection (VPN) to the server. The existing infrastructure of the hospital network has been used whenever possible, in order to prevent creating a parallel

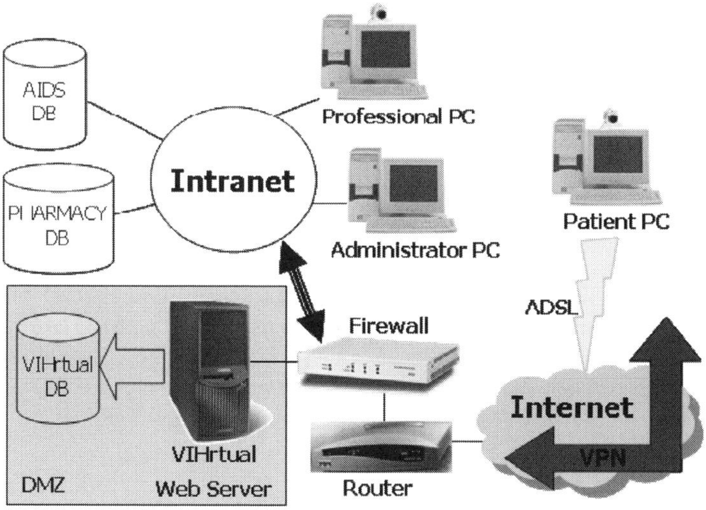

Figure 4. VIHrtual Hospital Architecture.

network exclusively dedicated to the project. Of critical importance in the system has been the connection of the server with three databases.

The VIHrtual database is the new database created for the telemedicine system, where the data of the patients involved in the trial are stored. This database is filled and synchronised with the HIV/AIDS database, which the Infectious Diseases Service of the Clínic Hospital has been using over the last 15 years where more than 3.000 HIV/AIDS patients are registered. Finally, the server is also connected to the Pharmacy database, where all the available drugs are recorded and kept up to date by the pharmacists.

This web-based system has been developed with a special effort in the selection of the equipment for the patients, trying to integrate them as much as possible in a home environment (size and "look and feel"). The graphical interface has also been carefully designed in order to ease its use for professionals and patients, as can be seen in Figs 1 and 2.

Other main goal has been developing a low cost system in order to being able to increase the number of patients for the clinical trial. Therefore, low price home web cams and ADSL were some of the chosen technologies for the implementation, with more than acceptable results.

Security has been one of the most carefully designed aspects of the project, mainly because of the experimental nature of the project and the characteristics of the disease it is dealing with. As well as securing the communications, as mentioned before, with VPN tunnelling, patient's data is also encrypted and anonymized (all personal identification data is removed by the user administration tool described in Section 2.5) so that any improbable break in the server will result to be harmless. Users have a complementary fingerprint recognition device that jointly with the login and password will be checked to access the system. All accesses to the system are being monitored and the system sends automatically an alert e-mail to the technical responsible in case of recurrent access, in order to estimate the risk of the situation and check the identity of the possible attacker.

4. Clinical Trial Description

For evaluation purposes, a randomised crossed open and prospective clinical trial has been developed, where 100 patients are involved. They have been randomised in two branches: A – controlled by telemedicine service (n=50) and B – controlled by the day hospital of HIV as usual (n=50). The length of the clinical trial is two years, taking into account that the group of patients with the telemedicine system and the control group of patients will cross in a year time. This evaluation is being carried out since January 2005 by the Infectious Diseases, Mental Health, Pharmacy, and Social Services of the Clínic Hospital of Barcelona (Spain), involving a total of 20 healthcare professionals (eleven HIV/AIDS specialist doctors, a psychologist, a psychiatrist, two nurses, four pharmacists, a social worker). The evaluation is being monitored by an independent quality of life expert and the maintenance of the system is guaranteed by the development team and a company responsible of the installation and maintenance of the patient's equipments.

5. Conclusions

Nowadays, caring chronic HIV/AIDS patients involves a tighter control that implies several visits a year for the blood analysis and clinical follow-up. These visits are complemented by other visits (psychological, social, prevention, doubts…). Even more, patient self empowerment [10] and the coordination of the care team are mandatory within these care models.

Integration of a new technological service in a hospital is always difficult and implies a great effort. The integration of this telemedicine service into the Hospital Information System network has created a new architecture that must deal to satisfy the necessities of the new service without generating any conflict with the existing services.

One of the most important aspects is the data access security, as clinical information needs the highest level of protection by the Spanish law [11]. This project has been exceedingly cautious about the security facts, due also to the nature of the disease.

The evaluation will show when telemedicine is feasible for HIV/AIDS home-care and when it is not, depending on the patient health status, location or knowledge, or coordination difficulties between the care team or even our own system limitations. The results will allow us to know if it is possible to follow certain chronic patients at home, reducing the number of visits to their reference hospital and improving care from every health professional (physical, psychological, social, prevention, etc. improvements).

To sum up, the telemedicine system described has achieved the goal of creating an architecture that fulfils the demanding security and integration requirements of the Informatics Service of the Clínic Hospital. An easy-to-use graphical interface for both patients and professionals has also been developed. The low costs of the system allow us to cover a wide range of patients, where we hope to get promising results about the use of telemedicine systems for improving the follow-up of chronic HIV/AIDS patients and for creating a new care model for this disease.

Acknowledgement

We would like to thank all researchers from the Bioengineering and Telemedicine Unit that have collaborated in this project for their participation and dedication. We also would like to thank Dr. Emilio Fumero, Dr. Jordi Blanch, Dra. Araceli Rousaud, Dr. Carlos Codina, Dra. Maite Martin, and Dr. Xavier Badia for their inputs and dedication to the project.

References

[1] F.J. Palella, K.M. Delaney, A.C. Moorman et al, "Declining morbidity and mortality among patients with advanced human immunodeficiency virus infection", *N Engl J Med*, 1998; 338:853–60.
[2] G.S. Reiter, "Comprehensive clinical care: Managing HIV as a chronic illness", *AIDS Clinical Care, Massachusets Medical Society*, 2000.
[3] F.J. Penedo et al, "Personality, quality of life and HAART adherence among men and women living with HIV/AIDS", *J Psychosom Res*, vol. 54, 3, 2003; pp. 271–278.
[4] S.R. Smith et al, "A medication self-management program to improve adherence to HIV therapy regimens", *Patient Education and Counseling*, vol. 50, 2003; pp. 187–199.
[5] M.H. Cohen et al, "Causes of death among women with human immunodeficiency virus infection in the era of combination antiretroviral therapy", *Am J Med*, vol. 113, 2002; pp. 91–98.
[6] Ministerio de trabajo y asuntos sociales de España, "Anexo I: Diagnósticos sobre la exclusión social en España", 2000.
[7] D.J. Martin, R.A. Brooks, D.J. Ortiz and R.C. Veniegas, "Perceived Employment Barriers and Their Relation to Workforce-Entry Intent Among People With HIV/AIDS", *J Occup Health Psychol*, vol. 8, 3, 2003; pp. 181–194.
[8] T. Winter, C.T. Le, K. Boyd, L. Ackerson, "HIV and managed care: cost-effectiveness of an interdisciplinary disease management team", *Int Conf AIDS*, 1998; 3; 12:857.
[9] G.K. Berland et al, "Health Information on the Internet", *JAMA*, vol. 285, 2001; p. 20.
[10] H.R. Holman and K.R. Lorig, "Patients as partners in managing chronic disease", *BMJ*, vol. 320, 2000; pp. 526–527.
[11] Spanish Organic Law 15/1999, December 13th 1999, for protecting personal data.

Medical and Care Compunetics 2
L. Bos et al. (Eds.)
IOS Press, 2005

Towards a Mobile Intelligent Information System with Application to HIV/AIDS

D. KOPEC[a], R. ECKHARDT[b], S. TAMANG[a] and D. REINHARTH[c]
[a]*Department of Computer and Information Science, Brooklyn College, CUNY, USA*
[b]*Department of Biology, Brooklyn College, CUNY, USA*
[c] *Long Island Jewish Medical Center, NY, USA*

Abstract. The United Nations Security Council reports HIV/AIDS as the fastest growing threat to human development. In addition, the World Health Organization [1] reports that nearly 5 million persons (4.3 million adults and 700,000 children) are newly infected with HIV each year; more than 95% of them found in developing countries. Since STDs as a group are a personal problem which few people feel comfortable discussing, we believe that hand-held PDAs can provide an opportunity for learning about this disease while insuring anonymity. This device will employ the newest technologies including Bluetooth wireless technology, which can transmit and receive data via a short-range radio link using a globally available frequency band (2.4 GHz ISM band), enabling rapid and accurate synchronous and asynchronous data communication. The first generation of Bluetooth permits exchange of data up to a rate of 1 Mbps, even in areas with much electromagnetic disturbance. This emerging technology can facilitate HIV/AIDS outreach around the globe.

Recent advances in learning have taken a particularly cognitive perspective and these findings have implications for education in general as well as for the development of intelligent tutoring systems in particular. In the past, effective SmartBooks™ have been developed for AIDS education to disseminate the critical knowledge relevant to this epidemic [2].

Since 1993, the proliferation of the World Wide Web has created a plethora of new opportunities for the delivery of electronic distance learning systems. However, we feel that it is important that a whatever technology is employed is based on a sound educational theory. A new, comprehensive, web-based learning system called SmartTutor has been developed, at Brooklyn College of The City University of New York [3]. This technology provides a user-friendly, self-paced, easy to modify, software environment intended to serve the user's learning needs and is based on a generic SmartTutor methodology organized around the use of concept mapping. Early assessment of SmartTutor has shown that it is well received by students and helps significantly in their learning processes. It is readily adaptable to the presentation of academic and more general subject matter such as the latest available information on HIV/AIDS. Our new HIV/AIDS SmartTutor will incorporate this SmartTutor paradigm. Our new SmartTutor would provide worldwide access to medical professionals as well as the general public to learn about HIV/AIDS. This new device could also provide a survey tool to facilitate HIV risk assessment. Demonstrations of the SmartTutor learning system will be presented and the continued development of the applications will be discussed.

Keywords. Intelligent tutring system, information systems, wireless technologies, HIV education, AIDS education, SmartBooks™, SmartTutor

Introduction: The Problem of HIV

Since 1981 [1] the world has been confronted with and aware of the tragedy AIDS. In the Unites States, the disease has changed from one which was proven to be almost universally fatal within 10 years, with the progression from HIV to full-blown AIDS, to one which has been more manageable as a long-term serious chronic illness. Since 1996, with the introduction of powerful anti-retroviral therapies, has dramatically prolonged the time between HIV infection to the development of AIDS [2]. Hence, focus (in the US) has been able to change somewhat from treating a terminal disease (AIDS), to living with HIV. The adult HIV prevalence rate is estimated to be around 0.6%2, but this is only an average figure, and the US has a very diverse population. The number of HIV+ people living in America varies between 900,000 and 1 million according to different estimates – the UN estimates it to be 950,000 [5].

In the United States we have been able to contain the devastation of AIDS through research, knowledge, and experience. Research has focused on the treatment of HIV/AIDS, knowledge has focused on establishing behaviors to prevent the transmission of disease (e.g. safe behaviors vis a vis sexual activity, blood transfusions, healthcare professionals and especially high-risk populations). However, in underdeveloped, Third World countries in Asia and Africa, and even in Eastern Europe, the tragic specter of HIV/AIDS immediately threatens an entire generation of people.

1. SmartBooks

Since 1993 the proliferation of the World Wide Web (WWW) has created a plethora of new opportunities for the delivery of electronic, distance learning systems. However, one might ask, "How many of these systems facilitated by the platform of the WWW have been proven and tested as sound educational tools?" Between 1988 and 1992 we developed a technology at the University of Maine for building what we called "SmartBooks" [6,7]. The basis of this approach was the use of "concept mapping", which has been demonstrated to be a sound paradigm for learning and education [8] The ability to navigate in any direction does create the opportunity for the improved effectiveness of the learning process. The actual effectiveness is determined by each individual learner. The domain of application was education of college-age populations about sexually transmitted diseases (STD's), specifically, AIDS [9]. The importance of developing an anonymous, correct, flexible, and up-to-date source of information and education about this killer disease does not need explanation. More recently, (1996) at the U.S. Coast Guard Academy in New London, CT. we applied the SmartBook methodology to develop an effective electronic system for educating about "Rules of the Road". All cadets at the Academy need to pass a course on Navigation where study of a book nearly 200 pages long is necessary. Cadets who used our "Rules of the Road SmartBook" responded quite favorably when asked to consider its effectiveness as a learning tool. SmartBooks were developed in essentially four stages:

1. Interviews with subject matter experts to develop an effective "concept map" for a domain (possibly involving a number of iterations over several months). Typically the maps would go through considerable revision before a "stable" map was settled upon. The process of creating the maps was worthy of study in itself and revealed the perspectives of subject matter experts on the hierarchical importance of topics in their domains.

2. Translation of the final concept map into the hypercard language on the Macintosh (later Toolbook for Windows was also used). The coding process proved fairly straightforward for a typical computer science undergraduate.
3. Implementation of a working SmartBook. After several years of development work we settled on a set a of standard features for the SmartBook interface and standard navigation tools (buttons).
4. Testing and revision of the working system with the target population, undergraduate students.

Concept maps are a graphical form of knowledge representation whereby all the important information in a domain can be embedded in nodes (rectangular buttons or nodes in this system) and arcs (the lines connecting nodes). At any time during interaction with the system a user can see how he/she arrived at where they are (the path taken through the SmartBook) and where it can lead to. This is indicated by a pictorial representation on the top of each card illustrating how the shaded circle (node) was reached and what circle(s) (nodes) it can lead to. Arrows without circles attached to them represent nodes which exist but are not shown in order to avoid cluttering the screen. These nodes can be found on subsequent screens. "General Text" refers to the node which is currently shaded in a graph on a visible screen. Typical additional navigation buttons would include a "Quiz" feature where learners can assess their knowledge of particular topic areas in the concept map, as well as obtain a comprehensive score [10].

Most people would probably agree that formal learning over the last centuries has been achieved through books. Books consist of words that comprise textual information or images that comprise graphical information. A well-written and well-structured book is naturally an excellent source of information on a subject for a student to learn from. Books tend to be complete and sequential in their presentation of material. There is also an implicit hierarchical structure for the knowledge in most books which attempt to present learning material. This structure entails the presentation of material in a top-down form. That is, the general overview of a subject is presented first and then details on specific relevant topics or methods will follow. A good text will have all the important subject information as well as a table of contents and index detailed enough to direct the reader as to where to find information on any topic of interest covered in the book. Key words may also be highlighted in some way. However, lacking in any text is flexibility in the order of presentation of information. This is due to the very static nature of this form of knowledge representation, the style and content being rigid and unchangeable once a book is published.

The primary advantage of a SmartBook is flexibility and the fact that it can developed about any domain using a sound educational methodology. It can be used and traversed in many ways. The order in which material to be learned is presented is the choice of the user. All information is represented in two forms: graphically and textually. Graphical information has been derived from a form of knowledge representation called concept maps. The structure of these maps can embellish the knowledge of experts in a domain. Typically any node (oval or button) on a screen can be "clicked" to proceed to the next screen with a new map segment and more information. The key to a SmartBook's flexibility is that one can move in many directions via the nodes and arcs in a graph. Concepts in nodes are connected by arcs. Importantly, at all times the user can quickly determine how the current node was reached and what are the possibilities for proceeding from the current node. Textual information is always presented in a brief, compact and clear form.

In essence, the SmartBook, represents a road map through any knowledge base. Transparency in form and function is fundamental to SmartBooks. In addition to existing pop up windows, there is the potential for linking to a glossary of terms, synonyms for key words, a retrace facility, expert advice, and video-based presentation of graphical information. As any good knowledge base, it is easy to modify, expand, and refine.

2. SmartTutor

SmartTutor is an innovative computer based or Personal Digital Assistant (PDA) based learning strategy originally created as an adjunct method for the learning of college level sciences. The original project at Brooklyn College created and tested on-line tutorials for a variety of gateway science courses including computer science, biology, chemistry and most recently physics [11,12]. The drop-out rate from science courses in four-year and two-year colleges has been of great concern for a number of years and tutoring in all forms is widely accepted on most college campuses as a primary tool for helping at-risk students. Brooklyn College of The City University of New York has a national reputation in the field of peer tutoring, with past programs funded by NSF, the Howard Hughes Medical Institute and the U.S. Department of Education.

The SmartTutor model builds on this work, using the best that is known about collaborative learning and computer-based instruction to respond to the needs of urban public college students in critical gateway science courses (for majors) and core courses (required for non-majors). The project employs insights from five years of campus research on on-line tutoring to ensure that students have available effective instructional materials to aid their science education. The original SmartTutor project was carried out by a team of faculty from biology, chemistry, physics, computer science, mathematics, psychology and economics. These faculty have had considerable experience with summer bridge programs, immersions and other support programs for non-traditional students. One of the important payoffs of the SmartTutor project is that our faculty have sought to understand the causes for student failure and then share what they learn with colleagues and the academic community in general. An important aspect of the project during the past five years has been the direct collaboration between faculty and two groups of students: one is a group of trained peer tutors who via direct experience have gained knowledge of the kinds of difficulties the other group has been comprised of a number of advanced students who gain experience by working on web design and computer graphics.

SmartTutor has been designed to promote ease of use, including concept maps, animated graphics, exercises and glossaries, content based on careful research into student learning, TutorTips, and answers to frequently asked questions (FAQs). Students seek help bringing with them varied levels of understanding and they follow their own idiosyncratic paths to learning. The SmartTutor project was designed to formulate a model that will support students working at their own initiative and at their own pace to integrate and synthesize scientific knowledge. It combines collaborative learning techniques with on-line tutoring techniques (individualized learning, coaching controlled by learner). It is intended to provide all students with access to the best possible content and to provide an alternate path for students who may otherwise be too busy or too intimidated to seek help in other ways.

Unlike more traditional forms of computer assisted instruction where the learner moves in lockstep through a structured hierarchically graded sequence of information,

SmartTutor is designed for students to go in and out of the website at any point during their learning sequence. A basic resource for organizing SmartTutor content is SmartBooks mentioned above, an intelligent tutoring component designed by Kopec and colleagues to facilitate exploration of a knowledge base. SmartTutor is based on the assumption that ideas are linked together in meaningful idiosyncratic relationships by the learner. Concept maps are a basic port of entry for every SmartTutor subject, used to guide the learner toward the information (s)he is seeking. Concept mapping has proven to be an effective strategy for helping students build a conceptual framework on a particular topic to elucidate the main features and clarify relationships. Also, the map helps students understand how topics relate to each other more effectively than a linear list. By simply clicking on topics at any level, students are immediately taken directly to the information offered on that subject. We have found that students do not always know the technical names or categories for information they are seeking. SmartTutor uses special strategies to guide students toward the information they are seeking. Students can easily access previews of what each topic contains by moving the cursor to the boxes on the map.

Based on the success that has been accumulated both in developing and implementing the SmartTutor system to the learning of college level science, it is anticipated that this tutorial model will prove to be an excellent system for the dissemination of information concerning diseases such as HIV and others to health professionals and even to individuals lacking extensive knowledge bases concerning disease processes. Following our experience in successfully transmitting diverse knowledge to students with widely varying levels of preparation and skill sets, we anticipate similar success in transferring information concerning disease processes to the general public.

3. Dissemination

The HIV/AIDS education system we are proposing is to be storable on hand-held, portable, devices exploiting Bluetooth wireless technologies. This will enable reception of data via short-range radio link using a globally available frequency band (2.4 GHz ISM band), enabling rapid and accurate synchronous and asynchronous data communication. Given that the first generation of Bluetooth permits exchange of data up to 1Mbps, even in areas with much electromagnetic disturbance, we can expect further speedup in the near future. This gives us great hope as to the possibility of developing a fully versatile system which can be used by at risk populations in Asia, Africa, and Eastern Europe. Such a device could effectively serve medical professionals as well as the general public.

As we know, awareness and education with regard to HIV/AIDS goes hand in hand with safe behavior practices, ultimately contributing to the goal of containing and ending the worldwide epidemic. The "AIDS Companion" could serve as an invaluable educational resource to adolescents, adults, and anyone who would potentially be at risk, while ensuring anonymity, and facilitating easy revisions, updates, and improvements. Such a device would be easy to maintain, would be portable, and yet fully comprehensive. The dynamically changing information regarding this disease and its containment, would be easy to update.

Evaluation

The AIDS Companion will be assessed for its effectiveness as a learning tool through regular interviews and surveys with relevant target populations. This will give us ample opportunities for feedback, analysis, and improvement of our system.

References

[1] World Health Organization [online] WHO HIV/AIDS Programme, [cited 2005-3-1]. Available from Internet: http://www.who.int/hiv/en/.

[2] MMWR Weekly (1981) 'Pneumocystis Pneumonia- Los Angeles', June 5, 30 (21); 1–3.

[3] Kopec, D. Brody,M.,Shi, C., and Wood, C. "Towards an Intelligent Tutoring System with Application to Sexually Transmitted Diseases" in Artificial Intelligence and Intelligent Tutoring Systems: Knowledge-based systems for learning and teaching, Ellis Horwood Publishers, Chichester, England, May, 1992, pp. 129–51.

[4] Presentation at, CUNY Conference for Information Technology, John Jay College, (Nov. 4, 2004).

[5] Centers for Disease Control, Department of HIV Control and Prevention http://www.cdc.gov/hiv/dhap.htm.

[6] Kopec, D, Wood, C. *Introduction to SmartBooks.* Booklet to accompany interactive educational software *AIDS SmartBook*, Jones and Bartlett Publishers, Boston, MA (1994). Also published as United States Coast Guard Academy, *Center for Advanced Studies Report No. 23–93, December*, 1993.

[7] Kopec, D., Wood, C. and Brody. (1991) An Educational Theory for Transferring Domain Expert Knowledge Towards the Development of an Intelligent Tutoring Systems for STDs. *Journal of Artificial Intelligence in Education* Vol. 2 (2), Winter, 1991, pp. 67–82.

[8] Novak, J.D. and Gowin, D.B., "*Learning How to Learn*", Cambridge University Press, Cambridge, England, 1985.

[9] Wood, Carol L., "*Use of Concept Maps in Micro-computer Based Program Design for an AIDS Knowledge Base.*, EDD Thesis, University of Maine, Orono, 1992.

[10] Kopec, D. "SmartBooks: A generic methodology to facilitate delivery of post-secondary education." in *Proceedings AMCIS 2001* (Association for Information Systems) *7th Americas Conference on Information Systems.* Boston, August 2–5, 2001, Curriculum and Learning Track; (CDROM).

[11] Kopec, D., Whitlock, P. and Kogen, M.. "SmartTutor: Combining SmartBooks™ and Peer Tutors for Multi-Media Online Instruction. " Proceedings of the International Conference on Engineering Education, University of Manchester, Manchester, England, (UMIST), CDROM, August 18–21, 2002.

[12] Kopec, D. Whitlock, P., and Kogen, M.. "Enhancing The First Computer Science Course With Peer Tutors, SmartBooks™ and SmartTutors in: *"Innovations – 2003": World Innovations in Engineering Education and Research*". (Eds. W. Aung, M.Hoffmann, et.al.) August, 2003, pp. 85–94.

Symposium on Virtual Hospitals

Medical and Care Compunetics 2
L. Bos et al. (Eds.)
IOS Press, 2005

VEMH – Virtual Euro-Mediterranean Hospital for Global Healthcare

G. GRASCHEW[a], T.A. ROELOFS[a], S. RAKOWSKY[a], P.M. SCHLAG[a], S. KAISER[b] and S. ALBAYRAK[b]
[a]*Surgical Research Unit OP 2000, Max-Delbrueck-Center and Robert-Roessle-Klinik, Charité – University Medicine Berlin, Lindenberger Weg 80, 13125 Berlin, Germany*
[b]*DAI-Labor, Agent Technologies in Business Applications and Telecommunication, Technical University Berlin, Germany*

Abstract. The Virtual Euro-Mediterranean Hospital (VEMH) aims to facilitate the interconnection of various medical services through real integration. VEMH will provide an integrated satellite-terrestrial platform and realize telemedical services such as e-learning, real-time telemedicine and medical assistance and offer individual grants to young medical doctors. The methodologies of the VEMH are medical-need-oriented instead of technology-oriented. VEMH will provide for medical professionals in the whole Euro-Mediterranean area access to the required quality of medical service. For the successful deployment of the services of the VEMH GRID technologies have to be implemented especially for evidence-based medicine. A Metagrid Service Engine implements an additional software layer between proprietary GRID engines and the different applications. The use of mobile code is envisioned in future GRIDs which allows service creation and deployment on arbitrary nodes of a GRID. Dynamic Grid structures become an important point for the use of mobile code.

1. Introduction

Telemedicine aims at equal access to medical expertise irrespective of the geographical location of the person in need. New developments in Information and Communication Technologies (ICT) have enabled the transmission of medical images in sufficiently high quality that allows for a reliable diagnosis to be determined by the expert at the receiving site [1–3]. At the same time, however, these innovative developments in ICT over the last decade bear the risk of creating and amplifying a digital divide in the world, creating a disparity between the northern and the southern Euro-Mediterranean area.

The digital divide in the field of health care has a direct impact in the daily life of the citizens and on their quality of life. In recent years, different institutions have launched several Euro-Mediterranean telemedicine projects. All of them aimed to encourage the Euro-Mediterranean cooperation between the European member states and the Mediterranean Countries.

All these projects have demonstrated how the digital divide is only a part of a more complex problem, the need for integration. Therefore, provision of the same advanced technologies to the European, to the Mediterranean and to the Adhering Countries should be the final goal for contributing to their better dialogue for integration.

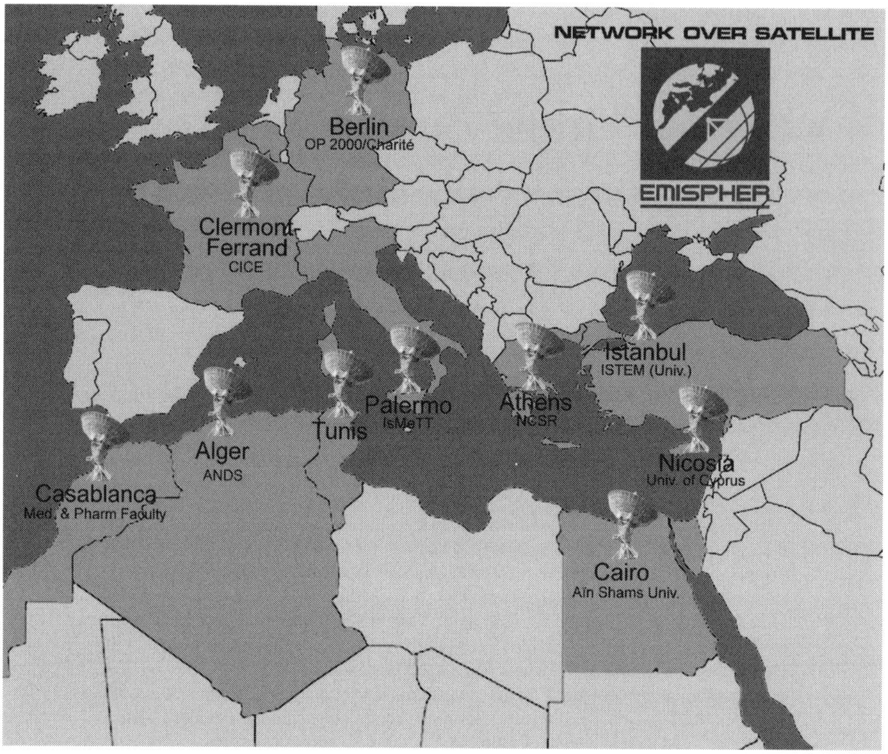

Figure 1. Centers of Excellence in the EMISPHER Network.

In the framework of the EMISPHER project (Euro-Mediterranean Internet-Satellite Platform for Health, medical Education and Research, EUMEDIS Pilot Project 110, see www.emispher.org/, 9/2002–12/2004, co-funded by the EC under the EUMEDIS Programme) a dedicated internet-satellite platform for Telemedicine in the Euro-Mediterranean area was deployed and put in operation [4]. The network currently consists of 10 sites in Morocco, Algeria, Tunisia, Egypt, Turkey, Italy, Greece, Cyprus, France and Germany, (see Fig. 1) and hosts key applications in the field of medical eLearning (courses for under-graduates, graduates, young medical professionals, etc., in real-time and asynchronous modes), real-time Telemedicine (second opinion, demonstration and spread of new techniques, Telementoring, etc.) and eHealth (medical assistance for tourists and expatriates). The EMISPHER network serves as a basis for the development and deployment of a Virtual Hospital for the Euro-Mediterranean region.

2. Virtual Euro-Mediterranean Hospital – VEMH

Due to the experience in the exploitation of previous European telemedicine projects and, in particular to activities carried out in the framework of the EUMEDIS programme, an open Euro-Mediterranean consortium would like to propose the Virtual Euro-Mediterranean Hospital (VEMH) initiative. *VEMH* aims to facilitate and accelerate the interconnection and interoperability of the various services being developed (by different organisation at different sites) through real integration. This integration must take into account the social, human and cultural dimensions; that strive towards common approaches but open and respectful of cultural differences: *multi-lateral cooperation instead of aid.*

VEMH is dedicated to bridging such a digital divide by establishing high quality equal access to real-time and on-line services for healthcare for all of the countries of the Euro-Mediterranean area. *VEMH* will provide a heterogeneous integrated platform consisting of a satellite link, such as in the EMISPHER project, and a terrestrial link, like in the EUMEDCONNECT project, for the application of various medical services.

2.1. VEMH Services and Activities

E-learning. In the project the **Me**diterranean **M**edical **U**niversity (**MeMU**) will be developed. The leading medical centres integrated in the network provide pedagogical material and modules for synchronous and asynchronous e-learning in their medical specialties. The central gateway to MeMU is an integrated satellite- and terrestrial-based platform and will provide the users with access to various contents in the network and support the participation in real-time e-learning events.

Real-time telemedicine. VEMH will offer the following categories of applications:

- second opinion,
- tele-teaching & tele-training (demonstration and spread of new techniques),
- tele-mentoring (enhancement of staff qualification),
- undergraduate teaching courses
- optimisation of the learning curve.

These real-time interactive tele-medical applications contribute to improved quality of patient care and to accelerated qualification of medical doctors in their respective specialty (see Fig. 2). Thus, this international network of distributed but integrated competence contributes directly and indirectly to improved healthcare.

Medical assistance. As tourism constitutes a substantial economical factor in the Mediterranean region and because of the increasing mobility of the population, continuity of care through improved medical assistance is of major importance for improved healthcare in the Euro-Mediterranean region. The introduction of standardised procedures, integration of the platform with the various local and national communication systems, and training of the medical staff involved in medical assistance allow for shared management of files related to medical assistance (medical images, diagnosis, workflow, financial management, etc.) and thus for improved care for travellers and expatriates in the Euro-Mediterranean region.

Fellowship programme. VEMH will offer individual grants to young medical doctors coming from the Mediterranean and from accession countries. Each fellow will be trained in one of the fields of the MeMU through the tele-teaching and tele-training VEMH services. This training programme will include an internship period in some of the clinical and scientific institutions of the VEMH consortium. The VEMH faculty will constantly monitor the progresses of the fellows and will evaluate them at the end

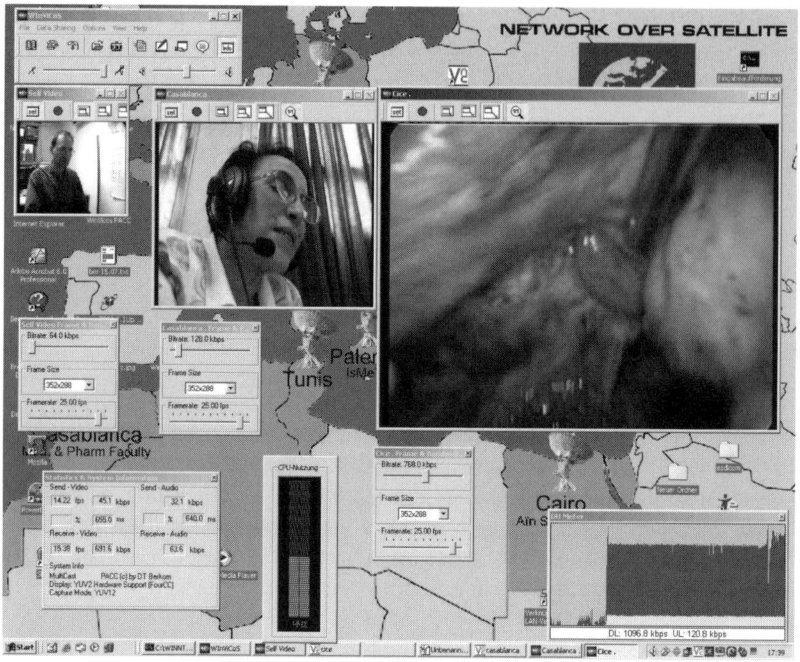

Figure 2. Interactive Multipoint Teleconsultation During Laparoscopy between OP 2000 – Berlin, FMPC – Casablanca and CICE – Clermont-Ferrand.

of the training period. The scope of the fellowship programme is to allow young medical doctors to develop and gain experience in a multicultural and multidisciplinary environment.

2.2. Methodology of the VEMH

The methodology in the VEMH medical network of competence will be improved by the realization of a management of the clinical outcomes. By the integration of different telemedical solutions in one platform it will be possible to support many different medical applications which can be arranged in a matrix structure where the individualisation of the user needs per country are represented as matrix columns and the applications with integrated technological solutions are represented as matrix rows. A criterium for the selection of applications are low access costs.

The VEMH provides a modular distributed medical network for integration and optimisation of various applications. The developed new methodologies and applications should be useable for more than one disease. The methodologies of the VEMH are medical-need-oriented instead of technology-oriented.

2.3. Evaluation and Assessment of VEMH Services and Applications

The justification of the various VEMH services and applications will be assessed by using a comprehensive evaluation methodology. This will in particular examine various outcomes including clinical, organisational, and economic as well as other relevant outcomes. The criteria under which such services can be evaluated are based upon the

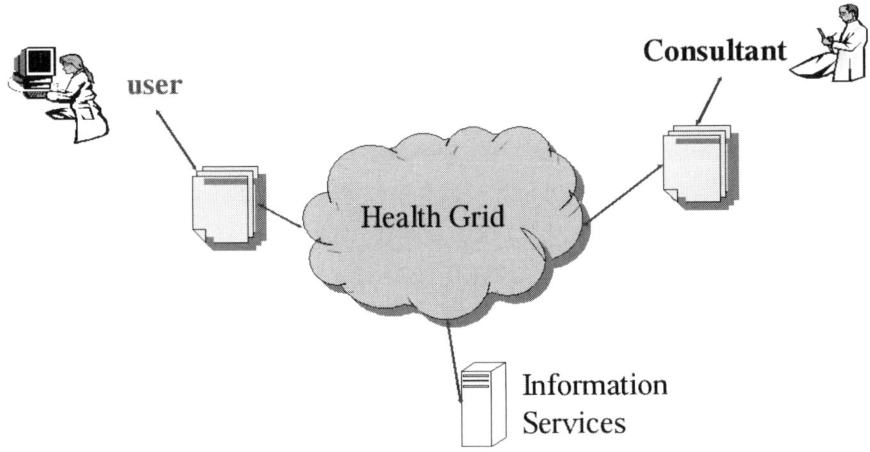

Figure 3. Health GRID for the VEMH.

work of Bashshur (1995) [5]. The rationale for using this type of methodology is to ensure that the services or applications are capable of having an immediate and positive impact upon patient care in the VEMH region.

2.4. VEMH Outcomes

VEMH will foster cross-Mediterranean cooperation between the leading medical centres of the participating countries by establishing a permanent medical and scientific link. Outcomes of the VEMH are guidelines for different diseases in the different medical fields presented in standardised way, education on this new standards for all users and future users, new e-learning interactive tools and quality control and score of quality. Benefits of the VEMH are increased effectiveness, accelerated decision making, improved quality of decisions via real-time global exchange between experts reducing the travel and integration of the human resources in this region.

3. GRID for Healthcare

For the successful deployment of the services of the VEMH like acquisition and processing of medical images, data storage, archiving and retrieval and data mining GRID technologies have to be implemented especially for evidence-based medicine (see Fig. 3) [6]. To achieve this conventional GRID technology has to be expanded to cover not only local computing resources but to a dimension of organisation spanning integrated networks. Among the challenges to be met are issues like heterogeneous computing systems, expectation of high privacy and trust levels as well as ease of use and general flexibility.

3.1. Metagrid Services

An agent-based Metagrid Service Engine (MGSE) implements an additional software layer between proprietary GRID engines and the applications and integrates the different approaches. The Metagrid Services should address the main issues of today's GRID Computing software. Low level GRIDs like the SUN Grid Engine provide scalable high performance GRIDs and need homogeneous GRID nodes because scheduled tasks contain only scripts designed to call the programs needed for the tasks.

3.2. Mobile Code

We envision the use of mobile code in future GRIDs which allows service creation and deployment on arbitrary nodes of a GRID giving a flexibility unknown by today's GRID technology. Services can be created and distributed in a Grid through mobile code, severely reducing the need for software installation in the Grids nodes.

The main objective is on the one hand an integration of low level concepts like the SUN Grid Engine in wide scale management like the Open Grid Service Architecture OGSA and on the other hand bringing more flexibility to systems based on the OGSA framework by integrating features like dynamic service distribution, mobile code, etc. The ultimate goal being the ability to distribute tasks over a secure and organization spanning dynamic GRID.

3.3. Dynamic Grid

By using platform independent software Grids can be extended to large scale networks, allowing the flexible use of computing resources from a vast number of Grid nodes. Here support for dynamic Grid structures becomes an important point. Meta-Grid Services have to be able to tolerate changes in the managed Grid, like the addition or removal of nodes at runtime. Fallback mechanisms have to go to work when tasks cannot be fulfilled because nodes they where assigned to drop out without returning the appropriate task results.

3.4. Experimental Environment

In co-operation between Sun Microsystems and the Technical University Berlin a GRID testbed has been set up. At start, the testbed consisted of seven multiprocessor nodes based on heterogeneous hardware configurations (see Fig. 4): Sun SPARC RISC Architecture, Intel-based 64-bit computers, and Intel-based 32-bit nodes. Additionally, a Sun StorEdge mass storage unit with nearly 1Terabyte of harddisk space is part of the network. All nodes are interconnected by an Gigabit network. The systems are configured to run Linux or Solaris operating systems and the Sun Grid engine (version 6.0) creating a heterogeneous system. The testbed has recently been extended by adding two more V44z model computers providing a Grid with nine nodes and a total of 24 CPUs.

4. Conclusions

Through the deployment and operation of an integrated interactive communication platform (satellite link, terrestrial, wireless, etc.), *VEMH* will provide for medical professionals in the whole Euro-Mediterranean area access to the required quality of medical service depending on the individual needs of each of the partner. The services such as E-learning, the applications in real-time telemedicine and the improved medical assis-

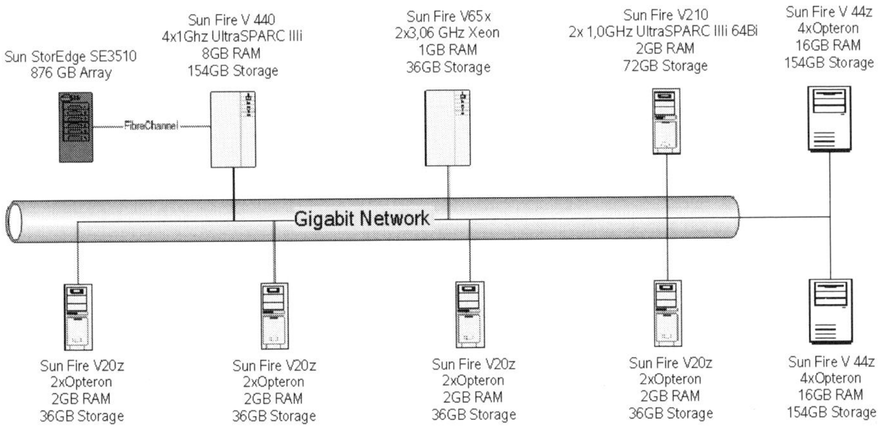

Figure 4. Experimental GRID infrastructure at the DAI laboratory.

tance contribute to an improved level of healthcare in the whole Euro-Mediterranean region and build the basis for the introduction of Evidence-Based Medicine. For the successful deployment of the various medical services in the VEMH the development and implementation of Health GRID technology appears crucial.

References

[1] G. Graschew, S. Rakowsky, P. Balanou, P.M. Schlag, Interactive telemedicine in the operating theatre of the future. J. Telemed. Telecare, 6, suppl 2 (2000) 20–24.

[2] R.U. Pande, Y. Patel, C.J. Powers, G. D'Ancona, H.L. Karamanoukian, The telecommunication revolution in the medical field: present applications and future perspective. Curr. Surg. 60 (2003) 636–640.

[3] G. Graschew, T.A. Roelofs, S. Rakowsky, P.M. Schlag, Broadband Networks for Interactive Telemedical Applications. APOC 2002, Applications of Broadband Optical and Wireless Networks, Shanghai 16.–17.10.2002, Proceedings of SPIE, 4912 (2002) 1–6.

[4] G. Graschew, T.A. Roelofs, S. Rakowsky, P.M. Schlag, Überbrückung der digitalen Teilung in der Euro-Mediterranen Gesundheitsversorgung – das EMISPHER-Projekt, In: A. Jäckel (Hrsg.) Telemedizinführer Deutschland, Ober-Mörlen, Ausgabe 2005, 231–236.

[5] R.L. Bashshur, On the definition and evaluation of telemedicine. Telemedicine Journal 1 (1995), 19–30.

[6] http://whitepaper.healthgrid.org/.

Medical and Care Compunetics 2
L. Bos et al. (Eds.)
IOS Press, 2005

A Distributed Database and a New Application for the DRG System

Liana STANESCU and Dumitru Dan BURDESCU
University of Craiova, Faculty of Automation, Computers and Electronics
stanescu@software.ucv.ro, burdescu@topedge.com

Abstract. The article presents a new solution for the implementation of the DRG classifying system used in Romania to finance hospitals. The new solution implies two proposals. The first one refers to the use of a fragmented and distributed database at level of each hospital, and the second refers to the management and the viewing of this database by means of an on-line application implemented in Java. The solution proposes that the distributed database should be managed by two powerful tools, meaning Oracle8 Server and Net8. Different types of users are proposed, each type with his own rights for managing and viewing the database. Excepting local users who use only their local database, there are also global users from National DRG Bureau who can see data from all local databases, at any time. This solution is more efficient, secure and modern, than the one used now.

Keywords. DRG, distributed database, Oracle8 Server, Net8, on-line application

1. The DRG System

The Romanian Government uses nowadays the DRG classification system as a base to finance 185 hospitals, and it plans to extend this number in the following years.

The DRG is a system which permits to classify the patients based on the diagnosis, the procedures and other information (the complexity of each case) and to link this type of patients that each hospital treats to the expenses needed [1].

The necessary data for the patient classification on the basis of the diagnosis and the procedures in DRG categories are: age, sex, hospitalization period, principal diagnosis, secondary diagnosis, procedures, health condition when leaving hospital, the birth weight (in the new-born child case). These data define the DRG classification system.

Through the system of the diagnosis group (DRG) the characteristics of each patient who left the hospital are analyzed, and in accordance with these, the patients are classified in a different category. This way, the DRG system makes an "image" to the hospital results, trying to standardize the results of this activity.

To be able to classify each patient that left the hospital in a diagnosis group one has to run through four phases:

1. the disponibility of the clinical data for the patients that left the hospital
2. the codification of the necessary data for the diagnosis and the procedures in order to have a standardized language for these variables and to be able to use them easily

3. gathering these data in an electronic manner
4. the automatic classification of each patient in a diagnosis group

Nowadays, to gather the information for the patients it is used the DRGNational v4.0 application that is delivered through the district agencies [1]. This application must be installed on every computer used for gathering data about the patients. The electronically registration for a patient, one for the whole period the patient stays in hospital, is in concordance with the new clinical observation form introduced by the Romanian Health and Family Ministry. Once collected, the data are added to a database which has to be sent monthly to the DRG department from the National Health Institute for Research and Development, Bucharest.

Nowadays, the application DRGNational v4.0 is delivered on a CD as a Runtime application implemented in Microsoft Access 2000, that collects information about the patients at the department level, encrypt them and after that send them to the DRG National Bureau using the e-mail. The data centralization from all departments on a single computer is also possible, where the application also has to be installed, and send them in this centralized manner to the DRG National Bureau.

2. The Description of the New Proposed Solution

2.1. The General Presentation

A new solution is proposed for the implementation of the DRGNational Application in order to eliminate the difficulties of the one used at present. The new solution supposes on the one hand the usage of a distributed database, and on the other hand an on-line application implemented in Java.

First of all, MS Access 2000 is an administration system for desktop databases and it administrates with efficiency a slightly reduced number of recordings: around 20000–30000 records, generally used in activity management in small companies. That is why, instead of using MS Access 2000 it is proposed a much stronger system of database administration, which offers distributed support, named Oracle8 [2].

A distributed database is a set of databases stored on multiple computers that typically appears to applications as a single database [3]. Consequently, an application can simultaneously access and modify the data in several databases in a network. Each Oracle database in the system is controlled by its local Oracle Server but cooperates to maintain the consistency of the global distributed database. A database server is the Oracle software managing a database, and a client is an application that requests information from a server. Each computer in a system is a node. A node in a distributed database system acts as a client, server, or both, depending on the situation.

All Oracle databases in a distributed database system use Oracle's networking software, Net8, to facilitate inter-database communication across a network [4]. Just as Net8 connects clients and servers that operate on different computers of a network, it also allows database servers to communicate across networks to support remote and distributed transactions in a distributed database [4]. Net8 makes transparent the connectivity that is necessary to transmit SQL requests and receive data for applications that use the system. Net8 takes SQL statements from a client and packages them for transmission to an Oracle server over a supported industry-standard communication protocol or programmatic interfaces.

The new solution offers more advantages:

- It cancels the encrypt phase of data and the transmission through the e-mail because it can bring a lot of problems; the data received by e-mail at the DRG National Bureau must be saved in a certain format, eventually a database, in order to be consulted either with visualization, or with the elaboration of some reports, statistics or graphics, this being the most efficient way; when adding in the same database information resulted from different sources there may be some problems; for example: the primary key values might be identical in several different files. In this case certain processing must be made before being saved in database; all these require a lot of time;
- The data that DRG National Bureau sees are always up to date; it is not necessary to wait for the end of a certain period of time to receive those data; anytime the up-to-day data can be seen as reports, statistics or graphics, which is a very important thing for the medical domain; these up-to-day data could be placed even at the disposal of some international medical institutes, an usual and absolutely necessary task.
- At the level of each hospital implied in the DRG network, the application, the database and the database server must be installed on a single computer (server); it will be accessible for any user from the hospital in the range of his rights from his own computer, using a browser; in this manner it is not needed to install the application on each client's computer; of course, the server's performances must be very high, as the capacity to transfer data in the network; at this level, the application is especially dedicated to the users from the departments who must insert in the database new observation sheets or to update the ones corresponding to the patients already hospitalized. So, for each hospital a database will be independently managed, which will function in a distributed database system.
- At the national level must use another part of the on-line application which allows the authorized users only the view in different forms of all the information in the independent databases existing at the hospital level. For this, there must be users' accounts which allow server-to-server connections, so that there could be performed distributed queries on all the existing databases al hospital level [4].

2.2. The Database Structure

Applying the normalization process [5,6], the database proposed for this on-line application will be described further on. First of all, there is a series of set-up tables which contain encoding. Each of these tables contains an id field which identifies uniquely the records and a name.

Table **tblStatus** allows encoding of the patient status by means of two fields status_id (primary key) and status name.

For encoding the diagnoses there are three tables **tblClass**, **tblSubclass** and **tblDiagnoses** connected by a 1:m relationship because in one class there are several subclasses, and in one subclass there are several diagnoses.

For encoding the XR investigations and the functional explorations there is the table **tblXr,** respectively **tblInvestFunct**

There is also a table which allows the encoding of the surgical procedures, **tblSurgical**

The table **tblInt** allows encoding of the different types of hospital registration

Some other tables in the database are:

In the table **tblHospital** there are data about the hospital from the DRG network: hospital_id (primary key), hospital name, county, city, number of beds.

In the table **tblDepart** there are data about the departments from each hospital: department_id (primary key), department name, hospital_id (foreign key) used to implement the relationship 1:m between the tables tblHospital and tblDepart.

In every department works a number of doctors about whom there are data in the table **tblDoctor**: doctor_id (primary key), name, specialty, department_id (foreign key) used to implement the relationship 1:m between the tables **tblDepart** and **tblDoctor**.

For a certain department and a certain doctor the patients who have a new sheet at every hospital record are registered. For their data a new table **tblPatient** was created having the following structure: sheet_id (primary key), personal_id, first name, last name, sex, birth weight in the new-born child case, data of registration, data of release from the hospital, doctor_id (foreign key) in order to know the doctor who attended the patient, the code of the first principal diagnosis, the code of the second principal diagnosis, the code of the secondary diagnosis, the code of the hospitalization type, the code of the patient status.

The database also contains a series of tables as the result of the implementation of some m:m relationships between the above tables.

The table **tblPatient_XR** stores for every observation sheet identified by sheet_id the codes of the effectuated XR investigations

The table **tblPatient_FuncExpl** stores for every observation sheet identified by sheet_id the codes of the effectuated functional explorations

The table **tblPatient_Surgical** stores for every observation sheet identified by sheet_id the codes of the surgical procedures made during the hospitalization time

The tables: tblHospitals, tblDepart, tblDoctor, tblPacient, tblPacient_XR, tblPacient-FuncExpl and tblPacient_Surgical were horizontally fragmented. In each site of the distributed database, namely at each hospital level, these tables contain only the records corresponding to the hospital departments. The other tables that contain encoding exist in each site.

Taking into consideration the necessity of data recovery in case of the system failure, it has to be considered the data replication. In such a special case a safety copy of the database can be used [3].

2.3. User Interface

The proposed user interface of the on-line application for the management and viewing the database follows on the whole the options of the currently used application. This can be for the benefit of the persons who are already familiar with the old application.

Obviously, there are also some differences that this new solution brings. Below, there are shortly presented the proposals for the user interface and for the operation mode.

The main menu of the application is: Patient File, Search, Reports and Exit. Each of these menus has few submenus. The first option groups the web pages managing the sheets of paper for the hospitalized, the second allows searching patient details or searching data through other tables (for example the diagnoses table), and the third allows to see the reports, statistical data, graphics.

After the user connects to the database (he enters the username and password) he can insert records for new patients, or modify existing ones.

If he adds a new record, he must write the name and surname of the patient, date and time of hospitalization. When he presses Submit button, the new record is inserted in tblPatient table. After that a new submenu with the following options is generated:

- General Information
- Diagnoses
- Surgical Interventions
- Functional Explorations
- XR Investigations

When General Information option is called, a new form appears allowing to enter general information about the patient: name, surname, birthday, sex, status (insured, uninsured, foreigner), personal ID, address, type of hospitalization, name of the doctor.

The Diagnoses option allows entering two main diagnoses, the diagnosis when leaving the hospital and other complications, if any. The other three options represent auxiliary information regarding surgery, radiography, analyses (if any).

As it can be seen, data about patients are added at different moments of time, so the update function is very used and therefore very important, as searching function matching one of several criteria. It is proposed to find information about patients searching for record number, or patient details: personal ID, name, surname. Once the user identifies the patient, he can update what he needs, using the option above.

To ease the operator's work filling the data, certain data can be selected from drop-down controls. For example, selecting a diagnosis or a type of analysis can be done in such a manner.

The data added in forms are validated. For example, it is checked if a field is date type or, if some fields aren't null (name, surname).

When the patient leave the hospital all the data needed now are added (diagnosis, health condition), and the flag which indicates this is set to true.

Regarding the reports, the user can get them for one department, hospital or even DRG National Bureau. In the first case the data reflect information only from that department, in the second case data from all departments in the hospital, and in the last case from all data in the distributed database.

The reports may consider the patients from a certain month in order to match the financial part of the application, or all the patients who have ever been (or still are) hospitalized in that department.

The application wants to make a few statistics regarding the number of patients with a certain diagnosis in every district, over a period of time, or in accordance with health condition when leaving the hospital.

When a user logs on, and tries to update the database, he will see only those data he has access rights to see. For example, a user from a department will see only the records with patients in his department.

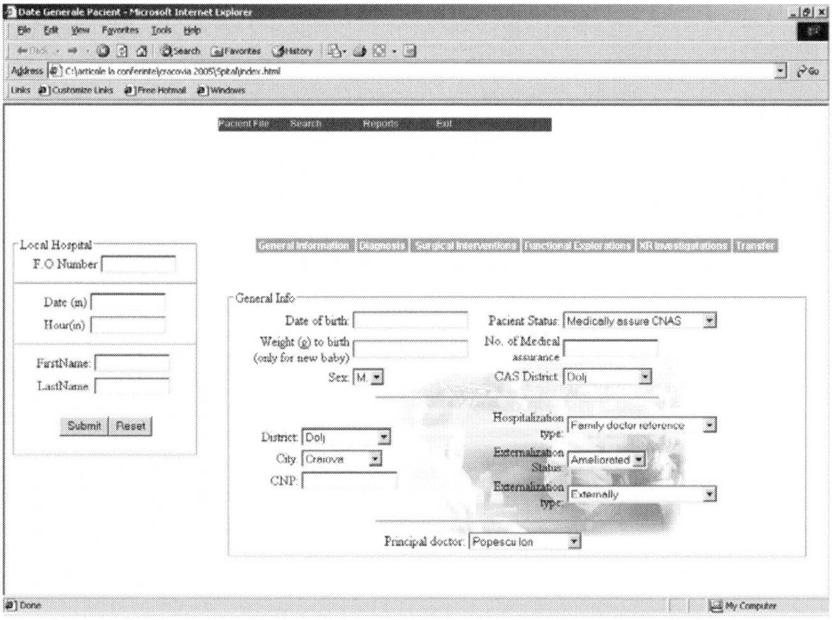

Figure 1. The application window allowing the insertion of a new observation sheet.

In Fig. 1 one can see the proposal for the application window opened for a user identified by name and password who can proceed to the insertion of a new observation sheet being entitled to this.

In Fig. 2 there is the proposed application window which allows the update of the data concerning the principal and secondary diagnoses of the patient.

2.4. Users and Rights

For this new proposed application there have been identified and proposed the following types of users:

- Department Level Users – they have rights to access only data at the department level. They can insert, update and delete records from data regarding only their department.
- Hospital Level Users – they have rights only for viewing data from all departments in their hospital. The managers of the hospital belong to this category.
- Hospital Level Administrators – they have rights to insert and update data about the hospital and the departments. They work with tblHospital and tblDepart tables; they have to make accounts for the department level users and hospital level users.
- National Level Users – they might have the right to view data from all local database using reports, graphics and statistics. They don't have any rights to modify data. The users from National DRG Bureau belong to this category.
- Main Administrator of the database who coordinates the whole activity

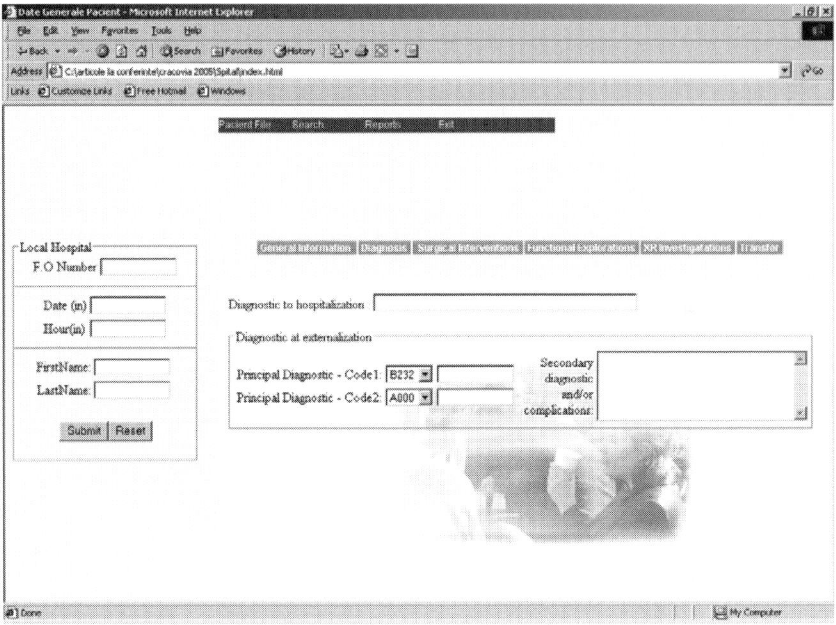

Figure 2. The application window allowing the updating the principal and secondary diagnoses.

3. Conclusion

This paper presents a new solution to implement the DRGNational application, used by the medical system in some hospitals in Romania as the basis for the establishment of the degree of finances they need. There are presented not only the drawbacks and the inconvenient of the used application, but also the proposed solution.

This new alternative supposes a distributed database consisting in several databases each one stored in a computer at the level of the hospital involved in the DRG network. A database management system Oracle8 was proposed and also Net8 to facilitate inter-database communication across a network. Each Oracle database in the system is controlled by its local Oracle Server. The users from each hospital department use a Java application [7–9] which manages the local database. Each of these users has very clearly established rights: some can update the database, others, for example the hospital management staff can only view the data. There is also another group of users, the ones at the national level, who have a different on-line application which allows the performance of distributed queries on all the databases existing in the distributed system. This makes it possible to view all the data in different forms (reports, statistics, plots).

The proposed solution is not a very cheap one, but it is probably the most effective. The existence of a database at the level of each hospital, allows a better management of it, a good performance speed for the users' requests, in comparison with the existence of a single national database, to which all users can connect. The distributed databases from DRG network, at hospital level are much smaller that a single national database. This is a benefit for local users for whom the response time for updating data is much faster.

The number of local users at hospital level is smaller than the number of users who might have to access a national database, so the concurrency access to the distributed databases is easier.

Taking into account these facts, the solution presented in this paper has much more benefits than the one used nowadays in Romania. Moreover it is better than the one which uses a central national database accessed on-line by users from all the hospitals and from the National DRG Bureau.

References

[1] DRG Romanian Oficial Page http://www.drg.ro, 2005.
[2] Oracle8 Server Distributed Database Systems, http://www-rohan.sdsu.edu/doc/oracle/server803/A54653_01/toc.htm, Oracle Corporation, 1997.
[3] Ozsu T., Valduriez P., Principles of Distributed Database Systems (2 edition), Prentice Hall, 1999.
[4] Net8(TM) Administrator's Guide, http://www-rohan.sdsu.edu/doc/oracle/network803/A51576_01/toc.htm, Oracle Corporation, 1997.
[5] Burdescu D, Ionescu A, Stanescu L. Databases, Universitaria, Craiova, 2004.
[6] Elmasri R, Navathe SB. Fundamentals of Database Systems. Addison – Wesley Publishing Company, second edition, 1994.
[7] Forta D,Smith E, Stirling S,Kim L, Kerr R,Aden D, Lei A. Dezvoltarea aplicatiilor JavaServer Pages, Teora, Bucuresti, 2001.
[8] Goodwill J. Pure JSP, Java Server Pages: A Code-Intensive Premium Reference, Smas, 2000.
[9] Matthews M, Cole J, Gradecki JD, Gradecki J. MySQL and Java Developer's Guide, Wiley, 2003.

Medical and Care Compunetics 2
L. Bos et al. (Eds.)
IOS Press, 2005

Incorporating the Sense of Smell into Haptic Surgical Simulators

Brandon S. SPENCER
Graduate School of Computer and Information Sciences, Nova Southeastern University 3301 College Avenue, Fort Lauderdale, FL 33314, USA

Abstract. It is widely recognized that the sense of smell plays an important role in the field of medicine. The sense of smell not only assists the physician in the diagnosis of certain disorders, but it also plays a surgical role as well. Historically, learning this skill was contingent upon some level of clinical exposure to medically related odors. The advent of computerized scent production devices could change this. This article proposes a hypothetical surgical simulation model that incorporates olfactory technologies into existing, haptic, surgical simulators. If incorporated into virtual educational settings such as these, computerized scent production devices could be used not only as a novel way to enhance the virtual experience, but also as a way for medical students to begin to recognize the important role that the sense of smell can play during surgery.

Keywords. Telemedicine, telesurgery, distance education, simulation, virtual reality, smell

Introduction

Patient simulators, which currently exist in nearly 1/3rd of all medical schools in the United States, are increasingly being used as educational tools for doctors, nurses, and other health care professionals [1]. In the quest to increase the realism of instructional simulators, enhancements to the physical, functional, and task fidelity aspects of simulation-based training continue to push the technological envelope [2]. Medical simulators run the gamut, from simulated patients, to distance educational, virtual reality simulators operating over high-speed networks [2,3].

As the length of medical training time decreases, and the expected knowledge base of health care providers increases, simulation is often being called upon as an educational supplement to real world experiences [2]. This is especially true in those cases where physical distance is a hindrance to receiving proper medical training [3,4]. Regardless of whether or not distance is the issue, haptic simulators have recently been shown to be efficacious, supplemental educational aids when it comes to teaching the complexities of surgery [5].

At advanced complex training levels, such as learning by way of the surgical simulator, it is important that the appropriate clinical clues are incorporated into simulated systems so as to support high-level decision making [2]. Students often complain that the lack of clinical realism associated with many medical simulators is an important limitation [1]. In order to create a strong sense of presence in the virtual environment, the traditional modalities of touch, hearing, and vision must be superceded. For these reasons, in addition to the fact that simulators play a supplemental role to real world, clinical experiences, it is important that virtual technologies provide the student with as much realism as possible, including details that have historically been considered technically out of reach, such as appealing to the human sense of smell.

The sense of smell plays an important role in the field of medicine [6–8]. Not only is the sense of smell often used as an aid in the diagnosis of various medical disorders, but it also plays a surgical role as well. The recent development of computerized, scent-producing devices makes the incorporation of smell into medically related simulators a natural transition. This paper proposes a hypothetical model whereby computerized, scent production devices are incorporated into existing, haptic, surgical simulators as a novel way to enhance the fidelity of the virtual experience, in addition to helping medical students begin to recognize the important role that the sense of smell can play during surgery.

1. Background

1.1. Smell and Memory

The connection between smell and memory has been well documented, in both context dependent and context non-dependent situations [9–13]. In addition, incorporating aromas in virtual learning environments has been demonstrated to be an affective memory enhancer. In one important study demonstrating this enhancement [14], a multi-sensory, virtual-reality office space experiment was conducted on 322 undergraduate students. This study demonstrated that by increasing the modalities of sensory input (tactile, olfactory, etc.), the sense of presence was increased, as well as the user's memory of the environment (and objects in that environment). In the "reception area" of their virtual reality office program, where there was a strategically placed coffee pot, the experimental group was exposed to the aroma of coffee via a small mask, while the control group was not. It was found that after post-testing, 95% of experimental subjects recalled the location of the coffee pot, versus a 59% recall rate for of the control group. Similar results would be expected from the inclusion of olfactory devices into haptic, surgical simulators.

1.2. Smell and Medicine

When it comes to detecting the presence of various odors, the nose is a very sensitive instrument [15]. In traditional Chinese medicine, the sense of smell has always been recognized as a valuable, medical diagnostic tool [8]. Doctors are taught to use the sense of smell to recognize disorders even before a patient begins exhibiting symptoms, and the importance of smell, for the purposes of diagnosis, can be universally applied to the practice of medicine in general [6,7].

For example, clinicians are trained to recognize the smell of pears (acetone) on a patient's breath as being indicative of diabetes [6,7,16]. Syphilis, kidney failure, abscesses of the lung, uremia, scurvy, liver failure, rheumatic fever, diphtheria, pneumonia, and scarlet fever are also just a few of the conditions described by clinicians as having distinctive odors.

In addition, odors that can be associated with surgery, such as infected wounds, human tissues, and human body fluids such as blood or bile, have also been considered in terms of tele-present surgical applications because of their importance to surgeons [17]. For example, in regards to tele-present surgical and tele-present battlefield surgical environments, Keller [17] proposed models that consisted of neural-network based electronic noses that had the ability to identify medical odors in remote surgical environments, electronically transmit the detected odor information over a computer network to a separate location, and then re-create the surgically related odors for the benefit of the coaching surgeon.

1.3. Computerized Olfactory Technologies

Appealing to one's sense of smell via multimedia applications is not a new idea, especially from an entertainment perspective. In the 1950's, the documentary *Behind the Great Wall* provided the audience with 72 scent cues that were piped through a theatre ventilation system [18]. In the early 1960's, Helig [19] created the "Sensorama Simulator," a simulated motorcycle ride through the streets of New York City that appealed to all the human senses except for the sense of taste. In the early 1980's, John Waters released *Polyester*, a movie in which audience members were provided with scratch and sniff cue cards to use at various times during the show [18]. It was not until the late 1990's that real progress was made in the development of computerized olfactory technologies [20].

One such late 1990's olfactory, computerized system was an electro-mechanical device created to produce various on-cue aromas that were activated by programmable personal computer (PC) events [21]. This early version of computer controlled scent technology made use of a mechanical design (stepper motor, solenoids, actuator, etc.) to provide atomized scent cues based on graphical user interface input. Other early olfactory systems used compressed air to disperse liquid scents or were waxed based [20]. As computerized olfactory technologies have become more commercially viable, new designs are seemingly less complicated and more sophisticated.

Some contemporary, computerized, olfactory technologies make use of a heated oil and fan system, such as the "Scent Dome," a device that is currently available for purchase from a Georgia based company called Trisenx [22]. The Scent Dome, which is approximately 5.5 inches wide, 8 inches long, and 2.5 inches tall, plugs into a standard COMM port and is powered by a re-chargeable 6-volt battery [23]. Each Scent Dome can be fitted with one interchangeable scent cartridge at any given time, and each scent cartridge contains 20 distinct chambers, with 20 distinct vials of scented oils, the combinations of which have the potential for creating thousands of aromas [22].

Much like the previously mentioned electro-mechanical olfactory device [21], the Scent Dome is also controlled by a graphical user interface. This proprietary software allows the user to mix and match aromas by way of a virtual beaker, and to specify their intensity [22]. After a scent is created, and the Scent Dome software (or third party software) activates it for dispersion, the software communicates with the Scent Dome via a serial connection, at which time the selected chambers are heated up and the aroma is blown out of the Scent Dome by way of a small fan.

In another contemporary design, Aerome, a German Company, has developed a valve dispersion system that makes use of six glass tubes filled with granulates that each store a customizable aroma [23]. After being activated by software, filtered and compressed air is forced through the selected glass tube via a serial connection. Unlike the Scent Dome, which was designed to generally interface directly with a standard PC, the Aerome system has been mostly incorporated into proprietary, commercialized designs, such as standard and desktop sized multimedia kiosks. Never the less, like most scent-technology manufacturers, systems can be customized to fit the needs of the customer.

Other companies currently developing computerized, olfactory technologies include Aromajet, British Telecom, Osmooze, AC2i, ScentIT, ScentAir, and DaleAir [20,25]. These designs are either inkjet systems, wax based systems, airbrush systems, microencapsulated systems, or are similar to the Trisenx heated oil and fan design.

In regards to the transmission of synthesized smell over the Internet, AromaJet successfully conducted such an experimental transmission in December of 2000 [26]. During this experiment, several distinct fragrances were transmitted from Sidney, Australia, to an AromaJet Scent Kiosk in Plano, Texas, where the fragrances were recreated using proprietary scent generation software and hardware.

For the purposes of this model, the successful transmission of synthesized smell over the Internet is an important accomplishment. This transmission demonstrates that incorporating computerized, olfactory technologies into virtual, surgical classroom environments is a real possibility.

1.4. The Virtual, Surgical Classroom

Simulation has been defined as "an educational technique that allows [for] interactive, and at times immersive, activity by recreating all or part of a clinical experience without exposing patients to the associated risks [2]." Early medical simulators, such as the "Sim One" from the 1960's, were used to teach anesthesia residents the basic skill of giving injections and performing endotracheal intubation [1]. The Sim One, which was computer controlled, was programmed to respond to intravenous anesthetic medications, the administration of inhaled oxygen, and the administration of nitrous oxide. The creators of the Sim One discovered that for those residents who used the simulator, proficiency was achieved more quickly and with fewer trials than their operating/emergency room training counterparts.

The achievements of Sim One students were attributed to four advantages of the patient simulator over traditional methods [1]: 1) there was a planned and gradual increase in the difficulty of tasks, 2) the procedure could be performed as many times a needed, 3) there was immediate feedback, and 4) students were able to work at their own pace. In addition to these attributes, which are inherent to all patient simulated environments, Maran and Glavin [2] describe additional benefits of the simulated environment as being no risk to patient or student, a reduction in interference from outside stimuli, and an enhancement in the ability to evaluate student performance.

Medical simulation systems have come a long way since the days of the Sim One, now pushing the bounds of virtual reality. Virtually reality, which was developed as a computerized tool intended to mimic the natural environment as accurately as possible, has been described as the ultimate computer based technology [2]. Patient simulators can be as simple as a mannequin on a table, to as complex as haptic, virtual reality simulators [2] running over computer networks [3].

In those countries with sparsely and unevenly populated regions, where students must often travel great distances to receive specialized surgical training, virtual reality simulators are being integrated into the classroom [4]. Advancements in networking technology are creating the ability to provide simulated medical training that spans continents, a fact recently demonstrated at the annual SimTecT simulation conference in Canberra, Australia [3].

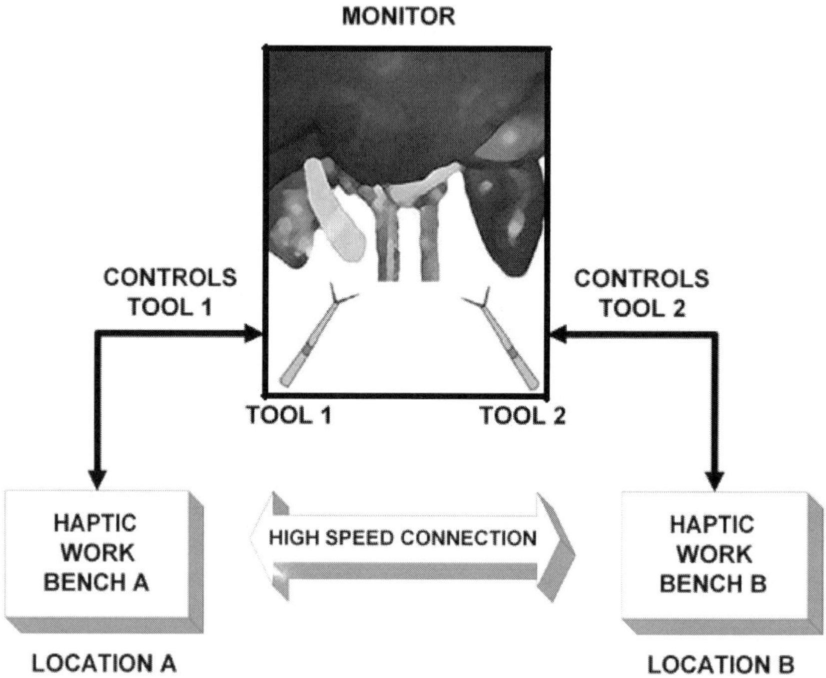

Figure 1. The haptic, surgical simulator.

Using a high-speed fiber network provided by the Center for Networking Technologies for the Information Economy (CeNTIE), representatives from the Stanford University School of Medicine (California) and the Commonwealth Scientific & Industrial Research Organization (CSIRO) of Australia, performed a virtual laparoscopic cholecystectomy (surgical removal of the gall bladder) using 3D haptic simulators [3,5]. This type of simulator, which provides haptic feedback to the user, is classified as a combination computer-generated image and part task trainer simulation model [2]. During this simulation, which was being viewed in 3D by audiences at each location, two surgeons, one playing the role of resident in training at the Canberra convention center in Australia, the other playing the role of instructor at Stanford University in the United States, simultaneously performed the simulated procedure on a stereo image of a gall bladder and surrounding organs [5]. Each having control of one of two virtual surgical tools at one time [3], as depicted in Fig. 1, the haptic simulators allowed each surgeon to not only see and hear what the other surgeon was doing in real time, but to also feel tissue resistance and the virtual manipulations (spatial retractions, organ dissection) being made by the other surgeon [4,5].

2. The Olfactory Incorporative Model

At the SimTecT interactive simulation demonstration, the surgical instructor illustrated how the haptic simulator dealt with surgical mistakes and mishaps [27]. During a normal laparoscopic cholecystectomy, the gall bladder is retracted just enough to allow for

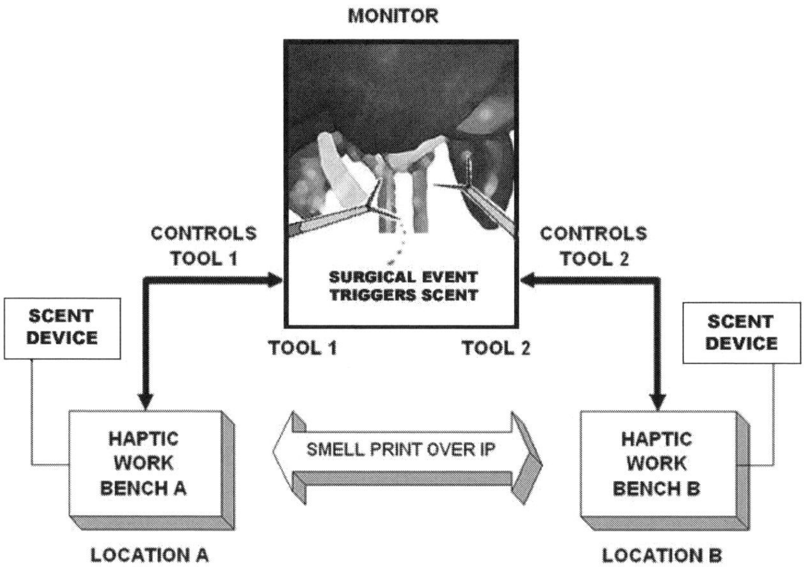

Figure 2. The olfactory incorporative model.

the proper dissection of the organ. In order to demonstrate the haptic effects of over retraction, the instructor used the surgical grasper to apply more force than was necessary, which ultimately resulted in the virtual rupturing of the gall bladder. This rupture in turn resulted in the simulated release of bile into the abdominal cavity. This event, in addition to any medically simulated surgical event, could be used to trigger the release of a virtual odor using a computerized olfactory device.

In order to accomplish the simulation of surgically related odors, such as fetid blood, bile, or an infection, some type of computerized olfactory device must be incorporated into each haptic simulator (see Fig. 2). Depending on the number of odors to be represented, any one of the commercially available computerized olfactory devices could be incorporated.

As previously mentioned, Aromajet demonstrated the ability to transmit synthesized smell over the Internet [26]. For their purposes, the smell print that was transmitted from one location, and recreated in another, was a novel aroma. In this case, the odors that would be recreated in medically simulated environments would not be novel, but instead predetermined based on a certain number of pre-defined medical events. For this reason, odors could either be activated by the complete smell print traveling over an IP network, or by some abbreviated code intended to trigger the embedded logic within each haptic simulator.

Referring to Fig. 3, assume the following situation has occurred during the simulation. The resident in training, at Haptic Workbench A and in control of Tool 1 (a grasper), has used excessive force in the retraction of the gall bladder (or some other organ as modeled). At the very moment when the tissue was virtually ruptured, the smell print (or abbreviated code) for bile (odor 1) is sent to both haptic simulators, which in turn activates the computerized scent device. Haptic Workbench A receives the smell print via a serial connection, while Haptic Workbench B receives the smell print via a high-speed network connection. At this point, the computerized olfactory

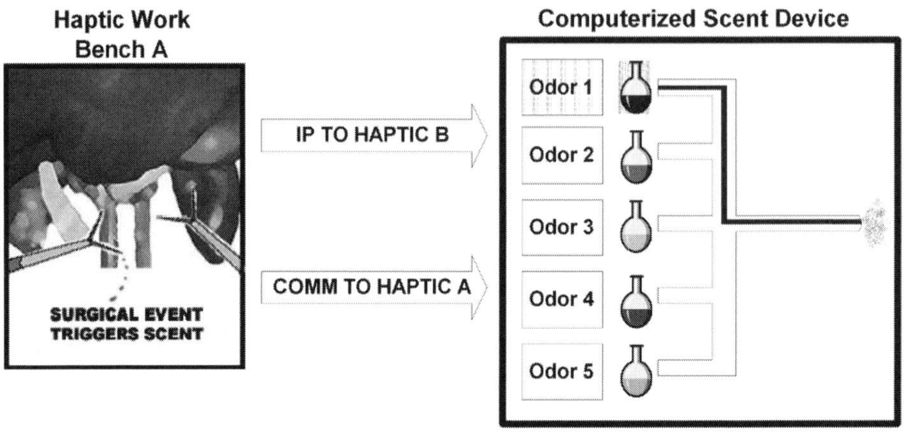

Figure 3. Activation of the scent device.

device, which has been incorporated into both haptic simulators, begins reproducing the odor of bile at both locations. Because the devices can control the intensity of the odor, and not all surgical damage is immediately apparent, differing levels of damage can be virtually represented. If a botched surgical event is not severe enough to render any apparent, visual damage, the faint odor of leaking body fluids should be indicative to a surgeon of a problem.

3. Discussion

Simulations, such as the model described here, should not be considered replacements for real world clinical training, but instead should be considered as educational enhancements to be used to teach or reinforce basic skills [1,2]. Maran and Glavin [2] discuss this in terms of experiential learning, whereby the learner constructs knowledge by matching new information, gleaned from new experiences, with previous knowledge. Simulations help to facilitate learning, via post reflection, by exposing the learner to challenging situations that differ from the norm.

Statistically it has been found that the average medical student will not encounter many of the more complex medical situations during supervised training, but instead through clinical experience [1]. For those students who are given the opportunity to experience the real thing, the severity of the problem usually demands immediate medical attention from the staff, leaving little room for education. Simulations provide an advantage to the student, in that learning to deal with complex medical situations can at least be virtually experienced, if not clinically experienced.

In addition, adding complexity to simulation systems, such as adding smell to the virtual, surgical environment, might help to not only eliminate the "adrenaline gap" often experienced by medical students in simulated environments, but the real world, stress related deterioration of performance as well. The adrenaline gap, which is described as the under-performance of a student during simulated medical scenarios due to the lack of stress typically associated with real world events [2], might be reduced by the increased virtual intensity realized by the introduction of medically related odors. On the other hand, as there is no risk to patient or student, real world, stress related performance deterioration, which is the result of too early an exposure to the clinical environment, might actually be reduced as well.

Smell is, in and of itself, a complicating factor in regards to this model, as people often interpret the same odor in different ways [15]. The science of smell is a complex issue, and little success has been achieved in creating adequate classification schemes [15,20]. The quality of any medically reproduced odor must be high. Getting a panel of experienced medical professionals to agree that a specific odor reproduction was indicative of a specific medical condition or body fluid could prove to be difficult. In addition to this, odor intensity and duration of presentation also play significant roles in the efficacy of scent delivery [15]. Never the less, there are companies in the business of designing customized odors, regardless of the nature of the request [28].

In addition to the incorporative, haptic simulator modeled here, computerized olfactory technologies have additional applicability to the field of medical education as well [29]. One potential application of the technology would be to incorporate it into all types of medically related simulators, whether they are static or networked, surgical or non-surgical. Depending on the application, exposing students to the odors associated with various medical disorders would be a major educational benefit to the student.

4. Conclusions

As the length of medical training time decreases, and the expected knowledge base of health care providers increases, simulation is being called upon as an educational supplement to real world experiences [2]. Advanced, complex training levels, such as those experienced by students using haptic, surgical simulators, require that appropriate clinical clues be incorporated into simulated systems, so as to support high-level decision making. This includes appealing to all five of the human senses as is appropriate and technologically feasible, including the sense of smell.

The ability to use one's sense of smell is widely recognized as an important skill when it comes to the field of medicine [6,7,16]. Not only does the sense of smell play a role in the diagnosis of various medical disorders, but it plays a surgical role as well [17]. Recent advances in computerized, olfactory technologies make appealing to the sense of smell in simulated environments a real possibility.

This article proposes a surgical simulation model, based on current haptic, surgical simulation technology [3], that incorporates computerized, olfactory devices into the simulation framework, intended for use as an educational supplement. This incorporation would not only enhance the realism of the virtual experience, but would also serve as a way for medical students to begin to recognize the important role that the sense of smell plays during surgery.

References

[1] M. Good, "Patient simulation for training and advanced clinical skills," *Medical Education*, Vol. 37(1), pp. 14–21, 2003.

[2] M. Maran and R. Glavin, "Low-to high-fidelity simulation – a continuum of medical education," *Medical Education*, Vol. 31(1), pp. 22–28, 2003.

[3] SimTecT. (2004, May). Health and medical simulation symposium: International haptic demonstration (medical link). Available at http://www.siaa.asn.au/simtect/2004/2004.htm.

[4] Internet 2. (2004). Health sciences news archive: Virtual surgery master class. Available at http://health.internet2.edu/news/archive.html#surgerymasterclass.

[5] HAVnet. (2003). Adding touch to web-based surgical training: A SimTecT–Stanford University live demonstration. Available at http://havnet.stanford.edu/events/simtect.html.
[6] R. Winter, *The Smell Book*. New York: J.B. Lippincott Company, 1976.
[7] D. Ackerman, *A Natural History of the Senses*. New York: Random House, 1991.
[8] Cranfield University. (2000). Institute of bioscience and technology. Available at http://www.cranfield.ac.uk/report2000/schools_ibst4.htm.
[9] A. Cann and D. Ross, "Olfactory stimuli as context cues in human memory," *American Journal of Psychology*, Vol. 102 (1), pp. 91–102, 1989.
[10] F. Schab, "Odors and the remembrance of things past," *Journal of Experimental Psychology: Learning, Memory, and Cognition*, Vol. 16 (4), pp. 648–655, 1990.
[11] D. Smith, L. Standing, and A. DeMan, "Verbal memory elicited by ambient odor," *Perceptual and Motor Skills*, Vol. 74, pp. 339–343, 1992.
[12] M. Larkin, "Sniffing out memories of holidays past," *Lancet (North American Edition)*, Vol. 354 (9196), p. 2142, 1999.
[13] Glaser, G. (2001). Past scents. *Health*, 15 (6), 128–134.
[14] D. Huong, N. Walker, C. Song, A. Kobayashi, and L. Hodges, "Evaluating the importance of multisensory input on memory and the sense of presence in virtual environments," in Proc. *IEEE Virtual Reality Conference,* 1999, p. 222.
[15] W. Barfield and E. Danas, "Comments on the use of olfactory displays in virtual environments," *Presence*, Vol. 5 (1), pp. 109–121, 1996.
[16] S. Green. (2004). Bad breath (Halitosis) facts. Available at http://www.qualitydentistry.com/dental/halitosis/facts.html.
[17] P. Keller, R. Kouzes, L. Kangas, and S. Hashem, "Transmission of olfactory information for telemedicine," in *Interactive Technology and the New Paradigm for Healthcare*, K. Morgan, R. Satava, H, Sieburg, R. Mateus, and J. Christensen, Eds. Washington, DC: IOS Press, 1995, pp. 168–172.
[18] C. Platt. (1999, Nov.). You've got smell! *Wired Magazine*. Issue 7.11, Available at www.wired.com/wired/archive/7.11/digiscent_pr.html.
[19] M. Heilig. (1962). United States Patent: 3050870. Available at http://patft.uspto.gov/netacgi/nph-Parser?Sect1=PTO2&Sect2=HITOFF&p=1&u=/netahtml/searchbool.html&r=1&f=G&l=50&co1=AND&d=ptxt&s1=3,050,870&OS=3,050,870&RS=3,050,870.
[20] J. Kaye, "Aromatic output for HCI," *ACM Interactions*, January/February, pp. 49–61, 2004.
[21] E. Tan, A. Wahab, and G. Goh, "PC-controlled scent system," *IEEE Transactions on Consumer Electronics,* Vol. 44 (1), pp. 130–136, 1998.
[22] Trisenx. (2004). Senx-Ware Scent Design Studio (SDS) technical overview. Available at http://www.trisenx.com/SenxWhitePaperRev3.0.x.pdf, (2004).
[23] B. Bonsor. (2001). How internet odors will work. Available at www.howstuffworks.com/internet-odor.htm.
[24] Aerome, Inc. (2004). Get in touch with scent. Available at http://www.aerome.de/english/home_english.html.
[25] J. Kaye, "Computer-controlled smell output," *Perfumer and Flavorist*, Vol. 28 (6), pp. 19–29, 2003.
[26] PRNewsWire. (2000, Dec). AromaJet.com announces fragrance synthesis over the internet. Available at http://www.aromajet.com/comp.htm.
[27] HAVnet. (2003) Videos from the SimTecT interactive demonstration. Available at http://havnet.stanford.edu/events/simtect_video.html.
[28] Dale Air. (2005). [Home Page]. Available at http://www.daleair.com/index.html.
[29] B. Spencer, "Using the sense of smell in telemedical environments," in *Studies in Health and Technology Informatics: Medical and Care Compunetics I*, L. Bos, S. Laxminarayan, and A. Marsh, Eds. Washington, DC: IOS Press, 2004, pp. 135–142.

e-Health Symposium

Medical and Care Compunetics 2
L. Bos et al. (Eds.)
IOS Press, 2005

"Joining Up" e-Health & e-Care Services: Meeting the Demographic Challenge

M. McKEON STOSUY and B.R.M. MANNING
European Federation for Medical Informatics:
Working Group on Planning and Modelling in Healthcare
Mary.McKeon@doh.state.nj.us, Bryan.manning@btinternet.com

Abstract. Substantial demographic changes in the number of elderly in the developed world are forcing a radical re-evaluation of how to deliver care more effectively. "Joined up" multi-disciplinary, multi-agency extended care co-ordination and support service centres are beginning to set the pace towards the establishment of "Virtual Service Utilities". The dual keys to this are the optimizing of end-to-end service process chains and real-time access to comprehensive records and relevant knowledge systems.

Keywords. One-stop-shops, customer relationship management [CRM], electronic healthcare/social care records [EHR], knowledge acquisition and management, genomaps, virtual enterprises, end-to-end processes

Introduction

Currently there is considerable activity across the spectrum of e-service provision across the public and associated private and voluntary sectors, following the path already laid down in terms of e-business and "virtual enterprises". These latter collaborative networks are based on supply chain integration by optimizing both end-to-end process chains and information flows.

Increasingly governments and their agencies have begun to adopt this approach for healthcare. Generally defined as e-Health the focus tends to follow a medical model with varying degrees of outreach into psycho-social and socio-economic domains. A number these initiatives are at varying stages of development across the US, Europe and the UK.

This paper compares and contrasts current strategic approaches to developing "one-stop-shop" multi-disciplinary, multi-agency extended care service client support centres found on both sides of the Atlantic. In the UK, EU and USA e-government 'joined-up' initiatives have led toward a 'one-stop-shop' Contact/Advice Centre approach combining new technology with traditional personal contact procedures. Its objective is to draw together the 'front office' functions of the multiple agencies involved in providing Health and Welfare/Human Services into a single entity that can deliver a coordinated response to most issues presented to them.

US – Aging and Disability Resource Centres

In the US the Aging and Disability Resource Center (ADRC) Grant Program is a joint operation involving HHS' Administration on Aging (AoA) and Centers for Medicare & Medicaid Services (CMS). This provides states with an opportunity to effectively integrate their long-term support resources for consumers into a single coordinated system.

The AoA and CMS initially funded twelve ADRC project states in October 2003, adding a further twelve in July 2004. Each program will serve older adults and individuals with disabilities, and will cover a three period [1].

The ADRC's are to serve as visible and trusted places where people can turn for information on the full range of long-term support options, as well as assistance in accessing those options. The centres will offer consumers reliable information to help them make appropriate choices for themselves and their families.

Some state programs will utilize a single agency serving as the entry point to all long-term supports while other states will establish multiple sites that are coordinated and standardized to ensure there is "no wrong door" for individuals trying to access the long-term care system.

The grants will assist states in their efforts to streamline access to multiple public programs and ensure that families can find the assistance they need through a single point of entry into the long-term support system.

EU – European e-Health Area

In Europe, European Community research programs [2–4] have been supporting e-Health for the last fifteen years with allocated co-financing reaching €500M. As a result a wide range of products, systems and services have now been tested and put into practice.

These include tools for both health authorities and professionals as well as personalized health systems for patients and citizens. Typically they cover a wide range of healthcare management systems that include telemedicine services and networked electronic health records, and others which support prevention, diagnosis, treatment, health monitoring, and lifestyle management.

Experience gained has shown that technology alone cannot deliver the full potential of e-health/e-care unless combined with process and organizational changes together with the development of new skills. Its goal is to provide the foundations for restructuring and improving, citizen-centered healthcare systems, whilst at the same time respecting the diversity of Europe's multi-cultural, multi-lingual health care traditions.

e-Care will be central to responding to the major challenges that the health sector– which employs 9% of Europe's workforce – is currently facing. These include the rising demand for health and social services, due to an ageing population and higher income and educational levels. In particular, by 2051, close to 40% of the Union's population will be older than 65 years old.

UK – National Program for IT

In the UK the National Health Service [NHS] is committed to a £6B country-wide e-health program interlinking all NHS service providers. The NHS Plan, published in

July 2000, is an action plan for 10 years setting out measures to put patients and people at the heart of the health service and promising increased funding over five years to 2004.

At the core of this NHS National Program for IT (NPfIT)[5] a "centralised" demographic records "spine" service not only maintains a national master patient/citizen index but also holds key clinical data that may be required to support treatment in an emergency. All NHS Hospital and Primary Care Trusts in turn hold a detailed Electronic Health Record [EHR] for each citizen.

The Programme will be implemented over a 7–10 year timeframe commencing in 2004 and will provide completely new IT infrastructure providing:

1. Electronic patient record services,
2. Electronic appointment bookings (eBookings),
3. Electronic transmission of prescriptions (ePrescribing),
4. Web-based access to patient records and other services.

Local application infrastructures will be provided across the five geographic clusters by its local service provider. Each cluster covers between 5–7 Strategic Health Authorities [SHAs] and includes all the NHS trusts within each SHA.

The new electronic patient records service is called the National Care Records Service. Patient records will be stored on the National Spine database but accessed and updated locally, using workstations and remote devices. This will include Picture Archiving Systems [PACS] which will hold all images taken by the NHS that traditionally were/are held on x-ray film, MRI, CT, Ultrasound etc.

NCRS is an electronic records management service that will provide the infrastructure for provision of healthcare information across the NHS. There will be a single, secure, national system connecting all Trusts and integrating all the diverse systems currently in use.

The aim of NpfIT is to provide a country-wide [England only] integrated electronic records service for all individual patients. These records, provided through links with each of the five LSP Clusters will be held on a single nation-wide service known as the "Spine" provided by the National Application Service Provider [NASP].

The NASP is responsible for creating and maintaining the national Master Patient Index [MPI] together with the "Spine" records service. The MPI acts as the single reference for all NHS information systems. The "Spine" holds an up-to-date summary of information and key events in the patient's life and care.

Access to more detailed patient-specific information held by other NHS Trusts will be provided by the system to the current point of treatment. Typically this could be in-patient medication records and anaesthetic records in the case of a hospital, or treatment or support services delivered in the community.

Linkages with other central, local government, private sector and voluntary agencies are currently in the early stage of development. A centrally-funded "one-stop-shop" initiative, whilst broadly confined to local government service provision, is becoming the standard means of interfacing with the citizen. Whilst currently based on a combination of Call Centre and Customer Relationship Management systems, web-services are beginning to emerge.

The next leap forward will be to inter-link the NPfIT system with local government as it matures.

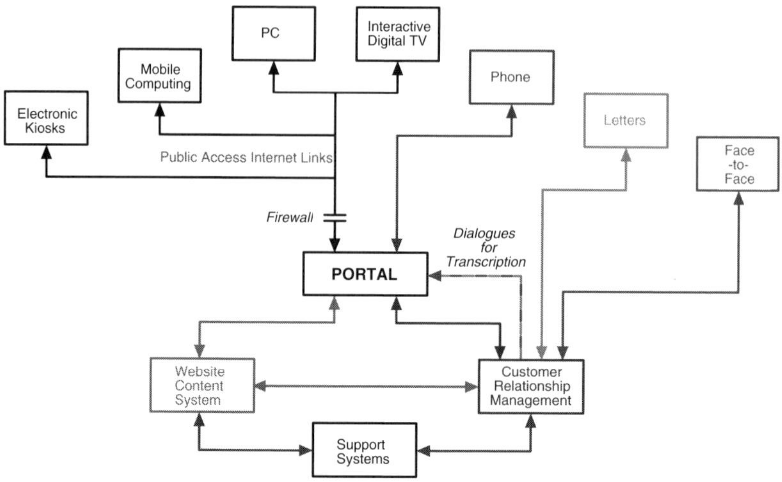

Figure 1. Generic e-Health Service Access Architecture.

Generic Multi-Mode e-Public Service Access

In the UK, EU and USA e-government 'joined-up' initiatives[6] have led toward a 'one-stop-shop' Contact/Advice Centre approach combining new technology with traditional personal contact procedures. Its objective is to draw together the 'front office' functions of the multiple agencies involved in providing Health and Welfare/Human Services into a single entity that can deliver a coordinated response to most issues presented to them.

A prototypical systems architecture, outlined in Fig. 1, provides for an interface with the citizenry that spans the spectrum of communications media ranging from 'face-to-face contact' through to current digital technologies. The resulting dialogues are supported either through Customer Relationship Management [CRM][7] systems or directly via an integrated set of agency Websites.

Although one of its major objectives is to provide comprehensive advice and guidance to a wide variety of questions, ranging from the seemingly trivial across to complex multi-disciplinary issues, it also has to arrange an equally diverse variety of follow-up actions. This can range from the relatively simple short duration care process involving only a single professional, to a lengthy and complex multi-professional one provided by a wide variety of agency service providers.

In both circumstances Contact Center staff need rapid, easy access to a variety of support systems, which hold relevant knowledge and case records. This has to be coupled with appropriate interaction with the very diverse set of agency management systems that are in place.

However this is not just a technology issue – it is significant business transformation one, as it involves the creation of a "Virtual Enterprise" that can deal with a complex mix of highly variable end-to-end care processes. In these circumstances it is important to recognize that whilst the creation of a fully integrated information infrastructure is the key enabler, it is only that. The key to this lies in the management of change, enabling far more effective and streamlined ways working that cut across the old boundaries between the many professional, departmental and agency "silos".

Inter-agency working inevitably raises major issues of security not only of personal data but also of system, content and commercial confidentiality risks, which have to be addressed as part of the transformation process.

Whilst the aim of these Centres is to respond to the wide spectrum of care problems that beset citizens from time to time, much of the focus and expenditure of resources will inevitably be on those with chronic conditions. As these types of cases almost invariable involve a complicated mix of health and social care issues combined with a host of psycho-social, socio-economic and other varied problems, Centre staff will have to deal with and be able to break down the presenting demand into a range of process streams.

These will typically involve:

- Care Needs Assessment leading on into individual Care Plans and Case Management and Coordination by the most appropriate Agency
- Financial Assessment leading on into the development of an appropriate package of advice and guidance, plus support in regards to Benefits claims
- Counselling services across a wide range of topic and problem areas
- Provision of a wide range of Support Services spanning the spectrum of other relevant goods and service, e.g. housing down-sizing/adaptations; meals-on-wheels; community support
- Monitoring Unmet Needs and initiating Follow-up action

Core Centre IT support will need to provide inter-agency service systems access and an IT infrastructure that supports Performance Monitoring, Resource Utilisation and Cost Controls. Resource development and training needs will have to be met as well.

One Stop Shop: Front Office System

Whilst still providing a direct person-to-person interface with customers, the ultimate goal is to make it easier for the public to save time and travel in resolving problems and issues via interactive e-services. Its basic design aim is to provide a single customer focused point of contact and multi-service care problem solving service.

The technology used to enable this shift from the traditional service "silo" centred approach to a customer-focused one is derived from Customer Relationship Management [CRM] systems used in the financial and utilities sectors. This gives CRM staff easy access via a Client Index not only to their consolidated multi-service records but also to the supporting service sector knowledge databases needed to establish an effective solution to the client's problems. These core systems are supported by a Geographical Information System [GIS] to automatically provide appropriate location information, as well as an e-forms based data collection/collation facility.

This direct person-to-person dialogue is supplemented by a parallel interactive Website e-CRM service providing similar functionality as well usual Content managed information services. However in this case there will be no access to individual personal records for confidentiality and security reasons.

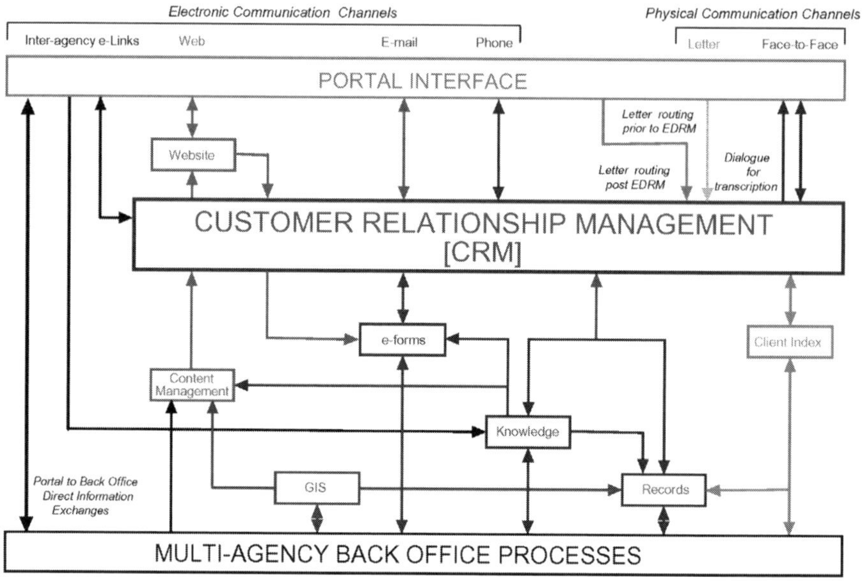

Figure 2. Customer Relationship Management Interface.

As shown above in Fig. 2, a Portal provides a single gateway hub to all communications, which also include all e-government/e-links not only with other relevant organisations. Where appropriate some case related information may be routed directly to CRM office environment from mobile staff working in the community served. However most will be directed straight through to specific back office departments for action and subsequent updating of records, etc.

Where appropriate face-to-face and phone call voice data can routed though the Portal for subsequent transcription to electronic record format. Similarly letters can be scanned transformed via EDRM into the same formats.

Knowledge Extraction System

Currently both CRM and website system content tends to remain inherently static after the long haul to get them up and running. Whilst this is partially due to scarce resources, the key constraint is the problems of knowledge acquisition, verification and content updates. However lack of on-going content currency will rapidly devalue the system and alienate users.

Leading-edge technology[8] now offers a way to move toward dynamic service updating by multi-media monitoring all communications traffic through the Portal interface shown in Fig. 3 below. Face-to-face and phone call voice data transcribed via the Portal to an appropriate common text format can be combined with all throughput from other channels and filtered through a concept extraction process. Rather than just providing a keyword indexing system this filtration process automatically then classifies the information content as required broadly into Summaries; Taxonomies; Categories; Contributor Profiles.

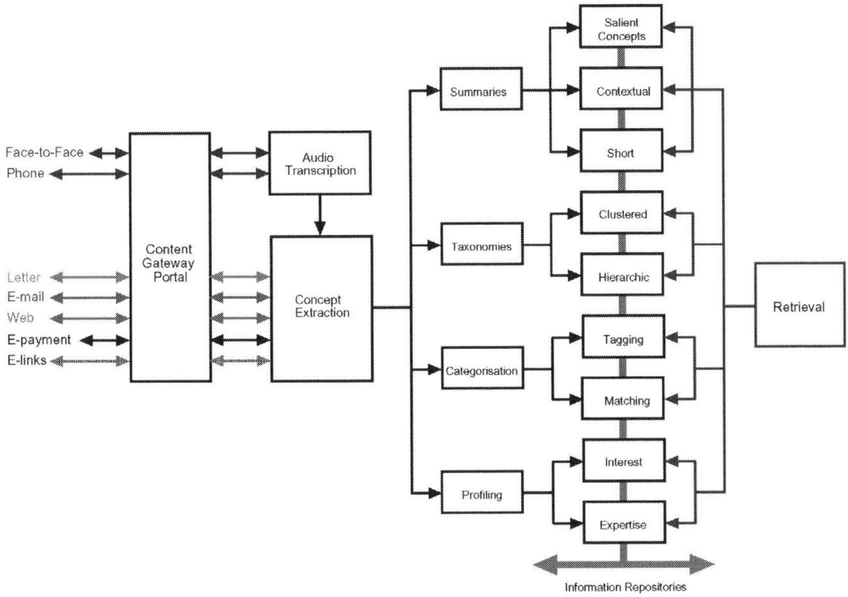

Figure 3. Knowledge Acquisition Access.

Summarisation can be used to compact content down to more a manageable scale for rapid assimilation, recognition of recurrent themes and trends, as well as adding valuable cues to hidden key contextual information. Automatically created taxonomies can minimise the work involved in organising content for easier intuitive navigation. They will also provide a useful aid to recognition of emergent patterns and trends.

Similarly automatic categorisation of content will enable hypertext and other linkage mechanisms required to support rapid searches though ever growing repositories of information. Since both the source and users of all throughput will be automatically logged, this will support both interest and expertise holder search criteria.

Overall One Stop Shop System Architecture

As discussed previously the overall aim is to provide individual members of the public, their families, caregivers or other parties acting on their behalf a single focal point to obtain help in resolving health and social care/support issues across the spectrum of services provided by governmental, private sector and voluntary bodies.

Experience gained across most professional disciplines indicates that lengthy "trawls" though detailed records is neither considered desirable nor necessary, except in complex cases. In order to speed the process of accessing relevant client information an "event index" is used not only to select and review specific records, but also to establish the sequence and pattern of events, as well as the various parties involved. The addition of a link to short key point summaries further reduces the need to wade though masses of detail to rapidly gain a comprehensive overview.

An additional and often a significant aspect in many cases in the complex is a clear and concise overview of the relationships involved in the presenting circumstances.

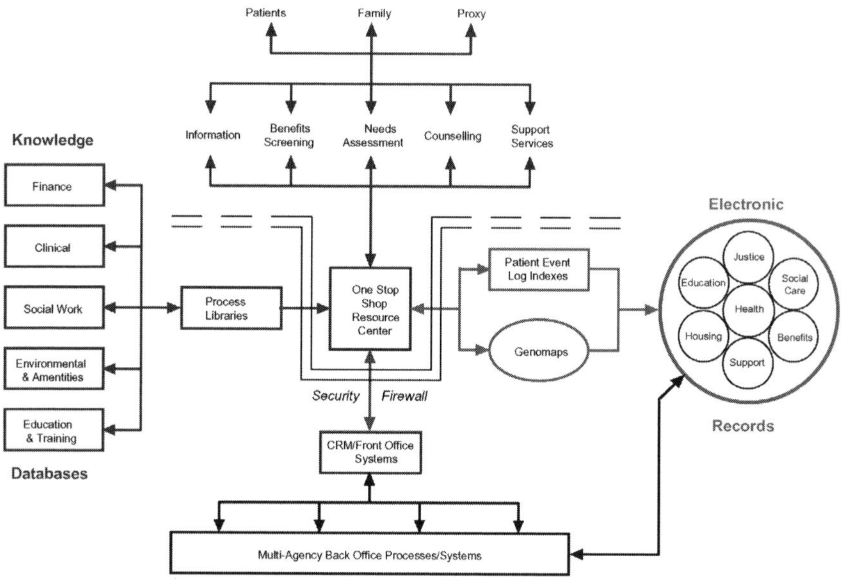

Figure 4. Community Care Resource Centre Service Structure.

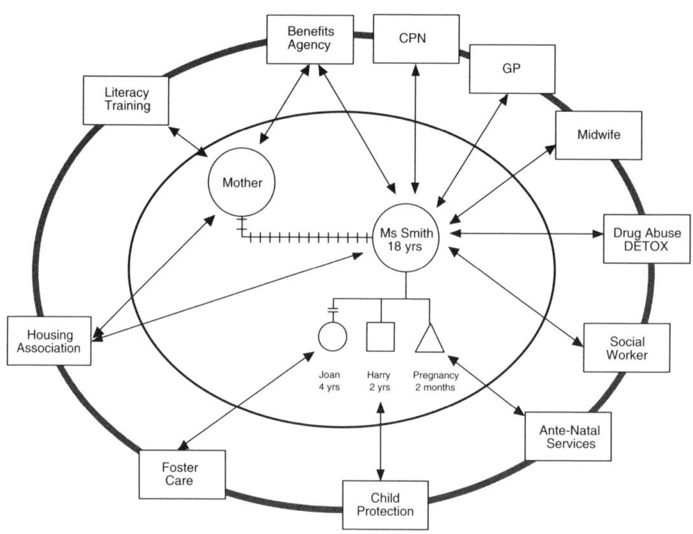

Figure 5. Genomap.

This together with the range of agencies and professions involved can be readily available diagrammatically via a Genomap.

Centre staff need to have appropriately validated/privileged access both to these personal Electronic Records, as well as to the supporting Knowledge databases required to enable them to answer a highly variable mix of enquiries effectively.

To ensure the currency, and hence effectiveness, of both core support database systems need to be dynamically updated from the multi-agency back office sources.

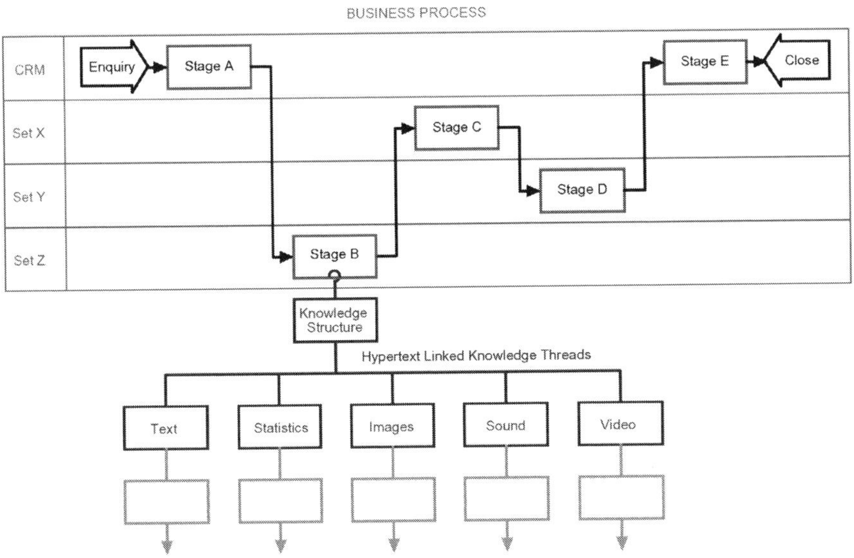

Figure 6. Process Linked Knowledge Access.

Genomapping

Increasingly it is being recognised that the complete healthcare cycle extends beyond the purely clinical treatment process. In these circumstances the wider psycho-social, socio-economic and care support/recovery-influencing factors need to be included.

This extended cycle adds a further layer of complexity to an already complex chain as it extends to include other agencies and professional disciplines. Whilst the generic approach outlined above is equally applicable, an addition layer is needed to identify and index the additional multiple agency process threads that are potentially involved.

The Genomap shown in Fig. 5 above fulfils this role, as well as adding significant information that can radically affect the viability of the health, treatment and recovery cycle, yet is often unavailable due to current inter-agency boundary issues.

This form of mapping shows the immediate family/home circumstances as well as the agencies and disciplines known to be involved. This approach can not only reveal key issues that can still remain hidden due to current cross-professional ethical considerations such as mental health problems, but also missing services that could have a major impact on cases.

Genomaps can provide a case co-ordination overview as well as the controls needed to ensure that the most appropriate inter-weaving, inter-dependent case-specific processes are properly integrated to provide an optimum route back towards a healthy life. The resulting "road map" not only provides a collaborative framework but also enables the sharing of knowledge/ expertise in support of well informed decision taking.

As this type of care process is no longer constrained to a single location or agency, timely, effective and information-rich communication between all professionals becomes evermore important. Whilst technology is increasingly able to provide this type of access through a combination wireless/landline linked PDAs, Laptops or PCs, it brings with it new sets of co-ordination, control and security problems.

Process Linked Knowledge Access

This process mapping based methodology has been developed out of approaches stemming from the use of Business Process Re-engineering techniques across a variety of economic sectors[9].

Transfer and adaptation of proven best practice tools and techniques from other domains to the potential benefit of the Care sector typifies the "out of the box" lateral thinking approach needed to successfully carry through the major transformation involved.

The Knowledge Management Support concept, discussed below, evolved in this way. In this case methods used to model and validate conformance of business procedures to regulatory criteria have been combined with those used to respond more effectively to complex enquiries requiring rapid access to specialist knowledge by Centre staff.

The basic approach is shown in simplistic terms in Fig. 6 above. In this a notional five stage sequential process is split between Customer Relationship Management System [CRM] multi-service access processes and activities within three separate Service Providers or Professions [Sets X – Y].

Knowledge structures of varying depth and complexity can be "hung" on complete stages or to individual steps within them as appropriate. This indexes sets of relevant knowledge to points where they are most likely to be needed, either as "aide memories" or to assist with decision processes.

Of necessity these structures are likely to be branching hierarchies with content spanning the full range of media types. These "knowledge sets" are analogous to the "Used Case" sets found in the Unified Modelling Language [UML][10]. As such they can potentially be used many times, being attached wherever relevant to process steps that can well be common to many different Care Pathways.

Whilst Care Pathways are mainly used to define the preferred procedural treatment route, in reality they are part of an "envelope" of acceptable alternative variations, which will share "knowledge sets". As alternative routes are often conditional branches off the primary one, decision options will need to be contained within these sets.

This approach is essentially generic and is equally applicable to administrative procedures. Here the main differences are in more formalised processes together with need for access to Care Records or management information which require specific security constraints.

Secure Multi-Mode Information System

In these circumstances secure access to both knowledge and care records is an essential feature of any technical solution[11]. A potential architecture is shown in Fig. 7 below.

This is based on two main lines of firewall access security. The first limits access rights to those with certificated Public Key Infrastructure [PKI] profiles. This can be either to "medical knowledge sets" via relevant Care Pathway maps, or to specific case data using the Genomap and the time and date sequenced Event Log Index to specific records

This first level access is focused primarily on providing read only access to approved users with personalised role dependent profiles. Write access profile permissions are limited to case workers who have reporting responsibilities for of their all patient/client related activities.

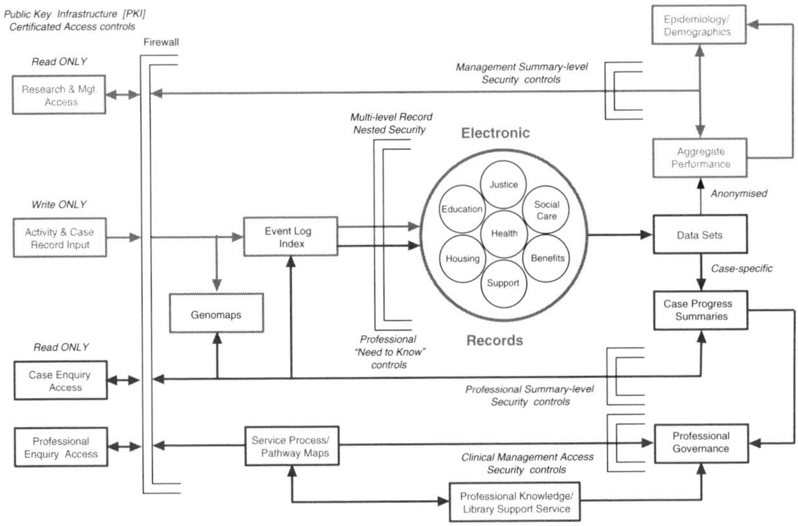

Figure 7. Secure Multi-Mode Information System.

The second firewall protects against unauthorised access both to Multi-Agency Electronic Care Record data and to derived management information. Write access profiles incorporate the ability to set subsequent multi-level read security on all entries to the record and can be set to lockout access right down to individual words, phrases to features within a document or media.

Read access profiles can either case-specific or anonymised for subsequent aggregation for research or management purposes. Case-specific access to the core records is controlled by "need to know" role dependent profiles via the Event Log Index. Somewhat less stringent profiles are used to control access both to Case Progress Summaries and to Professional Governance reviews, which compare actual practice against Care Pathway standards.

Customer Relationship Service Process

Almost without exception client/patient dialogues with the service broadly divide into:

- Queries – All aspects of provision of relevant services and/or necessary goods as well as likely implications of governmental procedures/issues
- Requests – Applications/Bookings for services which may be accompanied on occasion by incoming or outgoing payments
- Comments – All aspects of service provision

The response process for each of these three types of dialogue are all logged and the salient features/results of the dialogue added to the client Case Records. Current practice broadly follows Call Centre procedures, which are usually an intrinsic component in most CRM designs.

These are based on scripted question sequences, derived from an analysis of prior Frequently Asked Questions [FAQs] profiles and supplemented where necessary by reference to appropriate Knowledge systems. As speedy access to relevant content is important to maintain client/patient confidence within a dialogue, indexing it to the pertinent Service Process map steps can be a major aid as well as providing an immediate visual reminder of the potential sequence of events.

Where interaction with one or more specific services is involved in delivering a target outcome the procedures will extend to provide:

- Initial Appointment Booking/Referral to the appropriate agencies and professional staffs
- Ongoing service process availability/progress status reporting, especially where clients/patients have multi-agency dependencies

The essence of this 'one-stop-shop' approach is aimed at providing a single point of contact for case coordination and communication support not only to clients/patients but also to others who may be acting on their behalf.

It also aims to provide a similar support capability to the agencies and their professional staffs, without abrogating their overall responsibilities for case planning and management. This approach has begun to be replicated in web services, albeit with its interactivity limited to following the FAQ scripted sequences supplemented by hypertext links to appropriate Knowledge Content Management system pages.

Essentially the CRM and Interactive Website facilities are identically structured. The essential and obvious difference between the two is the absence of the human interface with the client in the latter.

Most of any dialogue between the client and the Centre will generally follow a scripted Question and Answer interaction with the client's responses recorded using an e-forms transaction logging process. Once again the difference is the lack of a human interface.

In both scenarios there may be the need to breakout of the Q&A sequence to consult the relevant Domain Knowledge and/or Regulatory Rules and Procedures. However in this case the client has direct access to these sources, where appropriate, as opposed to receiving input indirectly from Centre staff. Whilst direct access may be beneficial, it inevitably requires a fair measure of latent knowledge to interpret the nuances and subtleties involved.

In some respects website technology has run ahead of the ability of designers to assemble and give easily navigable access to relevant content. The general approach taken involves complex hierarchical structures that can be many levels deep and may spread laterally to almost resemble hedges rather than the more traditional tree format. Navigation is often less than intuitive, sometimes resorting to an alphabetical index in which the listings do not connect readily with the reader's own perceptions of the required topic headings.

However a greater problem lies in securing and then maintaining currency of site content. This demands a mix of editorial and librarianship coupled with the tenacity required to ensure contributors deliver appropriate copy to agreed deadlines. Whilst well-structured content management is the prime key, another significant influence is the need for visual arts skills to develop a recognisable layout style that actively supports and develops user interest.

However in this situation where media skills meet those of technology head on, they tend to do so with relatively little consideration for the variable abilities and tenacity of their potential audience, all of which highlight the need to consider strategic alternatives to current practices.

CREATION OF A SUSTAINABLE VIRTUAL ENTERPRISE

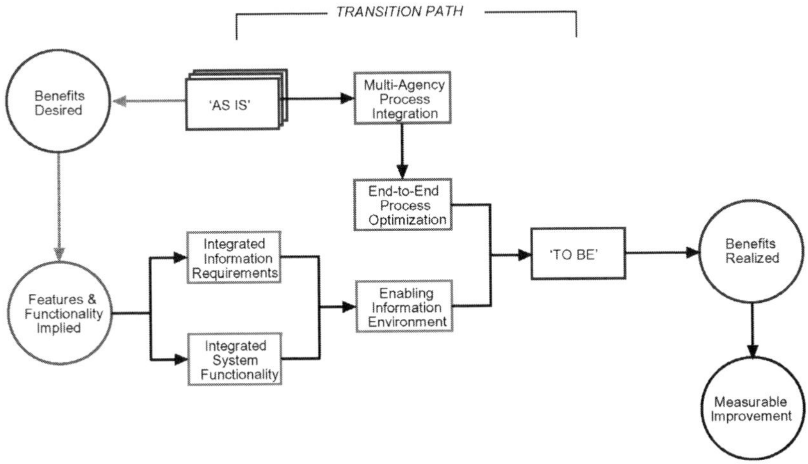

Figure 8. Benefits Realisation.

Delivering Measurable Benefits

All managed change is ideally focused on deriving some set of measurable benefits. The main problem this presents is how to transform the way any enterprise operates from the current "as is" condition to the desired "to be" situation. The scale of this inevitably is considerably magnified when it involves creating a multi-agency "Virtual Enterprise". However big this challenge may appear it is already underway in the UK as NpfIT] and in the US within the ADRCs.

The generic model for the transformation of any set of multiple entities into a "Virtual Enterprise" is shown above in Fig. 8. In essence it is a two part, two stage operation, the first of which involves two parallel activities. This involves planning both the re-configuration of a set of multiple disconnected business processes into a single optimised end-to-end process, together with the design of an integrated information environment that enables the re-configuration to function effectively.

The second stage focuses on implementing the transition to the full "to be" functionality through which the desired benefits can be realized. Whilst the technology is the key enabler, the success of the transformation and the attainment of its targeted benefits is critically dependent on achieving a major cultural change within the overall working environment. This in turn depends on creating conditions where all concerned see and wish to secure, palpable benefits both for themselves individually as well as for the complete enterprise.

Cost-Benefit Analysis

Concerted leadership by the health care and technology industries as well governmental units at all levels is needed to address a myriad of technical, administrative and other issues that would underlie a strong health information technology marketplace.

In the US, savings in the range of $140 billion per year, close to 10 percent of total U.S. health spending, could be achieved through health information technology – by reducing duplicative care, lowering health care administration costs, and avoiding errors in care[12].

For adoption of electronic health records in particular, the most commonly-cited barrier is insufficient resources and a perceived lack of evidence for a positive return on investment. Healthcare organizations are not adopting clinical information technology at a rapid rate due to the poor financial case, difficult modifications of clinical workflow and decision making processes, perceived legal barriers to sharing information among disparate organizations and limited capacity of health care organizations to organize regionally.

In the US, electronic systems are costly, and traditionally healthcare has spent proportionately less on them than most other industries. There is a need to encourage healthcare stakeholders to invest in IT. Incentives are necessary to counteract current economic realities that discourage investment in IT. Although providers in the US bear the cost and the risk of investments in IT, they often do not realize the full benefits because of financial incentives in the current system that rewards piecemeal and volume-based care.

The UK the picture has been somewhat similar, but will radically alter with the massive investment in the NPfIT program. The key difference is that this is funded by central government in accordance with its political commitments and its performance targets set by the NHS. Moreover the phased delivery of the program in terms of the IT system itself is provided free to all NHS Trust service providers. However all other implementation costs involved in service process transformation have to be funded by each NHS Trust, who have to justify this expenditure in accordance with Treasury rules for due diligence. It should be noted that this program is confined solely to the NHS and does not extend beyond its operations to social and other care services.

In order to effectively adopt IT, healthcare organizations must quantify and document detailed projections for developing and incorporating IT before making decisions as to how to proceed. Organizations must take a business-driven approach rather than proceed just on the basis of expectation of cost savings. Healthcare organizations need to develop a full Business Case that includes an analysis of the legal and organizational issues and barriers to health information exchange as well as a high-level qualitative financial analysis of healthcare IT application. The goal of this analysis should be to clarify and improve the understanding of the operational impact, risks and opportunities involved, together with a carefully considered, comprehensive implementation plan that secures the commitment of all concerned to achieving real benefits at all levels.

Among incentive vehicles, financial incentives have the greatest impact and can be designed as either direct (i.e. direct payment for adopting IT) or indirect (e.g., pay-for-performance for outcomes measures, care coordination or chronic care management)[13]. These should include support of interoperability among data sources and multiple provider types.

The return on investment for IT use is significantly improved when interoperability of information is considered, as much of the operational and clinical gain can be more fully realized with patient-centric data transparency. Incentives that promote IT adoption without emphasis on interoperability have the potential to fund IT approaches that fail to enable the full clinical quality and economic efficiency gains that IT has to offer, resulting in a weaker business case.

Sustainability – Creation of a Virtual Public Utility

The notion of procuring computer services from a utility is not new. Others have proposed an open source prototype of a *virtual public utility* for secure health care transactions[14]. Druseikis & Woods described a *virtual public utility* as a technical specification of a communications infrastructure with certain useful functional behaviours and specific security properties all of which are directed to risk management. The creation of the virtual public utility results in an operating entity, the *cooperative*. A virtual public utility enables a group of health care providers, plans, clearing houses, payors, or others to effectively share the cost of providing common infrastructure services and to bear shared risk. The functions of the virtual public utility could be those of transaction routing, security administration, auditing and control. When put into operation, the virtual public utility distributes responsibility for the implementation of common registration authority functions. The users of the utility must trust the actions of other members and jointly assume risk. Of central concern to such a virtual public utility would be the common security infrastructure to be provided to the entire health care enterprise cooperative.

The common infrastructure involves both extensional elements, such as its architecture and technology as manifested in software, as well as relational elements, such as laws, regulations, rights and traditions fulfilling expectations of groups, organizations, communities, and societies. The development of such a virtual public utility would need to address integration with existing information technologies while also creating and implementing comprehensive specifications and criteria for sustained use and attempting to minimize or mitigate the adverse impact of technological change over the entire health care enterprise over an extended period of years.

The creation of the "virtual public utility" is accomplished as follows. Contractual relationships and regulations governing the conduct of members of the cooperative which define the specific objectives for secure health care transactions must be clearly delineated. The ownership or pecuniary interest in the utility is vested in the cooperative which is directly owned or operated by a collection of members who each directly benefit from the intrinsic efficiencies provided by the cooperative and who directly bear the expense for operating it. The cooperative seeks to minimize costs and share risk in the interests of the members.

An additional function of the cooperative is to indemnify its members in the event that there are violations of the operating rules or regulations of the utility. Indemnification is a specific requirement needed to assure mutual support of required procedures for registering and authenticating users. These requirements must be supported by the software infrastructure of the utility. The fixed and variable costs for the cooperative are governed by specific choices for software engineering and processes for organizational development. Health care is almost always delivered locally and there will be certain health-economic regions that naturally lead to the formation locally-based healthcare cooperatives.

This model has support from the US federal government which envisions leveraging the cooperation and economies of scale from organizing regional healthcare players to facilitate administration of regional clinical initiatives and a transition to performance-based methods of paying for healthcare services[15].

The ordinary notion of a public utility often reflects the need for making capital investments that must necessarily be depreciated over long periods, and regulating the prices charged to consumers. However the hidden costs of protecting information in health care transactions at the point of breech leads to risk in the form of regulatory judgments with civil, and possibly criminal, penalties. This risk creates the opportunity to share[16] and mutually indemnify owners and stakeholders – who are also users – of the cooperative. The risk is created because individual organizations need to adapt to new workflows, significantly different from approaches in the past, and must additionally trust each other according to objective criteria that are not fully defined and not centrally controlled.

In its raw form the public internet fails to provide a means of user authentication in any meaningful form. Open networks such as the public internet are characterized by the ability for new users to join the network without much effort and no central administrative control.

Yet membership in a network supporting health care transactions is fundamentally not open to all. The cooperatives will need trustworthy authentication processes. Identity management, the processes of binding electronic credentials to individuals, is critical. In the terminology of PKI, there would be a registration authority, which would implement business processes to assure that credentials (key pairs) were issued only to legitimate participants. A valid transaction begins with a legitimate connection to the network, and beyond that arguably begins with network actions that authenticate the end-points before anything is sent.

In short, network end-points, providers and plans, need to trust the processes of the registration authority. Once the registration process becomes decentralized there becomes the problem of how to trust the registrations created by processes that are out of central control. We argue that such central control can never be totally dispensed with; therefore it is an intrinsic cost of doing business that must be managed and distributed among all members of the network. A cooperative model for sharing expense among the participants seems the most logical.

Conclusions

The concepts outlined within this paper combined with other evolving Telemedicine, Smart Home and Clinical/Care Assistive Technologies provide a potential answer to the forecast demographic imperatives.

References

[1] Administration on Aging: Aging & Disability Resource Centers. www.aoa.gov/prof/aging_dis/aging_dis.asp.

[2] Commission of the European Communities [COM(2004) 356]: e-Health - making healthcare better for European citizens: An action plan for a European e-Health Area.

[3] Commission of the European Communities [COM(2001) 723 Final]: The future of healthcare and care for the elderly: guaranteeing accessibility, quality and financial viability. 5/12/2001.

[4] Braun, A; Constantelou A, Karounou V, Ligtoet A & Burgelmann J-C. Prospecting e-health in the context of a Eurpean Ageing Society; Quantifying and qualifying needs. Final report November 2003 IPTS/ESTO: Sevilla, Spain.

[5] Department of Health. Delivering 21st Century IT Support for the NHS: National Strategic Programme. www.npfit.nhs.uk.

[6] G.A. Stosuy, J.P. Eaglin. The Community Services Network: Creating an integrated Service Delivery Network – The Baltimore open systems laboratory model. New Technology in the Human Services Vol 12 1/2 87–98. NTHS 1999.

[7] B.R.M. Manning. Consumer Relationship Management in the Community. International Consultants Guide. Feb 2002.
[8] Audentify: Contact Centre Solutions – White Paper. Audentify. 2003.
[9] B.R.M. Manning et al. Clinical Process Maps as an Indexing Link to Knowledge and Records. Proceedings HDL 2003: Healthcare Digital Libraries Workshop in conjunction with ECDL 2003, Trondheim, Norway, August 2003.
[10] Unified Modelling Language Specification. V.1.5. Object Oriented Group Inc. March 2003.
[11] Information Security Management. ISO/IEC 17799:2000.
[12] Agency for Healthcare Research & Quality Study. www.ahrq.gov.
[13] Achieving Electronic Connectivity in Healthcare: A Preliminary Roadmap from the Nation's Public and Private-Sector Healthcare Leaders July 2004, the Markle Foundation.
[14] Druseikis & Woods (USC, 2001).
[15] Burda, David. Building Blocks – The Formula for a successful Healthcare IT Network, Health IT Strategist. February 2005.
[16] Trusted 3rd Party Management: tScheme and Confidence in Online Identity. April 2004. www.tScheme.org.

Note

This paper was originally prepared to support a presentation entitled "e-Care Contact Centers: A Strategic Vision for Chronic Care" given at a Technology Workshop that was part of the 2005 Annual Programme Meeting of the [US] Council on Social Work & Education Conference, New York February 2005.

Medical and Care Compunetics 2
L. Bos et al. (Eds.)
IOS Press, 2005

Development and Deployment of a Health Information System in Transitional Countries (Croatian Experience)

Ranko STEVANOVIC[a], Ivan PRISTAS[a],
Ana IVICEVIC UHERNIK[a] and Arsen STANIC[b]
[a]*Croatian National Institute of Public Health, Rockefellerova 7, 10000 Zagreb, Croatia*
[b]*Orthopaedical Clinic in Lovran, Setaliste Marsala Tita 1, 51415 Lovran, Croatia*

Abstract. Croatian Primary Health Care Information System pilot project, conducted between 2001 and 2003, aimed to develop and deploy a health information system based on the latest technologies which would improve the quality of primary health care and rationalise the consumption. 60 primary health care teams (physician and nurse) were equipped with PCs and connected via central server to the main national health insurer, state treasury and public health institute. Developed information system enabled rapid retrieval of documents, replacement of manual data input and a real-time insight into needed information as well as prompt interventions within the system. The project also introduced electronic smart cards for physicians and nurses, so that at each medical check-up the information system verified both the ensuree's and the physician's or nurse's status and rights.

Based on the experiences from the pilot project, plan has been made for comprehensive health information system at national level which would connect primary health care teams, hospitals, laboratories, dentistries, health insurance companies, state treasury, public health institutes and electronic health records database. Its major goals are more rapid diagnostics, accuracy in prescribing therapy, standardisation of the good practice as well as better utilisation of capacities, shorter waiting times and shorter stays in hospitals, which would lead to improvement in overall health care quality and better control over the health care consumption. Estimated 5-year investment for installing such system would be 125 million EUR. However, information system could save substantially more and yield a return of investment in only two years.

As information system for primary health care should be a strategic component of every health care reform and development plan, we can recommend our model, based on the results of the pilot project, to other transitional countries.

1. Introduction

Between 2001 and 2003, a project conducted in Croatia aimed to develop and deploy a health information system based on the latest information and communication technology (ICT). 60 primary health care teams (physician and nurse) were equipped with PCs and connected via central server to the main national health insurer, state treasury and public health institute. The most important experience and idea applied in this project was based on the concepts developed by Professor Andrija Stampar. According to these, primary health care is a venue where the major health problems of a population are resolved, and a point at which outcomes of changes in the system are most significantly reflected. A central health information system should be developed and deployed in parallel with the primary health care activity. Results of the trial run give us the ground to recommend such approach to all transitional post-communist countries. The development of such systems is feasible in transitional countries because most of them are still having one main insurer. In the developed countries, however, developing those could be difficult for they have a number of insurance companies that do not find their business interest in the full integration of health information and data from health. Indeed, for countries with a single dominant basic insurance company the above is the only positive alternative. Subsequent linkups of supplemental, auxiliary and other future insurers with the single information system on the national level will be much simpler to make.

At the beginning of 2004, i.e. six months after a software for primary health care was tested in Croatia, the European Public Health Alliance (EPHA) (http://www.epha.org, http://www.epha.org/a/1211) published a document titled "Communication from the Commission to the Council, the European Parliament, the European Economic and Social Committee and the Committee of the Regions – e-Health – Making health care better for European citizens: An action plan for a European e-Health Area" (Text with EEA relevance), Commission of the European Communities, Brussels, 2004-04-30 COM (2004) 356 (full document is available on the web page http://www.epha.org/IMG/pdf/e-health_action_plan.pdf). As made clear there, EU member states will start implementing in 2007 the solution Croatia reached in 2003. Establishing and developing this information system in transitional countries is one of the strategic projects for the coming years. Without rapid, reliable and comprehensive information availability, developing, implementing and monitoring any health care development strategy and system reform woul be difficult. One would be unreasonable to expect of a poor health system to keep and «save» enough money for "computerisation to happen spontaneously". One should do exactly the opposite: computerisation should be installed in the system as a money-keeping tool and implemented with the aim of exerting total control over the consumption as well as rationalising it, in order to save substantially more money than the cost of installing the information system.

In fact, the share of investment in information systems is directly proportional to financial effectiveness of the system (e.g. banks and insurance systems spend 5–6% of the total budget on computerisation of business operations). Whereas EU member states spend at least 2–3% of the health budget on computerisation, in the US this share varies round 4–10% [1]. Among transitional countries, it is difficult to find one investing more than 0.2–0.5 % of its health budget. This raises the question whether this might be the starting point for the vicious circle of ineffectiveness in transitional countries' health systems.

Neither can the elements of new organisation (new business rules) be set, nor the foundation laid of a redesign without investing in the computerisation aligned with modern concepts [2,3] under which information (processed data) become a business resource [4]. At the same time, the information-communication system for primary health care warrants the confidentiality of the data on patients and the standardisation of the good practice for most common acute and chronic mass diseases [5]. The system should provide the basic contents for the establishment of an effective management.

2. Cost-Effectiveness

The main goal of computerisation is to rationalise health consumption, not make savings. It is estimated that at least 20–30% of the money spent in health could be used more rationally. In the case of Croatia, the amount involved is between 700–900 million USD annually. Computerisation should produce the data and indicators needed to achieve this rationalisation. Estimated 5-year investment for installing comprehensive information system would be 125 million EUR. It is estimated that the entire investment in primary health care information system could produce a benefit in less than two years merely on account of detecting irrational drug prescriptions and irrational referrals to specialist examinations. Primary health care information system is precisely the point of most effective consumption control (before users enter into system), because the insurers' present system does not permit prompt control and intervention, but usually merely finds the irrational consumption that has already happened.

3. Goals and Improvements

Ample help offered by computerisation relates to rapid retrieval of documents and ensurees [6,7], replacement of manual data input, typing on typewriters, writing of recipes, referral notes, invoices, individual forms and reports. The information system should give a real-time insight into the data and information, as well enable prompt interventions within the system.

Improving the overall care of patients and ensurees, more rapid diagnosis and accuracy in prescribing a therapy are the major goals of such approach. The system should enable better utilisation of the capacities, shorter waiting times, and shorter stays in health institutions [8].

- The project was the first to introduce smart cards technology here for all physicians and nurses. Thus at each medical check-up or hospital admission the new information system also verifies both the ensuree's and the physician's status and rights. Equally as authentication in banking or other card business, only a "linkup" between the magnetic card and the doctor's card makes the transaction possible.

3.1. Insurance Provider Benefits

BI (Business Intelligence), utilisation of accurate and comprehensive data and information required in health insurance management is one benefit. Health data and ICT data are standardised, and the input independent of the wishes, ambitions and interests of teams and institutions. It sets the insurer and physician free of worries about data collection and primary data processing, because information system takes care of this with standardised applications. Thus, they can devote all their energy to the execution of managerial and professional activities. Within the information system, performance monitoring accurately measures the effectiveness and outcomes, as well as teamwork coverage and contents.

3.2. Benefits for the Health Ministry and Public Health

The benefits include: PHI (Public Health Intelligence), use of accurate and comprehensive data and information needed to run the public health system and public health initiatives. HMI (Health Management Intelligence), utilisation of accurate and comprehensive data and information needed by the Ministry of Health, health managers and decision-makers for efficient guidance and running of the system is another benefit. Interoperability and integrational tool will enable full interoperability and integration of data and information from the health system and its environment. Selection of qualitative indicators – currently data on more than 500 parameters are collected from the primary health service with the aim of extracting from this just a few pieces of information, i.e. indicators (exclusively on the level of ratios or trends). The future system with a few standardised characteristics will offer the possibility of analysing a much greater number of indicators. In the reporting, i.e. statistics, registering with public health registries (obligatory notification of immunizations, infectious diseases, malignomas, psychotics, disabled, etc.) will be carried out automatically, interactively and proactively. Linkage makes the carrying out of coordinated and joint preventive and curative interventions feasible. Safety: the system guarantees the confidentiality and safety of personal information and of data on health and disease (VPN, PKI, encryption, smart cards, separate authentication servers, data servers and data repositories). Accident and Catastrophe Early Alert System: one can boot the whole system with all data and information in 24 hours.

3.3. Benefits for Physicians/Teams and Medical Chamber

Utilisation of guidelines, instructions and tools needed by physicians and ensurees in order for standardised quality care to be provided, more rapid diagnosis setting and selection of good and rational therapy in the treatment of disease is one benefit (Health Care Intelligence). Dissemination and utilisation of the knowledge necessary to provide good medical care is another (Knowledge Intelligence). Other benefit still is a linkage with other participants in the process of treatment and prevention of disease (on-line linkage of all care providers). Equally beneficial is the regulated and safe utilisation of all data on the health and disease in an ensuree in care, on-line consultations with networked experts, e-consultations with specialists, telemedicine, direct engagement in scientific and technical public health projects and programmes. The benefit of time and money savings on office, postal and other expenditures are worth to mention.

3.4. Benefits for the Citizen-Patient-Ensuree

First, there is EI (Equity Intelligence): equity or enabling all who are in the same medical, insurance (and market) position to avail themselves of the same conditions and quality. Then, there is continuity, irrevocability, transferability safe data storage on the care for an individual ensure. Next are the benefits of guaranteed confidentiality and security of identity and personal data. The final benefit is the communication option, i.e. two-way (or multiple) communication between a physician and citizen-patient-ensuree (e-information, e-active calling, e-instruction sending).

3.5. Data Standards

In software applications and central information system use has been made of the EU and certain engineering standards in order for this system to be open from the outset and built for Croatia as an EU member state. It should support international and EU data standards and classifications, e.g. HL7 version 3, ICPC-2, ICD-10, CEN TC 251 and others.

3.6. Technical Elements and Standards for the System and Applications

Technical elements and standards for the system and applications for transitional countries should include the following: one system in common, but several licensed applications; the Internet infrastructure (to enable «paperless» operation); XML/HL-7 standard; electronic signature system safety standards and infrastructure – PKI (Public Key Infrastructure); marking clinical and other documents with barcode; electronic health and medical file; global registration and ensuree database; global database on codebooks [9–14]; access to external databases; data integration into primary health care service's information system; direct linkage with insurance administration, public health and ministry of health; e-recipes, e-referral notes, e-business, etc; standardised, equitable and measurable use of guidelines [15,16].

4. Conclusions

1. The present technology makes feasible and encourages the introduction of comprehensive centralised applications with the use of data and information being local and rule-regulated. As a gatekeeper at the entry to a health system, primary health care should have an information system of its own that would also integrate every future health information system similarily as family medicine integrates information and data from every part of health system.
2. In transitional countries, information system for primary health care is a strategic component of the health reform. Its goal is to improve the quality of primary health care and rationalise the consumption.
3. Investments in primary health care information system have no alternative. They are strategic and they would yield a return of investment in two years.
4. In transitional countries, health informatisation projects should be defined (through measurable targets) in phases by priorities and conducted all the way down to their execution phase.
5. New concepts and proven methodologies of project management should be used to guarantee effectiveness of the project (investment).
6. In the countries in transition, the primary health service's information system should allow physicians and nurses to switch to the new, facilitated mode of operation that gives them more time for patients and practice management improvement.
7. A primary health care information system grants access to data to all authorised staff needing it, as well as proactive use of the knowledge, standards, guidelines, procedures and algorithms. It should enable direct IT communication between "wherever you may be" and hospitals, specialists, home care

service, home visiting service, diagnostic units, as well as all later linkages in the process of treatment.

8. The system should permit the utilisation of diagnostic and therapeutic guidelines, warrant equality in approaching the patients and make the necessary knowledge available on the physician's PC.
9. The system should permit association in interest groups for special research projects, and business/problem-related linking and networking.
10. Health informatisation projects that were started in transitional countries back in the early 90s by informatisation of the insurance business operations should immediately be resumed. Family medicine practices ought to be equipped systematically with computers, licensed applications and linked to form a single health information system.

References

[1] Bates DW, Ebell M, Gotlieb E, Zapp J, Mullins HC. A proposal for electronic medical records in U.S. primary care. JAMA 2003;10:1–10.
[2] Stevanovic R. Computer software for family medicine offices. Med Fam Croat 2002;9:30–3.
[3] Stevanovic R. Collection and managing of health data, the linkage of informatics systems and quality of health data. In: Cvoriscec D, Madaric V, editors. Quality Management Standards in Hospital Care. Koprivnica: MOH; 2003. p. 100–9.
[4] Krcmar N, Stevanovic R, Kovacic L, Merzel M. Health center, family medicine and community health care reform. In: Matreljan E, Grgurev Z, editors. 7th Congress on Family Medicine; 2001; Opatija, Croatia. Opatija: HUOM; 2001. p. 219–27.
[5] Stevanovic R, Erceg M. A Proposal for National Preventive Medicine Informatic & Communication System. In: Strnad M, editor. 1st Croatian Congress on Preventive Medicine and Health Promotion with International Participation; 2003; Zagreb, Croatia. Zagreb: HZJZ; 2003. p. 308.
[6] Varga S, Stevanovic R. Health Informatics System - preventive benefits. In: Strnad M, editor. 1st Croatian Congress on Preventive Medicine and Health Promotion with International Participation; 2003; Zagreb, Croatia. Zagreb: HZJZ; 2003. p. 295.
[7] Stevanovic R. ICT of the primary health care. In: Klapan I, editor. 1st Croatian Congress on Telemedicine with International Participation; 2002; Zagreb, Croatia. Zagreb: Croatian Telemedicine Society; 2002. p. 86–7.
[8] Booth N. Sharing patient information electronically throughout the NHS. BMJ 2003;327:114–5.
[9] WONCA, International Classification Committee. The International Classification of Primary Care. 2nd ed. Oxford: Oxford University Press; 1998.
[10] Lamberts H, Wood M, editors. ICPC: International Classification of Primary Care. Oxford: Oxford University Press; 1987.
[11] Lamberts H, Hofmans-Okkes I. Episode of care: a core concept in family practice. J Fam Pract 1996;42.
[12] WHO. International Statistical Classification of Diseases and Related Health Problems, Tenth Revision, Volume 3, Alphabetical Index. Geneva: WHO; 1994.
[13] Okkes IM, Oskam SK, Lamberts H. Van klacht naar Diagnose [From complaint to Diagnosis]. Bossum: Coutinho; 1998.
[14] Hoffmans-Okkes IM, Lamberts H. The international classification of primary care (ICPC): new applications in research and computer based patient records in family practice. Fam Pract 1996;42:294–302.
[15] Lamberts H, Wood M, Hofmans-Okkes I, editors. The international classification of primary care in the European Community. Oxford: Oxford University Press; 1993.
[16] Brage S, Bensten BG, Bjerkedal T, Nygard JF, Tellnes G. ICPC as a standard classification in Norway. Fam Pract 1996;13:391–6.

Medical and Care Compunetics 2
L. Bos et al. (Eds.)
IOS Press, 2005

The Surveillance of the People with Chronicle Diseases Making the Personal Electronic Folder in Pharmacies for these Patients

Delia Carmen MIHALACHE[a], Andrei ACHIMAS-CADARIU[a] and Richard MIHALACHE[b]
[a] *Medical Informatics and Biostatistics Dept., University of Medicine and Pharmacy "Iuliu Hatieganu", Cluj-Napoca, Romania*
[b] *Faculty of Pharmacy, University of Medicine and Pharmacy "Iuliu Hatieganu", Cluj-Napoca, Romania*

Abstract. The aim of the project is to create a database in pharmacy, which will include all the medications and treatment schedules of the supervised patients for increase the quality of the health services, identify the possible drug interaction of the chronicle diseases therapy with treatment for acute disease, the possible reaction which could appear during the therapy and avoid the self medication, which could harm results of the therapy instituted by the specialists.

Introduction

The health services management is the ensemble of the activities, which refers to the anticipation and satisfaction of the health services request with the exchange process. This study will offer specialists and pharmacists, dates about the patient's needs, the patient's evolution after a treatment schedule, positive or negative results about a special therapy and cost of the drugs [1]. Over the last several years, enhanced technology has stimulated health care practitioners and entrepreneurs alike to develop new ways to deliver products and services using the Internet as a communications conduit [2].

1. Background

The last decade has seen a surge in the use of computerized health care data to provide better health service for the patients and information for pharmacoepidemiology and pharmacovigilace.

Now, in the Romanian health system, the collaboration between specialists – general practitioners – pharmacist – patients is made just with the prescription, medical letter and health books. This system is wrong because it doesn't have good evidence about the all daily medication, for the patient with chronicle disease. And also, nobody is considering the input of the over-the-counter (OTC) drug (drug without medical prescription), which can have a bad influence for the base therapy.

Self-medication with OTC can make a bad impact in the recurrence of disease or for the good display of the treatment schedule in chronicle disease. The people with chronicle or recurrent disease must be informed about the necessity to choose a medical therapy because of the aggressive sales of the OTC drugs [3].

In the western countries and USA databases with all the medications for the supervised patients are used with success. These databases are making the conjunction between the physician-pharmacist-patients, to ensure a good supervision about each patient's therapy.

2. Material and Methods

2.1. Design

The databases will be created in pharmacies, and will contain all the schedule therapy from the specialists and the entire OTC drug, which are bought directly by the patients. This information will be send permanently to the specialists and to the physician for:

- Enhance the quality of the health services offered to patients;
- Identify the possible drug interaction of the chronically diseases therapy with treatment for acute disease;
- Identify the other possible reaction which will could appear during the therapy;
- Avoid the self-medication, problem who could damage for the therapy instituted by the specialists;
- Avoid the overdose and under dose because the patient unawareness;
- Identify the intermediate events that may provide more detailed information on the disease process.

Doctors can send prescriptions via Internet or wirelessly to the pharmacy (pharmacy receives it as a fax). Alternately, it can be printed via an infrared printer and given directly to the patient. This system removes the possibility of illegible prescriptions and patient tampering, increases efficiency and optimizes the time of physicians and pharmacists. In the same way, the pharmacists will send the information to the doctors [4].

For a good supervision of the patients, these people will be distributed to the specific pharmacy, where they will buy the all drugs, including the over-the -counter.

In every pharmacy, each patient will have his own electronic file, where the pharmacists have to mention all the medication delivered for a specific patient. We will supervise only the chronicle disease (e.g. cardiovascular diseases, asthma, hepatitis, epilepsy, Parkinson disease, ulcer, diabetes etc.). In this cases are huge risks for medical interactions with the base therapy that can be omitted by the specialists, pharmacists and patients. These personal electronic files will be sending periodically to the clinics for a good supervision of the patient's evolution during the therapy.

The pilot program will be display in the pharmacies from Cluj-Napoca. The electronic cards will contain these rubrics:

- Name
- Surname
- Age

- Sex
- Address
- Personal physician and specialist
- Medical antecedents
- The therapy for the chronicle disease(s)
- The manner of the administration
- Therapy length
- Acute disease occurred
- Other drug consumed without recommendation
- The mode of administration of these OTC
- The quantity of these OTC
- Side effects
- Periodical medical examination
- results of laboratory tests
- demographic information

Thus, the patients are permanently supervised because of the directly contact with the pharmacist; contact witch is more frequently than with the physician or specialists. So, the conjunction between the physician and the patient is stronger and safer now, because of the special pharmacist's supervision. For us is important to enhance the safety and the self-consciousness about the patient, and, with the specialists, to ensure the best medical service.

2.1.1. Manage Patient Databases

The great advantage of these databases is:

- ✓ Easily input new patient records into patient database;
- ✓ Access critical patient information, such as insurer, age, height, weight, contact details, as well as any drugs or notes;
- ✓ Search patient database by writing the patient's last name in the search field;
- ✓ Access all of your past prescriptions with a tap of a button;

The pharmacists are trained to use this electronic files, how to make the patients with chronicle disease from their area to cooperate with them. The patients can be, probably, reticent in the beginning.

Every week, the full personal electronic files will be send to the physician and specialists, who can follow the drug interactions, adverse events and the good development of the therapy for that chronicle disease [5].

2.1.2. Patients

Patient agreed to participate by giving their free informed consent allowing access to all relevant clinical and medication data and storage analyses of these data. Patients from any age and gender category, smoker, alcohol intake, various diagnoses and underlying disease participate in the study, as in daily practice. No additional in- or exclusion criteria were considered. This illustrates once more the additional value of this study because in clinical trials are excluded:

- ➢ Patients with low and high age,
- ➢ Pregnant women,
- ➢ Patients with more chronicle diseases or complicated disease. [6]

The actual medical databases from the hospital include only inpatient information. In contrast to these databases, one of the primary purposes of pharmacies databases recording is the daily clinical management of all their patients.

3. Results

The remarks of this study provide practical dates for biostatisticians. The databases can provide detailed data about the prevalence and incidence of diseases, distribution of risk and preventive factors, and patterns of drug utilization. In addition, observational data from the general population are vital for adequately assessing unmet medical needs and planning areas where support is needed to improve public health conditions (basic research, clinical development, health care utilization studies, etc.).

The number of side effects was tabulated in absolute value and percentages. Incidence densities were calculated during follow-up as the number of reported adverse events per 1000 patients' months of exposure. The exposure period was defined as the period from start of therapy until end of the therapy or end of follow-up when still on therapy. All analyses were performed using statistical package.

This study is following the dynamics of the use of medication in time, for a known population. In this way, we can identify the people who use the new generation of drugs and the quantity of the drugs that are consumed. It is possible to see the ratio between the use of a new generation of the drug and old drugs.

4. Discussion

Using this system the pharmacists can informed all the time the patients how to incorporate the medication into your daily lifestyle, how to manage side effects, when to seek medical help and how to keep track of important information for the doctor and pharmacist. Many people forget 50% of what the doctor told them about the treatment schedule, so the pharmacist will provide all the instructions again, when the patients take their drugs from the pharmacy. We are trying to avoid limits situations when the patient is confused: he is not able to remember the therapy, the hours for the administration, the period of the therapy [7]. Pharmacists can help patients with chronicle disease make the best use of their medication – and decrease the risks of using medications. The management of the drug therapy is absolutely necessary, since more and more patients are dependent on drug therapy to sustain and improve their lives [8].

Besides data from clinical trials, estimates of the "real world" safety profile of many drugs were and still are scarce. This is one of the reasons to set up a large study follow-up different treatment schedule used in daily clinical practice, with the aim to assess the safety, efficacy and pattern of the drugs. Another objective therefore was to investigate whether reporting rates of adverse events change in time and to improve the balance of benefits and risks.

In epidemiological and medical research, one frequently has to analyze data that measure the time until the occurrence of some event. Examples are time to recurrence for peptic ulcer (related to the presence of etiological risk factors), the time to leukemia relapse after bone marrow transplantation, etc. [9] Data collected allowed to researchers to efficiently study rare outcomes, with an incidence rate of less than one per

10,000 persons per year, as well as chronic disorders, and conditions with short- or medium term incubation periods.

The patients keep going to give a great attention for own assistance (self-medication). The big number of the OTC is given a significant enhancing of the drug input and the people number, too. An application of this project is to enhance the awareness of the pharmacists, to train them about the new drugs, therapy plans and diagnostics. It is important for the pharmacist to be informed, as soon as possible, about the new drugs, he will be able to train the patient about their usage, to stop irrational usage and to supervise the patient during the therapy. The drug's dealers must be able to see that the drug marketing is not a commercial activity, but a medical activity with commercial tent [10].

5. Conclusion

Results of this study may be compared with clinical trial data and the limited published data from observational studies. In general practice it is know that unlabelled drug related adverse events are more frequently reported compared to labeled events.

Strategies to provide better health services are:

- ✓ To make a comparison of the ability for the different treatment schedule applied in clinics. To choose the best treatment schedule for each patient, in private, concerning safety profile and the incidence of side effects;
- ✓ To find the best length for the treatment schedule for each patient, in private;
- ✓ To dignify the best treatment schedule taking care about the ratio benefits/side effects/costs.

References

[1] Babb VJ, Babb J. Pharmacist involvement in Healthy People 2010. J Am Pharm Assoc, 2003 Jan-Feb;43(1):56–60.

[2] Menighan TE. Hot Topics in Pharmacy, in WEDI National Conference. 2003, Available: http://www.wedi.org/cmsUploads [cited at May 2004].

[3] Hondrea AM. Imbunatatirea managementului institutiilor sanitare prin introducerea marketingului serviciilor de sanatate. Management in sanatate. 2001 (2):25–7.

[4] BlueFish Rx Prescription Writer Software. Palm one – home page. Available to: http://www.store.palmone.com/product/index. [cited at May 2004].

[5] Chaffee BW, Bonasso J. Strategies for Pharmacy Integration and Pharmacy Information System Interfaces. Medscape from WebMD – home page. Available to: http://www.medscape.com/viewarticle/471252_1 [cited at October 2004].

[6] Salvador Rosa A, Moreno Perez JC, Sonego D, Garcia Rodriguez LA, Iglesias Abaj FJ. The BIFAP project: database for pharmaco-epidemiological research in primary care. Aten Primaria, 2002, Dec; 30(10):655–61.

[7] Smith LD. Steps Consumers Can Take To Be Informed About Their Medicines. Safe Medical Treatments: Everyone Has A Role. Consumer Health Information Corporation. 2000. Available to: http://www.consumer-health.com/services/cons_takecontrol2.htm.

[8] Shane R, Gouveia WA. Expanding Pharmacy's Reach Across the Care Continuum. American Journal of Health-System Pharmacy. 2005; 62 (4): 430–431.

[9] Bodewes-Claessens AC. Postmarketing Surveillance of Proton Pomp Inhibitors in Perspective. The Case of Lansoprazole. Den Haag, 2000. Available to: http://www.library.uu.nl/digiarchief/dip/diss/1924109/c1.pdf [cited at January 2005].

[10] Pradel FG et al. Physician over-the-counter drug prescribing patterns-an analysis of the National Ambulatory Medical Care Survey. Ann Pharmacother, 2002, Oct;33(4):400–5.

Medical and Care Compunetics 2
L. Bos et al. (Eds.)
IOS Press, 2005

Improving End of Life Care: An Information Systems Approach to Reducing Medical Errors

S. TAMANG[a,b], D. KOPEC[a], G. SHAGAS[a] and K. LEVY[a]
[a]*Department of Computer and Information Science, Brooklyn College, CUNY, USA*
[b]*Department of Research, Metropolitan Jewish Health System, NY, USA*

Abstract. Chronic and terminally ill patients are disproportionately affected by medical errors. In addition, the elderly suffer more preventable adverse events than younger patients. Targeting system wide "error-reducing" reforms to vulnerable populations can significantly reduce the incidence and prevalence of human error in medical practice. Recent developments in health informatics, particularly the application of artificial intelligence (AI) techniques such as data mining, neural networks, and case-based reasoning (CBR), presents tremendous opportunities for mitigating error in disease diagnosis and patient management. Additionally, the ubiquity of the Internet creates the possibility of an almost ideal network for the dissemination of medical information. We explore the capacity and limitations of web-based palliative information systems (IS) to transform the delivery of care, streamline processes and improve the efficiency and appropriateness of medical treatment. As a result, medical error(s) that occur with patients dealing with severe, chronic illness and the frail elderly can be reduced.

The palliative model grew out of the need for pain relief and comfort measures for patients diagnosed with cancer. Applied definitions of palliative care extend this convention, but there is no widely accepted definition. This research will discuss the development life cycle of two palliative information systems: the CONFER QOLP management information system (MIS), currently used by a community-based palliative care program in Brooklyn, New York, and the CAREN case-based reasoning prototype. CONFER is a web platform based on the idea of "eCare". CONFER uses XML (extensible mark-up language), a W3C-endorced standard mark up to define systems data. The second system, CAREN, is a CBR prototype designed for palliative care patients in the cancer trajectory. CBR is a technique, which tries to exploit the similarities of two situations and match decision-making to the best-known precedent cases. The prototype uses the open-source CASPIAN shell developed by the University of Aberystwyth, Wales and is available by anonymous FTP. We will discuss and analyze the preliminary results we have obtained using this CBR tool. Our research suggests that automated information systems can be used to improve the quality of care at the end of life and disseminate expert level 'know how' to palliative care clinicians. We will present how our CBR prototype can be successfully deployed, capable of securely transferring information using a Secure File Transfer Protocol (SFTP) and using a JAVA CBR engine.

Keywords. Information systems, palliative care, management information systems, case-based reasoning, palliative care, quality of care, end of life, electronic health records

Introduction

This research will evaluate the ways in which information systems can improve the quality of care for patients and caregivers who are dealing with severe, life-threatening illnesses. The palliative care model is relatively new and continues to be refined, especially when healthcare interventions are provided outside the physical confines of a hospital [1,2]. Community-based models, which incorporate intensive case management, are initiating chronic disease interventions "up-stream" in the course of illness. The Quality of Life (QOL) program, in Brooklyn, New York is an example of this approach [3].

CONFER QOL is a palliative information system that was developed for the QOL program. The development team consisted of both researchers and information services professionals. CONFER QOL is primarily used as a management information system (MIS). Development of this system began in 2002, and we are currently testing the integration of a new care planning form.

Our second palliative information system, CAREN, is a case-based reasoning (CBR) application. The information in the case library was obtained from the QOL program's clinical data forms and informal case notes, which are found in the patients' charts. These charts are maintained by the QOL program's Quality of Care Coordinators.

1. Patients with Chronic and Terminal Illnesses

Medical errors are alarmingly common, costly, and often preventable [4]. Chronic and terminally ill patients are disproportionately affected by medical errors [5–9]. In addition, the elderly suffer more preventable adverse events than younger patients. Myers and Lynn [6] suggest three key factors that make individuals who are nearing the end of life more vulnerable to medical errors, and the resulting adverse events:

1. These patients interact more with the health care system. This leads both to more medications and to more procedures overall. For example, on average, people with one chronic condition see three different physicians and fill six prescriptions per year, and people with five or more chronic conditions have an average of almost 15 physician visits and fill almost 50 prescriptions per year [9].
2. As a result of their poor health, errors that occur during the course of care are more harmful to the patient's overall health. In addition, these patients are often the least likely to recover from more serious medical error(s).
3. Patients with chronic illnesses are often exposed to organizational or habitual "process" patterns of patient care that, although repeatedly used, run counter to well-substantiated "best practices." Best practices are documented in the literature and establish the evidence-base for clinical pathways.

We have identified a fourth factor that contributes to the vulnerability of these patients who are confronting serious, life-threatening illnesses:

4. These patients are least able to monitor their own care, especially when they live alone or have no primary caregiver.

Patients confronted with chronic, and life-threatening illnesses are in dire need of safe, reliable and well-coordinated care. Currently, health care and community services are not organized to meet the needs of the growing population of people facing a long period of progressive illness and disability before death [10,11].

Worldwide, people are harmed as a direct result of medical errors that can occur while receiving medical treatment. How can information systems be used to improve the quality of care for patients who are dealing with chronic and terminal illnesses? Does the use of patient data for quality assurance purposes require special measures to protect a patient's privacy? Minimizing potential risks to patient privacy and confidentiality are not only an organizational obligation, but also mandated in the Unites States [12].

1.1. Palliative Care Expertise

Deficiencies in medical education about end of life care are widely recognized [13,14]. Sustaining leadership and disseminating practice guidelines for palliative care requires several approaches including: developing palliative care leaders, improving palliative care curricula, creating standards for competence, and creating and enhancing educational resources for end of life education [1,13,14].

Cases provide a flexible framework for illustrating the lessons of experience and the dilemmas requiring careful judgment [15,16]. We have carefully selected cases and created our palliative care library to comprise a "real life" clinical curriculum. The casework of the palliative care team is the foundation for the automated consultation in the CBR system we developed. Successful CBR systems have been used to simulate the reasoning of medical experts, for example FLORENCE [17], a care planner for nurses, MEDIC [18] a case-based physician and CASEY [19], a case-based diagnostician. CBR is particularly effective in managing the implicit knowledge that specialized healthcare professionals gain through experience.

2. Palliative Information Systems

Lessons learned from the palliative care databases in Hamilton and Halifax, Canada point to the following planning guidelines and system requirements for the software development life cycle of a future palliative information system [20]. We have also expanded this list of requirements to encompass our development experience with palliative information systems and the new government directives in the United States:

- have a clear definition of the uses for which the data is being collected
- decide on a clear set of goals and objectives
- have a short-term and a strategic plan
- select the data you will collect
- allocate the time and resources to collect and enter data
- provide fiscal support for the system's initial and continued system development
- state ownership of and responsibility for the database
- use a relational database system, such as Access, ODBC, or SQL to house the database

- provide the ability to merge information into other databases
- ensure data accuracy and integrity
- communicate with other palliative care programs and services
- enforce HIPAA compliance

2.1. System 1: CONFER: "eCare" Solutions

Different characteristics are associated with different levels of automation within an organization. Automated information systems allow for an organization to do the following tasks: collect detailed computerized patient information, record data, use decision support tools, standardize coding, standardize extraction tools and access a knowledge base via the web. CONFER [21] is based on the idea of "eCare," a process-based application for care management. The CONFER web platform uses XML (extensible mark-up language) to define the systems data. XML is a W3C-endorsed standard document mark up [22]. It defines a generic syntax used to mark up data with simple, "human-readable" tags. Users access CONFER via the company intranet. The application allows the QOL program to store and analyze various data types, and it is robust enough to support enormous quantities of information.

The initial QOL system consisted of two user forms, linked to multiple database tables, built with the SQL language. Continued development in the Research Department included the addition of two user forms, the Referral Log to track referral reasons and outcomes, and the Hospital Log to record and analyze data on participant hospitalizations. Additional changes to the prototype included modifications of the initial two forms, Patient Demographics and Action Log. The Research Department used requirements discovery prototyping to develop the system from the initial prototype. This development methodology is a "quick and dirty" way to develop an information system [23]. It falls into a rapid applications development methodology, which is a fast track to developing a system, usually through use of a working prototype built with code generating tools, that is refined to meet the stakeholders' needs.

2.2. System 2: CAREN Case-Based Reasoning (CBR) Prototype

Practice-based tools, to assist palliative care professionals would be a valuable asset for training novices and care planning. Development of the 'CAREN' palliative care prototype, developed with the CASPIAN CBR shell [24], was inspired by this growing need.

CBR came from research in the cognitive sciences, particularly the work of Schank and Abelson in 1977 [25]. Their group proposed that knowledge about situations is stored in the brain as scripts, which describe information about stereotypical events such as visiting the doctor. However, a weakness of scripts is their inability to provide a complete theory of memory representation. Schank went on to further explore the role of memory in problem-solving and situation patterns or MOPs (Memory Organization Packets) [25].

In the medical domain two knowledge types can be found: explicit or formalized knowledge and implicit or operative knowledge. The formalized knowledge is the knowledge that can be found in textbooks and clinical guidelines. This kind of knowledge is very suitable for rule representation. The operative knowledge consists of individual expertise, organizational practices and past cases. CBR has proved to be a well-suited paradigm for managing knowledge of the operative or implicit type [26,27]. Implicit knowledge is commonly employed by professionals for medical decision-making. Characteristics of CBR systems include [27]:

- the recognize-act cycle
- the use of domain specific knowledge
- a knowledge representation which allows a flexible modification of the knowledge base
- the use of expert lines of reasoning
- the capability of explaining the reasoning process
- inter-disciplinary knowledge in solving a problem

2.2.1. Indexing Cases and Computing Similarity

The ability to understand the new case in terms of old cases consists of two parts, recalling and interpreting. This first part is known as the indexing problem. This problem concerns the proper assignment of indices and ensures that the relevant cases are stored in memory and are called under the appropriate circumstances. The purpose of building an index scheme is to speed up searching. Here, searching means to find a set of cases from the case-base, which are similar to the new case. The final goal of the system is to find the case with the maximum similarity to the new input case. Our design consisted of a final index definition that is found in Appendix A. The definition we incorporated in our final prototype resulted after the evaluation of alternate indexing strategies.

CASPIAN uses the nearest neighbor matching algorithm (NNM). At the conceptual level, the nearest neighbor technique is simple. This algorithm compares the attribute value of each non-indexed case feature in the set of similar cases to every corresponding feature in the new input case. Attribute values used in CAREN include: secondary condition, age, income, advanced directives, visual, speech and hearing status, weight, and the presence or absence of disease-related symptoms. The comparison values are calculated for each feature and then summed for each case to get the total comparison value. NNM can be made more accurate by weighting attributes that are not defined as indices. In CAREN we weighted several case features including: weight, age, income, secondary condition. After the total comparison value is determined for each similar case, the algorithm selects the case with the highest value for similarity to be the best case match [28].

2.2.2. Case Adaptation and Learning

It is rare that a retrieved case is exactly the same as an existing case in the case library. Adaptation is the process of fixing an old solution to meet the demands of the new situations [27]. CASPIANs adaptation rules are divided into global rules, which are checked first, and local repair rules. Several strategies for adapting cases have been implemented in CBR systems [29].

CBR differs from other AI learning techniques in that it integrates the reasoning mechanism with the learning mechanism. For example, in the CASPIAN system the modified case is stored in the case-base by adding the new case to the case library. Inductive formation of reasoning is only responsible for some of the learning in the case-based reasoner. Most of a case-based reasoner's learning occurs through the accumulation of new cases, through the assignment of good indices, case attributes and weight values. Generally, as the caseload accumulates, so does the accuracy of the CBR. The system becomes more knowledgeable because it has acquired more cases, and thus new knowledge, through the automated reasoning process.

3. Research Methods

CONFER QOL and the CAREN case-based reasoner are designed for patients appropriate for palliative care, but are not hospice ready. Patients ready for hospice are referred directly to hospice. A nurse/social work team screens participants and the QOL program's Project Manager approves intake. CONFER QOL is designed for patients in different disease trajectories and also tracks referrals and patients with a 'bridge' status. The current design of the CAREN prototype is more exclusive, and was designed for a subset of the palliative care population.

The target population for the CBR application was individuals in the cancer trajectory. This group of QOL patients was sampled in a purposive manner. The QOL program manager suggested 17 specific cases she believed provided the best characteristics in regard to sample size and improved outcomes. Before the cases were translated into the CASL language, the test case, Patient 178, was selected randomly. Data was obtained through the use of CONFER QOL management information system and by manual chart review. In total, 22 field values were recorded for the 17 patients in the study sample.

3.1. CASPIAN CBR Shell

CASPIAN comes with its own language for defining cases, called CASL. The general syntax of a case is comprised of the following elements:

- Introduction
- Case Definition
- Index Definition
- Modification Definition
- Pre-processing Rule Definition
- Repair Rule Definition
- Case Instance

The case definition provides the key fields in a palliative care case. The weights of case attributes are assigned in the case definition. We have defined weights on the following case features: secondary condition, (4), age (1), income, (4), dyspnea (3), weight, (1), the presence disease related weight loss, (3), presence of pressure ulcers, (1), observer behavioral problems, (2), and the presence of any other disease related symptoms, (2). Any field that is not an index can be assigned a weight value. The case attributes defined in the CAREN case-based reasoner are found in Appendix A.

The index definition consists of the constraints for the retrieved case. All fields defined in the index definition must be an exact match; there is no weighting for similar attributes. After consulting with domain experts from the QOL program, we have identified the following indices as essential features for this prototype: primary diagnosis, living status (does the he/she live alone?), hospice status (is he/she hospice ready?), adl status (what activities of daily living are compromised?), pain symptoms (presence or absence?), and gender.

The rules in the repair rule definition are used in case adaptation. The rules are examined in turn, and if the condition(s) are met by the input case the repair rule's associated actions will be executed. When a repair rule is fired it is flagged, and once all rules have been examined, CASPIAN reviews the rules again. This is repeated until no new rules fire. In the prototype, we have developed preprocessor rules for income status, advanced care planning, and to ensure safety in the patient's home.

A case instance is an individual case definition with a solution. The instance is flexible in that every parameter is not a requirement for validation. The solution in each case instance is comprised of two main case management units, the goals and the suggested intervention strategies. The compiled case library is subjective to the Quality Care Coordinators who provided the documented consultation services. Each goal has at least one intervention strategy.

4. Findings and Results

Web-enabled, real-time information management systems like CONFER QOL can facilitate the process of participant tracking. Iterative improvements are periodically made to improve patient tracking and outcome measurement. CONFER QOL's main contribution has been its efficient and accurate reporting capabilities. Currently, the system provides formal reports that are viewed through a report editor including: participant demographics, patient process histories, participants program status, referral sources, diagnoses, hospitalizations, service referrals and palliative care resource intensity (e.g., types of contact, goals of contact, duration of contact, and types of actions by different care constituents including nurses, social workers, interns and physicians). Ad hoc reporting is also used to report detailed service utilization, referral outcomes and site of death research. Conifer's reports have been used to support management decision-making and assign organizational value to the "black-box" of social interventions in a predominantly "medically" oriented healthcare system.

To assess the application of automated case-based reasoning in the palliative care domain, we entered 16 participant cases. One of these cases did not have a primary diagnosis of cancer, and this was used as a control marker. If this case was ever returned by the system, we knew something was definitely wrong. These 16 cases comprise the expert knowledge base for which the CBR application will calculate the cases best match given the index definition and the assigned attribute weights.

4.1. Applying Automated CBR for Palliative Care Consultation

In the first phase of the case-based reasoning cycle, CAREN retrieved the case that was most similar to our randomly selected test case, Patient 178. The best case match in the CAREN case library was Patient 171. In the second phase of the CBR cycle, the prototype applied the preprocessing rules and then reused the solution part of Patient 171's case definition.

Patient_171 matched on all indices (primary diagnosis, gender, pain status, living status, and activity of daily living status), income group, advanced care, speech and hearing, oxygen, cpap, insulin, weight changes, absence of pressure ulcers and hospice readiness. The new case differs in secondary condition, 18 years of age, visual limitations (not a weighted attribute), presence of additional disease symptoms and behavioral problems (Patient 171 had compliance issues with her medication), and the advanced directives. One other case matched all index constraints, but after the similarity calculation patient 171 was determined as the most similar case.

To evaluate the potential of CBR as a tool for automating decision-making in the palliative care domain we compared CAREN's prospective consultation to a retrospective chart review. In addition, notable features about the test case, Patient 178, were also retrieved form the CONFER QOL information system.

The test patient's closest match, calculated and retrieved from the case base of cancer patients who are appropriate for palliative care, is also a female who lives alone. In addition, Patient 171 and 178 are both burdened by the increasing complexity of their life threatening illness. The solution part directly derived from patient_171's case instance includes: a brief patient sketch, which is mainly a summary of the indexed fields and can be used for debugging, as well as four goals with their corresponding intervention strategies. The first goal is psychosocial support, achieved through the interventions of individual support therapy by the care managers, telephone check-in support, assistance with the activities of daily living, and coordinating access to available social services. The second is the monitoring of the patient's disease status, achieved with the interventions of the program's medical and social assessment and establishing a relationship with patient_171's primary care physician. The third is effective pain management, achieved through medication review by the program's nurse and contact with the patient's primary care physician and the fourth goal is of advanced care planning.

After reviewing Patient 178's case history and comparing the results with CAREN's palliative care consultation, we conclude that automated CBR can be applied effectively in the palliative care domain. The automated case-based reasoner created a care plan with many of the goals executed in the field. Goals that CAREN identifies that are confirmed in Patient 178's chart are:

Goal 1: to facilitate entitlements or coverage
Goal 2: psychosocial support
Goal 3: monitoring disease status
Goal 4: to ensure safety in the home
Goal 5: effective pain management

The adaptation rules modified the most similar case, Patient 171, to fit the new case. This complemented the new care consultation for Patient 178 with an additional goal to research entitlements and coverage due to their self-reported annual income. This goal was not documented in the case history of Patient 178 by the care managers.

These preliminary results suggest CBR can be used to disseminate domain-specific knowledge. The CAREN application can be used to identify care goals and suggest appropriate interventions for patients dealing with life-threatening illnesses; however, we do feel it is not as comprehensive as the human expert after the in-depth chart review.

The CAREN case-based reasoner did not identify goals or interventions directly related to the patient's needs of self-care and medication education. In addition, it is noteworthy that the patient was suffering from clinical depression. The human reasoner addressed the patient's mental and physical decline in relation to a traumatic life experience; the automated reasoner did not. CAREN's results consisted of an applicable care plan, but results suggest that the CAREN application could be improved to more extensively incorporate the "know how" of a palliative care expert.

Conclusions

The CONFER QOLP palliative information system makes past palliative information systems appear simplistic. All the necessary components and requirements defined by the Halifax system [20] are integrated, but CONFER is a HIPPA compliant, XML-based, "eCare" version. CONFER has followed many similar logical and software development guidelines learned by adhering to the shortcomings of past systems. Many of the same goals were identified to meet problems that are generated by the complex nature of healthcare delivery. These problematic issues include: inadequate tracking, compromised data integrity, decentralized data and inefficient access and retrieval. Implementation of CONFER shows that information-gathering methods must also be addressed, to ensure that the system is monitoring valid and relevant actions and events. A method of quality control should also be incorporated into a palliative information system development guideline.

We have focused on how different IS can be used to improve the quality of care delivered to patients with severe chronic illness. Information systems like CONFER can play a critical role in measuring and reporting quality, but lack 'intelligence'. AI techniques can be used to design intelligent systems like CAREN. The CAREN CBR system can be used to disseminate guidelines for best practice and appropriate treatment and have the potential to be used in palliative care educational initiatives for novices and healthcare professionals unfamiliar with the concepts of palliative care. An ideal palliative information system would be web-enabled, efficient, accurate, reliable, user-friendly, and intelligent, merging many of the important features of the systems we have analyzed.

Future Directions

The experimental results of the CAREN CBR prototype suggest CBR can be used to disseminate domain-specific knowledge. The CAREN application can be used to identify care goals and suggest appropriate interventions for patients dealing with life-threatening illnesses; however, we do feel it is not as comprehensive as the human expert after the in-depth chart review.

Our next phase with the CAREN prototype is deploying the program on a secure web-based platform using opensource software. To transfer the individual patient cases, or electronic health records, and decided to use secure file transfer by encrypting the data (FTPS/SFTP). We considered several options, and we tested one of them. Company Bitvise Limited provides a product WinSSHD version 3.31, which is a SSH server for Windows with secure remote access and file transfer. It supports public key authentication, SCP, SFTP [30]. We can use any SSH client, which supports SSH protocol version 2, to log into WinSSHD. We tested the file transfer using CuteFTP Pro and PuTTY clients, but choose the Java client, which we found easy to install and use for Windows and MacOS, the most popular OS among Internet users.

The Java client has been built on a Secure FTP Factory from JSCAPE: a set of Java based client components for exchanging data between machines. It includes FTP (File Transfer Protocol), FTPS (FTP over SSL) and SFTP (FTP over SSH) components. The Java client has features such as ability to resume interrupted file transfers, progress monitor, and a built in event listeners to track the progress of file transfers [31].

Currently we are assessing Java CBR engines to implement the case-based reasoning cycle. Our future research will be to develop and evaluate and discuss the potential value a web-base case-based reasoner for palliative care consultation. We will describe how any collection of palliative care cases, or other electronic health record coded in XML format, can be incorporated into the framework we have defined in the CAREN prototype.

References

[1] Lynn, J., Schuster, J.L. & Kabcenell, A. Improving Care for the End-of-Life: A Sourcebook for Health Care Managers and Clinicians, U.K.: Oxford University Press, 2000.

[2] Nidetz, A., Fishman, E., Jacobs, M., Daniels, C. & Tamang, S. "Palliative Care Management Services in a Medicare Social HMO", Journal of Pain and Symptom Management, 1, 85–99, 2005.

[3] Hopper, S.S. A Special Report form the United Hospital Fund: Moving Palliative Care into the Community: New Services, New Strategies, New York: United Hospital Fund, 2004.

[4] Kopec, D., Kabir, M.H., Reinharth, D., Rothschild, O. & Castiglione, J.A. "Human Errors in Medical Practice: Systematic Classification and Reduction with Automated Information Systems", Journal of Medical Systems, 27(4), 297–313.

[5] Lynn, J. & Goldstein, N. "Advanced Care Planning for Fatal Chronic Illness: Avoiding Commonplace Errors and Unwarranted Suffering", Annals of Internal Medicine, 2003, 138(18), 812–820.

[6] Myers, S. & Lynn, J. "The Center of Patient Safety at the End of Life: Seeking Reliability and Safety in the Care of Individuals Nearing the End of Life with Serious Illness", Top Health Information Management, 2001, 23(2), 13–21.

[7] Myers, S. & Lynn, J. "Patients with Eventually Fatal Chronic Illness: Their Importance within a National Research Agenda on Improving Patient Safety and Reducing Medical Errors" Journal of Palliative Medicine, 2001, 4(3), 325–332.

[8] Desbiens, N.A. & Wu, A.W. "Pain and Suffering in Seriously Ill Hospitalized Patients", Journal of the American Geriatrics Society, 2000, 45(5), 183–186.

[9] Johns Hopkins University, Chronic Conditions: Making the Case for Ongoing Care, retrieved August 8, 2004 from http://www.partnershipforsolutions.org/.

[10] Lynn, J. & Adamson, D. "White Paper: Living Well at the End of Life: Adapting Health Care to Serious Chronic Illness in Old Age", Rand Health, retrieved on November 30, 2004, from http://www.medicaring.org/whitepaper/.

[11] Myers, S. & Lynn, J. "Patients with Eventually Fatal Chronic Illness: Their Importance within a National Research Agenda on Improving Patient Safety and Reducing Medical Errors" Journal of Palliative Medicine, 2001, 4(3), 325–332.

[12] Fusile, J.P., Arges, G.S., Barrett, L.B., "Straight Talk: New Approaches in Health Care. HIPAA: Deadlines are Looming. Are Providers Prepared?", Mod Healthc., 2002, 32: 37–40.

[13] Block S.D. "Medical Education in End-of-Life Care: The Status of Reform", Journal of Palliative Medicine, 2002, 5(2), 243–248.

[14] Brumley, R. "Future of End-of-Life Care: The Managed Care Organization Perspective", Journal of Palliative Medicine, 2002, 5(2), 263–270.

[15] Blustein, J., Post, L., & Dubler, N.N. Ethics for Health Care Organizations: Theory, Case Studies, and Tools, New York: United Hospital Fund, 2002.

[16] Cox, K. "Stories as Case Knowledge: Case Knowledge as Stories", Medical Education, 2001, 35; 862–866.

[17] Bradburn, C., Zeleznikow, J., & Adams, A. "FLORENCE: Synthesis of Case-Based and Model-Based Reasoning in a Nursing Care Planning System", Comput. Nurs., 1993, 11(1), 20–24.

[18] Gierl, L., Steffen, D., Ihracky, D. & Schmidt, R. "Methods, Architecture, Evaluation and Usability of a Case-Based Antibiotics Advisor", Computer Methods and Programs in Biomedicine, 2003, 72; 138–154.

[19] Koton, P.A. "A Medical Reasoning Program that Improves with Experience", Symposium on Computer Applications in Medical Care Conference, 1998, pp. 32–37.

[20] Critchley, P., Lohfeld, L., Maxwell, D., McIntyre, P. & Reyno, L. "The Challenge of Developing a Regional Palliative Care Information System: a Tale of Two Cities", Journal of Palliative Care, 2002, 18(1), 7–14.

[21] CONFER eCare Solution. Corporate Overview: Making eCare a Reality. Retrieved Sept 6, 2004 http://www.confer.com/.

[22] Harold, E.R., Means, W.S. XML in a Nutshell, O'Reilly and Associates, Inc., Sebastipol, CA., 2001.
[23] Martin, E.W., Brown, C.V., DeHauges, D.W., Hoffer, J.A. & Perkins, W.C. Managing Information Technology (4th ed.). Prentice Hall, Upper Saddle River, New Jersey.
[24] Anonymous, CASPIAN Case-Based Reasoning Shell, retrieved: November 18, 2003, from http://www.aber.ac.uk/compsci/Research/mbsg/cbrprojects/getting_caspian.shtml.
[25] Luger, G.F. Artificial Intelligence: Structures and Strategies for Complex Problem Solving (4th ed.). London: Addison-Wesley, 2002.
[26] Lee, J.K. & Kyeong, J.K. "A Case-Based Reasoning Approach for Building a Decision Model", Expert Systems, 2002, 19(3), 123–135.
[27] Kolodner J. Case-Based Reasoning, San Francisco, CA: Morgan Kaufmann, 1992.
[28] Price, C.J. & Pegler, I.S. "Deciding Parameter Values with Case-Based Reasoning", 1st UK Workshop on Case-Based Reasoning, Salford, UK, 1995, retrieved October 10, 2004, from http://www.informatik.uni-trier.de/~ley/db/conf/ukcbr/ukcbr1995.html.
[29] Watson, I. Applying Case-Based Reasoning, San Francisco, CA: Morgan Kaufmann, 1997.
[30] Bitvise limited, retrieved March 12, 2005, http://www.bitvise.com/winsshd.html. Page visited at March 12, 2005.
[31] JSCAPE. Secure file transfer. http://www.jscape.com/sftp/ Page visited at March 12, 2005.

Appendix A: CAREN CASL Case Attribute Definition

```
case definition is

field prim_diagnosis type is (CA, CHF, CVA, Dementia, DM, ASHD, HTN, FX,
               CVA_or_CHF, CVA_or_ASHD, ASHD_or_CHF)
               prompt is ['Primary Diagnosis:'];
field sec_condition type is (CA, CHF, CVA, ASHD, Dementia, DM, HTN,
               Seizures, Retardation, Pancreatitis, NA) weight is 4
               prompt is ['Secondary Condition:'];
       field gender type is (male, female, transgender)
               prompt is ['Gender Identification:'];
       field age type is number weight is 1
               prompt is ['Patient Age:'];
       field pain_sympt type is (yes, no)
               prompt is ['Symptoms of Pain?'];
       field income type is number weight is 4
               prompt is ['Income Group:'];
       field adv_care type is (yes, no)
               prompt is ['Advanced Directives:'];
       field lives_alone type is (yes, no)
               prompt is ['Does Patient Live Alone?'];
       field visual type is (yes, no)
               prompt is ['Visual Limitations:'];
       field speech type is (yes, no)
               prompt is ['Speech Limitations:'];
       field hearing type is (yes, no)
               prompt is ['Hearing Limitations:'];
       field dyspnea type is (yes, no) weight is 3
               prompt is ['Symptom of Dyspnea?'];
       field oxygen type is (yes, no)
               prompt is ['Patient uses Oxygen?'];
       field cpap type is (yes, no)
               prompt is ['Patient CPAP or BICP?'];
       field pat_weight type is number weight is 1
               prompt is ['Patient Weight:'];
       field weightchange type is (yes, no) weight is 3
               prompt is ['Recent Weight Changes?'];
       field insulin type is (yes, no)
               prompt is ['Insulin Dependent?'];
       field pu type is (yes, no) weight is 1
               prompt is ['Presence of Press Ulcers?'];
```

```
        field adl type is (yes, no)
                prompt is ['Compromised ADLs?'];
        field behavior type is (yes, no) weight is 2
                prompt is ['Behavior Problems?'];
        field other type is (yes, no) weight is 2
                prompt is ['Other Symptoms Evident?'];
        field hospice type is (yes, no)
                prompt is ['Patient Hospice Ready?'];

end;
```

Medical and Care Compunetics 2
L. Bos et al. (Eds.)
IOS Press, 2005

Standardized Semantic Markup for Reference Terminologies, Thesauri and Coding Systems: Benefits for distributed E-Health Applications

Simon Hoelzer MD[1,2], Ralf K. Schweiger PhD[1,2], Raymond Liu[3]
Dirk Rudolf[1], Joerg Rieger[1], Joachim Dudeck MD[1,2]

[1]Institute of Medical Informatics, Justus-Liebig-University of Giessen, Germany; [2]HL7 User Group, Germany; [3]University of California, Department of Medicine, San Francisco, USA

With the introduction of the ICD-10 as the standard for diagnosis, the development of an electronic representation of its complete content, inherent semantics and coding rules is necessary. Our concept refers to current efforts of the CEN/TC 251 to establish a European standard for hierarchical classification systems in healthcare. We have developed an electronic representation of the ICD-10 with the extensible Markup Language (XML) that facilitates the integration in current information systems or coding software taking into account different languages and versions. In this context, XML offers a complete framework of related technologies and standard tools for processing that helps to develop interoperable applications.

INTRODUCTION

The International Statistical Classification of Diseases and Related Health Problems, Tenth Revision (ICD-10), which is developed, maintained and published by the World Health Organization, has been fast becoming the world standard (http://www.who.int/whosis/icd10/). It represents the broadest scope of any previous ICD revision to date. ICD-10 is more comprehensive than current standards and extends well beyond the traditional causes of death and hospital admission. For example, ICD-10 supports the gathering of information on conditions that are not diseases but represent risk factors to health- lifestyle, life-management and psycho-social circumstances.

Structural changes introduced in ICD-10 should contribute to its effectiveness. Significant enhancements to the system's structure and presentation include an enlarged coding frame, hierarchic and logical presentation of codes, and increased use of combination codes.

Adaptability, maintenance and updating are critical if a classification system is to be dynamic enough to be used in our rapidly changing world. Unlike previous revisions, ICD-10 allows for enhancements to accommodate newly discovered diseases, such as AIDS. WHO has established an ongoing maintenance and updating process that ensures input from member states as well as from interested professional bodies. This enhances the long-term viability of the classification system.

With the introduction of the ICD-10 as the standard for diagnosis, the development of an electronic representation of its complete content, inherent semantics and coding rules is necessary. The electronic version should facilitate the integration of the ICD-10 in current information systems, coding software, analyzing tools, etc. taking into account different languages, versions (revisions) and other features that are relevant for different purposes (medical statistics and epidemiology, patient classification systems, etc.).

OBJECTIVES

Based on a project of the healthcare department of the Swiss Federal Statistical Office, we developed a concept of an electronic representation of this hierarchical classification system that fulfills the above mentioned requirements. In the future, the Swiss government wants to provide an official electronic version of the ICD-10 in the three national languages (German, French, Italian). To face this problem in a pragmatic way, our approach consisted in analyzing the available electronic resources that are provided by different national agencies of the World Health Organization (WHO Collaborating Centres). In Germany, for instance, the DIMDI (Deutsches Institut für Medizinische Dokumentation und Information), which is part of the German

Federal Ministry of Health, has the legal obligation for the provision and maintenance of the ICD-10 and other medical classification systems (www.dimdi.de). It takes in part the responsibility for developing and publishing the national coding rules and documentation standards within the scope of the requirements of statistical as well as financial applications. A consistent and comprehensive use of diagnostic terms becomes more and more crucial for the purpose of billing in the hospital care setting within the scope patient classification systems (e.g., German Diagnoses related Groups – G-DRGs).

On the other hand we decided to take into account current efforts of standardization in the frame of the Working Group II (terminology and knowledge bases) of the European Committee for Standardization (CEN/TC 251). The main scope of the so called Classification Markup Language (ClaML) as a European Prestandard based on the eXtensible Markup Language (XML) technology is to support the transfer of the majority of hierarchical healthcare classification systems between organizations and dissimilar software products [1].

Based on our experience with conceptual models and applications with XML we tried to use existing electronic representations of the ICD-10 (e.g. DIMDI files) and transfer them into a common XML structure [2]. This structure has been defined by an XML schema.

METHODS

XML is a subset or restricted form of SGML, the Standard Generalized Markup Language (ISO 8879). The goal of XML is to enable generic SGML to be served, received, and processed on the Web in the way that is now possible with HTML. XML has been designed for ease of implementation and for interoperability with both SGML and HTML (semantic markup). Today XML is a World Wide Web Consortium Recommendation [3].

XML Schema

There are two syntactical ways to describe an XML document type, the Document Type Definition (DTD) and the XML Schema. The biggest advantage of XML schemas over DTDs is probably the fact that XML schemas are XML documents. As a consequence, we can use existing XML tools such as parsers and transformation engines to process an XML schema. Another valuable feature of XML schemas is the expressiveness of the syntax, e.g., in terms of the documentation of the model.

Available electronic formats of the ICD-10

Currently, the industry is faced with a variety of formats in which classification systems are delivered. The ICD-10 is distributed by several national institutions in ASCII text, MS Word, HTML, etc.. But all these formats don't allow for the sufficient representation while merging content, structure, and the information for the presentation. Many different parsers have to be maintained, and yet, due to the informal nature of texts, a 100% guarantee for correct parsing into more formal structures is hard to give. A neutral format like plain ASCII files with comma separated value fields is widely used, but has insufficient structuring capabilities. In addition, the maintenance can be difficult because unwanted and unnoticed mistakes are easily made. For example, the accidental deletion of a tab, makes a sibling rubric into a parent.

A relational database is often used as a source to generate above mentioned electronic formats. Whereas a direct integration of these sources into a target application may be possible a complete representation of the content of, e.g., the first Volume (Tabular List) of the ICD-10 (including footnotes, links, explanations, remarks etc.) remains difficult. In addition, for an efficient browsing in the ICD-10 the user often needs the layout information inherent in the printed version. This information has to be assigned in order to maintain readability.

We assume that the comprehensive representation of the content, hierarchical structure, inherent semantics and layout can be achieved by a document-oriented approach. In this context, XML offers a complete framework of related technologies (www.w3.org/xml) and standard tools for processing that facilitates the development of interoperable applications [4].

RESULTS

Conceptual Model – XML Schema

After careful analysis of the current electronic version of the ICD-10 as well as the available print media we developed an XML schema to represent this specific document type. The model refers to a defined part of the tabular list of the hierarchical classification. We have chosen to split the complete tabular list at the hierarchical level of the three-digit codes. This way, the XML schema defines related XML documents that contain the information of the three-, four-, and five-digit codes and their relation and dependencies to superordinated classes (chapter, group, and subgroup).

The resulting XML structure (figure 1) allows for the representation of:

- all codes, their hierarchy (relationships), and related clinical terms
- internal links and dependencies:
  - dagger/asterisk system (this concept of the dual classification of certain conditions by the etiology (+) and manifestation (*) was first introduced in ICD-9)
  - information of excluded terms
  - included terms
  - general and code-specific remarks
  - footnotes
- definition of officially (nationally) accepted codes
- etc.

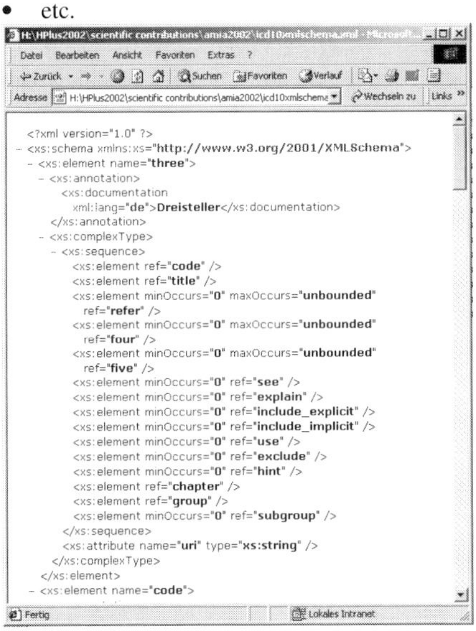
H:\HPlus2002\scientific contributions\amia2002\icd10xmlschema.xml - Microsoft ...
<?xml version="1.0" ?>
- <xs:schema xmlns:xs="http://www.w3.org/2001/XMLSchema">
- <xs:element name="three">
- <xs:annotation>
<xs:documentation xml:lang="de">Dreisteller</xs:documentation>
</xs:annotation>
- <xs:complexType>
- <xs:sequence>
<xs:element ref="code" />
<xs:element ref="title" />
<xs:element minOccurs="0" maxOccurs="unbounded" ref="refer" />
<xs:element minOccurs="0" maxOccurs="unbounded" ref="four" />
<xs:element minOccurs="0" maxOccurs="unbounded" ref="five" />
<xs:element minOccurs="0" ref="see" />
<xs:element minOccurs="0" ref="explain" />
<xs:element minOccurs="0" ref="include_explicit" />
<xs:element minOccurs="0" ref="include_implicit" />
<xs:element minOccurs="0" ref="use" />
<xs:element minOccurs="0" ref="exclude" />
<xs:element minOccurs="0" ref="hint" />
<xs:element ref="chapter" />
<xs:element ref="group" />
<xs:element minOccurs="0" ref="subgroup" />
</xs:sequence>
<xs:attribute name="uri" type="xs:string" />
</xs:complexType>
</xs:element>
- <xs:element name="code">

figure 1: *part of the XML schema*

Browsing the XML Schema

With our "XML Schema browser" the user is able to take any XML schema or DTD and to view and navigate the associated document model using an HTML browser (www.xsbrowser.com). This way, the user needn't understand the XML Schema syntax in order to understand the structure of the XML document type [5]. The screenshots within this article are based on the user front end of the xsbrowser. On the left hand side the elements and attributes of a certain node (defined on the upper line by XPath) within the schema are displayed. The right column (Meaning) shows a short textual description of each data item. This documentation can be provided in different languages. In our examples the used self-explanatory English data items are supplemented by a German documentation.

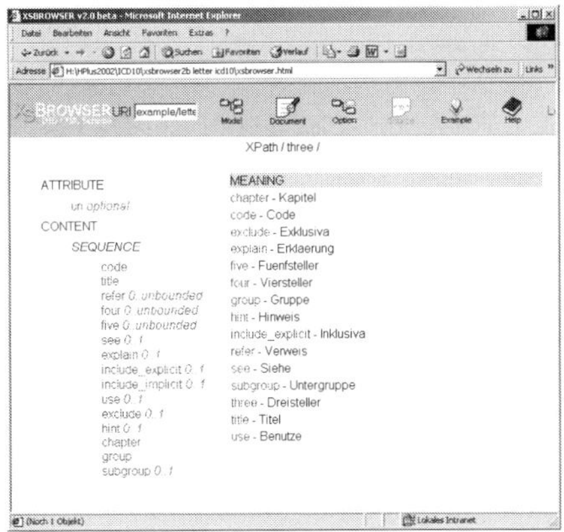

figure 2: *XML schema: three-digit code*

Figure 2 shows the elements that can be used on the level of a three-digit code. E.g., we are able to assign the code, title, included and excluded codes as well as the corresponding chapter, group and subgroup. Subsequent (four- and five-digit ...) codes contain a subset of the elements of the three-digit codes. Each group and subgroup itself can be characterized by a set of elements (figure 3). The attributes (first and last code) define the upper and lower border of the code range. The same applies for the "chapter" element that contains a title and a code range. The attribute URI (Uniform Resource Identifier) is used to point to referenced documents, such as a document that contains the information of an excluded code.

Conversion to XML

As outlined in the previous section, the DIMDI in Germany provides several electronic formats. We used an SGML representation of the German ICD-10 and similar ASCII file of the official French version. These resources are currently the most structured "raw materials" and are expected to be more or less continuously maintained. The structure of both linguistic sets aren't identical but can be converted into each other.

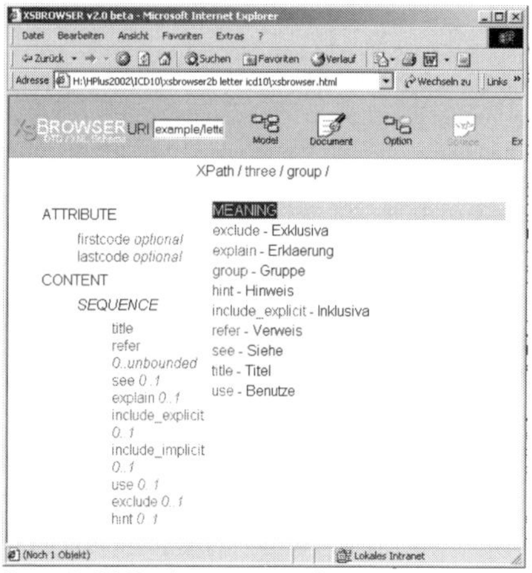

figure 3: *XML schema: group element*

In several steps, we converted the SGML / text files into XML. Subsequently, we split these files on the level of the three-digit codes into independent fragments (see above) and added the described structure defined by the XML schema. This conversion can be automated in order to be able to integrate updates of the different ICD-10 versions efficiently. Figure 4 shows an example of the generated XML document that represents the ICD-10 code D05 (carcinoma in situ of the breast).

```
<?xml version="1.0" encoding="ISO-8859-1"?>
<?xml:stylesheet type="text/xsl" href="http://simon.informatik.med.uni-giessen.de/lumrix/icd10-v2-de/icd10-ie5.xsl"?>
<?xml-stylesheet type="text/xsl" href="http://simon.informatik.med.uni-giessen.de/lumrix/icd10-v2-de/icd10-ns6.xsl"?>
<three uri="D/D05" xmlns:xsi="http://www.w3.org/2001/XMLSchema-instance"
xsi:noNamespaceSchemaLocation="http://simon.informatik.med.uni-giessen.de/lumrix/icd10-v2-de/icd10.xsd">
 <code>D05</code>
 <title xml:lang="de">Carcinoma in situ der Brustdrüse [Mamma]</title>
 <exclude>
  <item>Carcinoma in situ der Brustdrüsenhaut
   <refer uri="D/D04" fragment="45">D04.5</refer>
  </item>
  <item>Melanoma in situ der Brustdrüse (Haut)
   <refer uri="D/D03" fragment="35">D03.5</refer>
  </item>
 </exclude>
 <four uri="D/D050">
  <code>D05.0</code>
  <title xml:lang="de">Lobuläres Carcinoma in situ der Brustdrüse</title>
 </four>
 <four uri="D/D051">
  <code>D05.1</code>
  <title xml:lang="de">Carcinoma in situ der Milchgänge</title>
 </four>
 <four uri="D/D057">
  <code>D05.7</code>
  <title xml:lang="de">Sonstiges Carcinoma in situ der Brustdrüse</title>
 </four>
 <four uri="D/D059">
  <code>D05.9</code>
  <title xml:lang="de">Carcinoma in situ der Brustdrüse, nicht näher bezeichnet</title>
 </four>
 <chapter firstcode="C00" lastcode="D48">
  <title xml:lang="de">Neubildungen</title>
 </chapter>
 <group firstcode="D00" lastcode="D09">
  <title xml:lang="de">In-situ-Neubildungen</title>
  <hint xml:lang="de" />
  <include_explicit>
   <item>Bowen-Krankheit</item>
   <item>Erythroplasie</item>
   <item>Morphologieschlüsselnummern mit Malignitätsgrad /2</item>
   <item>Erythroplasie Queyrat</item>
  </include_explicit>
 </group>
</three>
```

figure 4: *XML document: D05*

Back end functionality and front end applications

The resulting XML documents (repository) are indexed and stored on the file system of a web server. For each version and linguistic set a subdirectory is assigned (see example: German version 2.0 - icd10-v2-de). These XML resources can be searched by using a generic XML search engine that has been developed at our institute. This tool allows for the context-sensitive retrieval of information contained in XML files according to a corresponding XML schema. For more details on this project please visit the following web site: www.lumrix.com

We developed a first prototype of a user interface that allows for different search strategies (web site: icd10.myelon.de). Beside full-text retrieval, the user is able to search for one or more specific terms in the titles and included codes of the ICD-10 (context-sensitive), in the ICD codes as well as in synonyms / associated terms by means of a German ICD-10 thesaurus. The "advanced search" offers the possibility to self-define the context of the structured retrieval.

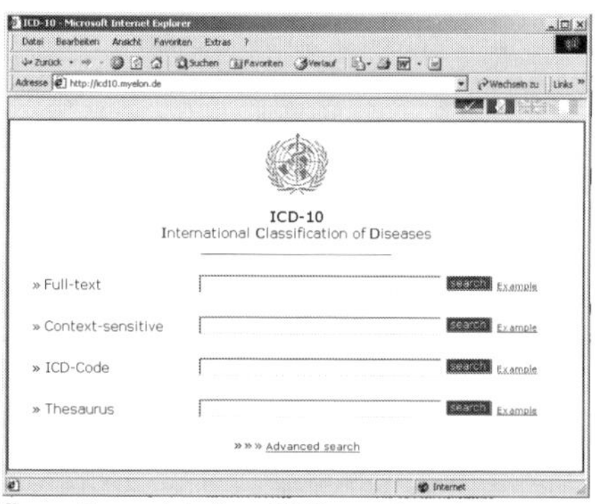

figure 5: user interface: *XML search engine*

The results are displayed in a standard web browser (e.g., Internet Explorer 5.5 and higher) using XML stylesheet language (see figure 4: ../../icd10-ie5.xsl). Once a retrieved document has been selected, the user is able to browse the complete ICD-10 using the links (URIs) to information (e.g., included codes, excluded codes, dagger codes etc.) in the referenced documents. Stylesheets are used for rendition and presentation of the selected XML document from the retrieved set of resources (ICD codes).

DISCUSSION

A consistent and comprehensive use of medical terms (such as the diagnosis) is crucial to ensure the quality of clinical coding and documentation for diverse purposes [6,7]. This implies that there is a strong need to store and transfer medical classification system in a standardized way. Currently, the industry is faced with a variety of formats in which classification systems are delivered. The Classification Markup Language (ClaML), a European prestandard provided by the Working Group II of the CEN/TC 251, wants to support the transfer of the majority of hierarchical healthcare classification systems between organizations and dissimilar software products. Based on these efforts we have developed a conceptual model for the representation of the hierarchical system of the WHO ICD-10. We decided to use an XML schema to describe this specific type of document because the expressiveness of XML schemas is superior to the expressiveness of DTDs. XML Schema provides data types that can be used to restrict and validate the content of both, XML elements and XML attributes. In addition, XML schemas allow a better reuse of already defined model concepts and provide therefore a greater "composite power" than DTDs.

Our XML schema of the ICD-10 differs from the CEN ClaML standard in that way that it extends the model with regard to specific informational needs (see results). Nevertheless, despite this additional granularity it is possible to transform our XML model into the CEN standard and vice versa.

As already mentioned, the content of the different versions and linguistic sets of the ICD-10 is maintained by national organizations. We are able to automate the conversion of these different electronic formats of the ICD-10 into the XML representation while leaving the provision of updates and errata to these established institutions.

Furthermore, our so-called XML framework, that includes an XML search engine, builds a technical solution that facilitates the developments of web-based services and user interfaces [4]. A pilot implementation of such services has been described that uses XML stylesheets for the rendition and presentation of ICD-10 content. The stylesheets apply the same "look & feel" as the print media of the ICD-10 to the electronic output.

The above mentioned concept allows for the fast provision of a multilingual ICD-10 and the possibility of the direct processing of XML output in clinical information systems and coding software (machine interfaces). In order to be able to enhance and speed-up the distribution of new or updated electronic versions we regard this web-based infrastructure to be an ideal solution. The XML- (web-) interface is the core component based on the concept of the Uniform Resource Identifier (URI). All communication between the target systems and the web server (ICD-10 repository) can be realized by standard URI requests. The results of the query are sent back in XML format allowing for further processing. But there is still a need of developing or adapting the application logic of front-end applications in order to process all the information that is inherent in the electronic representation.

Acknowledgment

This project is supported in part by the German Federal Ministry of Health.

The author can be reached by e-mail at:
simon.hoelzer@informatik.med.uni-giessen.de

References

1. http://www.centc251.org/WGII/N-01/WGII-N01-03rev%20_2_.pdf
2. Hoelzer S, Schweiger RK, Boettcher HA, Tafazzoli AG, Dudeck J. Value of XML in the implementation of clinical practice guidelines--the issue of content retrieval and presentation. Med Inform Internet Med. 2001 Apr-Jun;26(2):131-46.
3. http://www.w3.org/TR/1998/REC-xml-19980210
4. Schweiger R, Hoelzer S, Altmann U, Rieger J, Dudeck J. Plug-and-Play XML: A Health Care Perspective. J Am Med Inform Assoc. 2002 Jan;9(1):37-48.
5. Schweiger R, Hoelzer S, Heitmann KU, Dudeck J. DTDs go XML schema--a tools perspective. Med Inform Internet Med. 2001 Oct-Dec;26(4):297-308.
6. e Lusignan S, Minmagh C, Kennedy J, Zeimet M, Bommezijn H, Bryant J. A survey to identify the clinical coding and classification systems currently in use across Europe. Medinfo. 2001;10:86-9.
7. Cimino JJ. Terminology tools: state of the art and practical lessons. Methods Inf Med. 2001;40(4):298-306.

Medical and Care Compunetics 2
L. Bos et al. (Eds.)
IOS Press, 2005

Development of an Expert System for Classification of Medical Errors

D. KOPEC[a], K. LEVY[a], M. KABIR[b],
D. REINHARTH[c] and G. SHAGAS[a]

[a]*Department of Computer and Information Science, Brooklyn College, New York, USA*
[b]*Department of Health Informatics, Dalhousie University, Halifax, Ontario, Canada*
[c]*Long Island Jewish Medical Center, New Hyde Park, New York, USA*

Abstract. The 1999 report published by the Institute of Medicine (IOM) indicated that between 44,000 and 98,000 unnecessary deaths per year occurred in hospitals alone, as a result of errors committed by medical professionals in the United States. There has been considerable speculation that these figures are either overestimated or underestimated. For example, the possibility that they focus on isolated injuries rather than error, or the majority of surveyed respondents did not know what constitutes a (medical) error. These disagreements have led experts to challenge the estimates of patient harm attributable to error, as well as the methodologies used to enumerate them. Of particular concern is the process used in the identification, classification and prevention of medical errors. There have been numerous attempts to develop classifications of medical errors, and currently an abundance of taxonomies exist to describe their mechanism.

In previous research, (Kopec, Kabir, Reinharth, Rothschild & Castiglione, 2003) a new taxonomy of Medical Errors was designed by expanding the IOM classification. This model and its extension can be used as a blueprint for future design, development and implementation of an expert system for classification of medical errors. Effective classification can facilitate pattern recognition, and pattern recognition will help in understanding the nature, background and abatement of medical errors. Such a system's goal will be to perform convincingly as an advisory consultant, exhibiting expertise on a par with and beyond human experts in specified domains. Despite substantial disagreement on the validity of the published figures for fatalities in hospitals in the IOM report, what is of importance is that the number of deaths caused by such errors is nonetheless alarming. The identification and classification of errors in medical care delivery is a very complex process, and this process can be facilitated and simplified by the implementation of an effective classification system.

Keywords. Medical errors, expert systems, error theory, CLIPS, taxonomy

Introduction

Since the publication of the famous 1999 report by the Institute of Medicine (IOM) [1] there has been continued concern about the effective identification and classification of human medical errors. A number of papers have been published in the field, addressing the validity of the manner in which the estimated range of the number of deaths per annum due to medical errors was obtained [2–6]. Despite disagreements concerning the accuracy of the quoted figures, it is evident that it is impossible to quantify the full magnitude of the challenges to safety with certainty, as the health care sector does not routinely identify and collect information on errors[7]. It is clear that even with discrepancies between the estimates, the mortality rates strongly suggest that effective strategies need to be employed to reliably identify and classify errors. The development of an effective classification system will aid in reducing the occurrence of errors and thereby assist in improving the quality of patient care for the American Health Care System.

1. Research Goal

In previous research, the original IOM taxonomy was extended and a new approach to the classification, distribution and updating of medical information was recommended[7]. The goal of this study is to design an Expert System, utilizing this extended taxonomy, which will effectively classify medical errors and serve as a testbed for healthcare practitioners.

2. Taxonomy of Medical Errors

There have been numerous attempts to develop classifications of medical errors, and currently an abundance of taxonomies exist to describe the mechanism behind the types of medical errors.

The following etiology of categories of medication errors was given by the American Hospital Association[7]:

a) Incomplete patient information
b) Unavailable drug information
c) Miscommunication of drug orders
d) Lack of appropriate labeling
e) Environmental factors

The five error types most often observed and reported by U.S. family physicians were[8]:

a) Errors in prescribing medications
b) Errors in getting the right laboratory test done for the right patient at the right time
c) Filing system errors
d) Errors in dispensing medications
e) Errors in responding to abnormal laboratory test results

"Errors in prescribing medications" was the only one of these five error types that was also commonly reported by family physicians in other countries [9].

In an influential 1993 report, Kohn et al.[2] developed a classification of medical errors. This report classifies medication-related errors under "Treatment Error, etc.", but in our analysis we found that medication-related errors and errors related to clerical procedure are abundant in medical practice. Therefore, we altered the original IOM classification by specifically identifying and addressing these two types of errors, by including the NCC MERP[10] taxonomy. We also classified 'Errors Related to Diagnosis' into three clinical subgroups ("delayed", "missed", and "wrong", as opposed to the four subgroups of the IOM). Specifically, we have divided each type into subtypes, numbered according to the NCC MERP[10].

Human error[11] can be subdivided as follows: "A knowledge error referred to as a *mistake* occurs from inadequate or incorrect information. If the information is correct, but the wrong method of application is chosen, a rule error occurs, termed a *lapse*. An example of such an error would be an incorrect diagnosis. Finally, the plan may be good, but the performance is faulty, often from distraction or inattention. This is a skill-based error, termed a *slip*[11]. Reason[11] distinguishes between two kinds of human error – active and latent. Active errors are the ones which are immediately discernible, whereas latent errors are much harder to detect and may require considerable analysis to discover or understand." Based on our previous research[7], following is the classification of human errors in Medical practice:

1) Errors in prescribing medication:
   - Misuse by incorrect: medication, route, dose, administration
   - Overuse – using too much of a drug or prescribing a drug when not indicated
   - Underuse – failure to provide medication
2) Treatment Procedure(s) – other than by medication
3) Errors related to Clerical Procedures
4) Errors related to Diagnosis
   - Delayed Diagnosis
   - Missed Diagnosis
   - Wrong Diagnosis
5) Preventative errors – delayed or no follow-up treatment are examples
6) Other
   - Communication Failure
   - Administration Problems

The above approach for distinguishing between errors will be used in the design of the Expert System for the Classification of Medical Errors.

3. Cases of Errors

The study of more than 235,000 error reports submitted in 2003 by 570 health care facilities was the largest ever performed by the U.S. Pharmacopeia[12]. In their findings, as the number of reported errors goes up, the percentage that causes patient harm has gone down. However, the findings that were remarkable are those indicating that electronic prescribing is creating new types of errors. "Computer entry" was the 4th leading cause of errors accounting for 13% (27,711) of the medication errors reported in 2003[12]. In contrast, illegible or unclear handwriting was the 15th leading cause and accounted for 2.9% (6,134) of reported errors[12]. It might be expected that handwriting would move down the list as computerization becomes more widely implemented, however what was occurring was a new type of error. So we can see that information systems and the medical field present a double-edged sword. On one hand they offer the possibility of tremendous improvements in terms of memory capacity, speed and general processing power, but if coupled with arcane data entry systems, serious new problems are created. Can we return to manual data entry? Not at all. More important, is that data entry systems develop "anti-debugging" components to reduce human error.

Another example that emphasizes the enormity of the medical error scenario is seen in the article by, Myhre and D. McRure[7,13], which compares studies of errors in blood transfusions presented as Table 1 below.

Table 1 illustrates that errors occurred due to drawing specimens from the wrong patient (error by medical technologist), change of specimen in the laboratory (error by laboratory staff or medical technologist), and transfusion of blood into the wrong patient (errors by physician/nurse). Figure 2 below Table 1 illustrates the same data in a pie chart format. The numbers in the columns of the Table should add up to 100% since they are percentages of fatal error in Blood Transfusions, but they did not in the original published table[13]. Hence we have determined that the second row labeled "Other" should have the figures shifted one column to the left, for example, under "Mythre", the second row labeled "Other" should read 8(10%), under Honig & Bove it should read 4(10%) etc. This type of error can be committed by anyone including a variety of medical practitioners, in addition to physicians.

Another incident involved the assessment of the impact on ordering errors when

Table 1. Summary and Comparison of Various Reports of Fatal Errors in Blood Transfusions.

Summary and Comparison of Various Reports of Fatal Errors in Blood Transfusion.								
	Schmidt	Myhre	Honig & Bove	Camp & Monagha	Sazama	Linden	McClelland & Phillips	
Drawing Specimen								
Wrong Specimen	0	7(10%)	7(16%)	1(1%)	13(5%)	10(19%)	23(20%)	
Other	0							
Laboratory								
Specimen Exchange	5(16%)	9(12%)	9(21%)	10(8%)	25(10%)	10(19%)	6(5%)	
Other			8(10%)	4(10%)	27(22%)	20(8%)	7(13%)	
Transfusion								
Wrong patient	17(55%)	30(39%)	17(38%)	25(20%)	77(30%)	24(44%)	82(75%)	
Other	3(10%)	1(1%)	1(2%)	1(1%)	10(4%)			
Other causes	19%	28%	13%	48%	43%	NS	NS	
Total	31	77	44	126	256	54	111	699

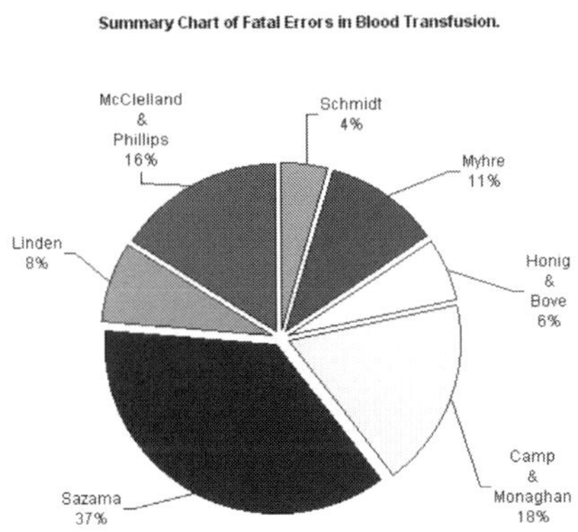

Figure 1. Pie Chart representation of the information in Table 1.

physicians stopped writing patient identifiers on requests for blood transfusions by hand[14]. Physicians, frustrated by the amount of time required to complete forms to order blood, wanted to eliminate the need for their handwritten patient identifiers, which were in addition to such information "stamped" on blood requests. This change was implemented, the blood ordering forms were modified accordingly, and after elimination of the handwritten identifiers in 1997, ordering errors increased from an annual rate of 1 in 10,000 to 6 in 10,000 blood requests by late 1999. Subsequently, clinicians were alerted by newsletter and the rate decreased to 3 in 10,000. However, the error rate did not decrease to its previous level of 1 in 10, 000 requests until mid-2001, approximately 2.5 years after reinstitution of the requirement for handwritten patient identifiers. The conclusion of this study [14] was that an obligatory second entry of demographic identifiers on a blood order requires ordering physicians to be given careful consideration to the identity of the patient receiving the blood transfusion, thereby reducing the likelihood of transfusion of an unintended recipient.

4. The Design, Development and Implementation of an Expert System for Classification of Medical Errors

As seen from examination of the above scenarios, errors in the medical field can occur in many different ways, with potentially diverse, wide-ranging and hazardous effects. Just review of the varied errors related to fundamental areas such as medication, diagnosis, treatment procedures and clerical procedures in terms of their number, etiology and possible ramifications, is a complex domain. Consideration of the number of possible permutations of specific elements or actions in a health-related setting that might be classified as error(s), coupled with the large variety of "system" type errors, leads us to conclude that we are dealing with an enormous range of possibilities. Which expert in the medical field will be able to hold in his or her head all the possible combinations of signs, symptoms and treatments that have occurred for all possible medical conditions?

Expert systems can be used for effective classification of a diverse range of possibilities, and many have been built to solve different types of problems. These systems are unique in that they can draw conclusions from a store of task-specific knowledge principally through logic or plausible inference[15,16]. They are also called knowledge-based systems because they contain the same kind of rules used by human experts when they make decisions in their field of expertise[15]. The heart of an expert system is the powerful corpus of knowledge that accumulates during system building. The knowledge is explicit and organized to simplify decision-making; and the accumulation and codification of knowledge is one of the most important aspects[15]. These systems are not locked into any specific decision path and as a result can select from alternative paths in their search for a conclusion[16].

When there are domain experts and a substantial number of rules, more than the human mind can effectively recall with speed and accuracy, such a situation can be remedied by building an expert system. We intend to use the Expert System shell CLIPS to design this system. The system will classify errors based on a set of production or decision rules. Rule-based programming is one of the most commonly used techniques for developing expert systems. In the programming paradigm, rules are used as heuristics or rules-of-thumb, which specify a set of actions to be performed for a given situation. In the event that two rules match a given problem situation, the system

Assume a patient had been admitted to a hospital due to complications with influenza, however, after what was considered an acceptable amount of recovery time, the patient showed no signs of improvement, and after assessment was found to be physically worse than he had been upon admission. Some of the questions that the system might ask would be as follows:

Q Is the patient male or female?
A male
Q What is the patient's age?
A 43
Q Did the patient stay overnight in the hospital?
A yes
Q How many days was the patient in hospital?
A 7
Q Give the number of medical staff that were exposed to the patient during his stay?
A 22
Q Did the patient come into contact with staff through: medical devices, food trays,
medicine dispensation?
A yes
Q Does the hospital have a hand-cleansing protocol for staff?
A no

The system, based on the rule constraints that it is designed with might continue with more questions to get more information from the user, and might respond with the following summary:

The patient is likely to have contracted a hospital-acquired infection due to the absence of a protocol for the effective practice of regular hand washing by staff. This determination is based on a 75% degree of certainty based on the following elements:

- *Patient was in the hospital overnight*
- *Patient was exposed to more than five members of staff*
- *Patient was exposed to staff through medical devices, food trays, etc.*
- *No hand-washing protocol for staff exists*

Figure 2. Medical error scenario and possible outcome on running through our Medical Errors Classification System.

will utilize a conflict resolution strategy to best resolve the tie based on the specified decision rules. For example, it could break a tie based on which rule is more specific, or which rule is shorter or based on "refreshing", that is, rules, which had recently been done after conflict resolution, might not be used again for some time in favor of new rules.

Figure 2 illustrates how this Expert System could assist in recognizing and classifying what is considered a typical problem in hospitals, that of not implementing a proper hand-cleansing protocol for medical personnel.

Conclusion and Further Research

The identification and classification of errors in medical care delivery is a very complex process, and this process may be simplified by the implementation of an effective classification system[7]. In order to reach a consensus on the classification of medical errors, it is necessary to develop a generally accepted international medical error classification system. Findings have indicated that errors are likely to affect patients in similar ways in countries with similar healthcare systems[17]. With this taxonomy, the major types of errors can be categorized and each major type can then be associated with a specific underlying mechanism. This can explain why and even predict when and where an error will occur[18], which in turn will assist in the generation of intervention strategies for each type of error, and also assist in the reduction and abatement of medical errors.

References

[1] Brennan T.A., The Institute of Medicine Report on Medical Errors: Could It Do Harm? *Tex Med.* 96(6), 13–15, 2000.
[2] Kohn, L.T., Corrigan, J.M., and Donaldson, M.S. (eds.), To Err is Human: Building a Safer Health System, National Academy Press, Washington, DC, 2000.
[3] Spencer, F.C., Human Error in Hospitals and Industrial Accidents: Current Concepts, *Amer. Col. Of Surgeons* 191:410–418, 2000.
[4] Ballas, E.A., Information systems can prevent errors and quality. *J. Am. Med. Inf. Assoc.* 8:398–99, 2001.
[5] Bates, D.W., Reducing the frequency of errors in medicine using information technology, *J. Amer. Med. Inf. Assoc.*, 8: 299–308, 2001.
[6] Richardson, W.C., The Institute of Medicine report on medical errors, *N. Eng. J. Med.* 343:663–65, 2000.
[7] Kopec, D., Kabir, M.H., Reinharth, D., Rothschild, O. & Castiglione, J.A., Human Errors in Medical Practice: Systematic Classification and Reduction with Automated Information Systems, *Journal of Medical Systems,* 27(4), 297–313, 2003.
[8] Kopec, D., Shagas, G., Kabir, M.H., Reinharth, D., Castiglione, J.A. & Tamang, S., Errors in Medical Practice?: Identification, Classification and Steps toward Reduction, Medical and Care Compunetics 1 (Eds. Lodewijk Bos, Swamy Laxminarayan and Andy Marsh). Proceedings of the 1st ICMCC (International Congress on Medical Care Compunetics), The Hague, The Netherlands, June 2–4, 2004, pp. 126–134.
[9] Dovey, S.M., Meyers D.S., Phillips R.L., Green L.A., et al, A preliminary taxonomy of medical errors in family practice. Qual. Saf. Health Care 11:233–238, 2002.
[10] National Coordinating Council for Medication Error Reporting and Prevention. *NCC MERP taxonomy of medication error*. http://www.nccmerp.org/pdf/taxo1999-05-14.pdf
[11] Reason, J. Human error, Cambridge: Cambridge University Press; 1990.
[12] Robeznieks, A., Data Entry is a top cause of Rx Errors, *American Medical News*, pp. 14–15, January 24, 2005.
[13] Myhre, B.A., and McRure, D. "Human error- A significant cause of transfusion mortality". Transfusion, 40:879–885, 2000.
[14] Moore, SB., Floss, ML., Ordering Blood for the Wrong Patient – Getting Inside the Minds of Ordering Physicians, *Mayo Clin Proc.* 78:1337–1339, 2003.
[15] Waterman, D., A Guide to Expert Systems.
[16] Webster, R., Miner, L., ExpertSystems – Programming Problem Solving, 1982.
[17] Makeham, M.A.B., Dovey, S.M., County, M., Kidd, M.R., An international taxonomy of errors in general practice: A pilot study, *Med. J. Australia* 177: 68–72, 2002.
[18] Zhang, J., Patel, V., Johnson, T. and Shortliffe, E., A cognitive taxonomy of medical errors, *Journal of Biomedical Informatics* 37: 193–204, 2004.

Medical and Care Compunetics 2
L. Bos et al. (Eds.)
IOS Press, 2005

Model of Good Practice Tools for Risk Reduction and Clinical Governance

D. SMAGGHE[a], M. SEGERS[b], P.-J. SPY-ANDERSON[c], N. BENAMOU[a] and N. EDDABBEH[a]
[a]*Business Flow Consulting - 196 rue Houdan, 92330 Sceaux, France*
[b]*GFI-OIS - 54 Chaussée des Collines, 1300 WAVRE, Belgium*
[c]*Airial Conseil - 3 rue Bellini, 92806 Puteaux, France*

Abstract. Information and Communication Technologies (ICT) are expected to support Healthcare Professionals in reducing medical errors, making the most relevant decisions and finding the most appropriate procedure for each patient. In particular, Knowledge Management and Decision Support Systems provide access to high quality information and to appropriate protocols. The present paper aims at comparing the approaches used in three ongoing R&D projects in order to support risk reduction and clinical governance. This comparison will lead to the presentation of a generic model of Decision Support Tools that transform shared and documented "Good Practices" into software entities that can pro-actively advice users in their daily work or when they encounter difficult situations.

Keywords. Good practices, healthcare, risk reduction, knowledge management, decision support, clinical governance

Introduction

An increasing challenge in today's healthcare environment is to manage risk and reduce medical errors. Indeed, Risk Management plays a crucial role in fulfilling the commitments of healthcare professionals to provide the best quality of care possible as well as the continuous assessment and improvement of the quality of care and the services rendered to patients.

Changes in the healthcare sector have made it more important than ever for healthcare providers to be proactive in identifying risks and taking appropriate preventative measures. New developments in medicine, combined with heightened regulatory and legal requirements have introduced new, unexpected and sometimes complex risk issues for healthcare providers. The responsibilities of risk managers are as broad as ever and include financial, legal and operational dimensions that frame the contemporary practice of medicine. In this context, physicians and hospitals are increasingly requested to assess the costs and quality of care received under various treatment protocols.

Information and Communication Technologies (ICT) are expected to contribute to this evolution and to help healthcare professionals in reducing medical errors, making the most relevant decisions and finding the most appropriate procedure for each patient. In particular, Knowledge Management and Decision Support Systems will help healthcare professionals in their assessment and management of risk. Access to high quality information has also been identified as being essential for good clinical governance. Better information would support the use of the best evidence and provide more accurate assessment of the quality of service to support clinical governance. Moreover, Decision Support Systems should provide ready access to appropriate knowledge or protocols. They should also provide a rational aid to diagnosis or probable outcome on the basis of patient specific data. By this way, the maintenance of protocol based on evidence can be ensured.

The paper compares the approaches used in various recent R&D projects[1] in order to support risk reduction and clinical governance. It emphasises the difference between ICT tools for:

- Collaborative practices: The IST PALLIANET [1] Project illustrates in Palliative care the emergence of knowledge driven collaborative practices in healthcare networks.
- Co-ordinated care: The IST CARE-PATHS [2] Project illustrates how the strict implementation of Clinical Pathways can contribute to the continuous improvement of the quality of care.
- Decision support: The IST NOESIS [3] Project illustrates how an advanced knowledge management platform coupled with a decision support framework can support healthcare professionals in the field of cardiovascular diseases.

1. Description of the Projects Objectives and Results

Each project aims at developing and implementing ICT tools that will support healthcare professionals in the improvement of care delivered to patients. The three projects are presented using a common framework:

- Objectives of the project and how they meet user needs
- Description of the ICT tool being developed
- Pilot implementations in order to demonstrate the benefits of the solution.

1.1. Pallianet

The PALLIANET project focuses on the improvement of collaborative practices in palliative care networks. It aims at improving communications and real time access to information amongst palliative care networks, in order to improve the quality of care services. The Information & Communication system that will be set up will enable a Palliative Care Team to support allied professional care providers, both medical practitioners and non-medical professionals. The project will lead to two major results:

- Better understanding the patient's context (clinical, psychological and social dimensions);
- Making information available to support decision making processes, in a complex and unusual context, thus providing quality of care.

---

[1] These projects have been partially funded by the European Commission under the IST initiative.

In order to extract knowledge and identify Best Practices, a *"Knowledge Generation"* module provides capabilities of mining both text (e.g. cases discussion, emails, chats, forums, etc…) and data (Patients' Records). It enables the transforming of experience and exchanged information (implicit information) into explicit knowledge stored as Best Practice Guides.

Thus the existing Patients Medical files are external to the *PALLIANET* system and can be shared and exchanged between healthcare professionals, which get semantic access to them through a "Care delivery context" database. In particular, Patient records will be automatically scanned by *Best Practice agents* and used in *Case discussions*.

A "Community & Knowledge Management Service" allows collaborative practices by sharing the experience and knowledge among the different actors involved around the patient. Specific tools will permit to support the actors of the palliative care team in their daily work:

- Communication tools such as "Forums", emails and chats are provided to healthcare professionals, patients and families to enable experience and information exchange.
- "*Case discussions*" enables the caregivers to get support from the palliative care co-ordination team; it might be useful for complex cases and whenever the caregiver feels the psychological need for "mentor" support.
- Certified knowledge is accessible as well through access to specific databases of relevant "Documents" (that have been validated by competent actors) and "Best Practices Guides" prepared by the co-ordination team.
- "Best Practice Agents" advises medical doctors when dealing with a given patient; they takes into account the patient's record and scan "Best Practice Guides" to support practitioners in making the best decision.

Two pilot implementations demonstrate the benefits of PALLIANET in supporting healthcare professionals:

- The palliative care team at Guys' and St Thomas' Hospital (UK) provides the context of an integrated service offered by hospital staff both in and out of the hospital.
- The Nepale network (France) provides the context of a light palliative care team coordinating the activity of city care providers in delivering palliative care in a geographic area.

1.2. Care-Paths

CARE-PATHS project's goal is to set up an intelligent operational environment for making clinical governance effective, to support health professionals, clinicians and care operators, in continually improving the quality of services and safeguarding high standards of care.

CARE-PATHS leans upon the concept of clinical pathways, with are plans of care that is applied to patients with a known diagnosis and a predictable clinical outcome. The aim of a clinical pathway is to coordinate and define the extent and quality of care that is provided. Clinical pathways are in fact strategies for handling complex treatment procedures. Their objective is to improve the quality and/or reduce the cost of a given product or service, while ensuring its timely execution.

The CARE-PATHS project major result will be a web-based software solution enabling healthcare institutions to implement and manage clinical pathways, thus covering the whole cycle of:

- Clinical pathway authoring
- Putting clinical pathways in practice
- Monitoring and managing patients' variance

The CARE-PATHS software solution consists of a set of intelligent tools for supporting health professionals, which can be used and combined at different degrees and adjusted to different clinical pathway contexts:

- A Semantic based knowledge system enabling the authoring of clinical pathways. The CARE-PATHS knowledge system covers both clinical pathways definition, document repositories internal to the healthcare institution and access to external medical document repositories, existing and authorised by accredited medical organisations and medical profession unions.
- Decision Support Tools for care givers to put in practice clinical pathways, i.e. enabling to develop a specific patient plan, evaluate a patient's condition, and promote the use of alternative solutions at each stage of the pathway. These Decision Support Tools gets access to patient records databases and more generally with the workflow of clinical documents at the specific site.
- Monitoring and analytical tools for clinical pathways' variance: historical data gathering with regards the patient application, evaluation of a patient's variance, which can be used by the Decision Support Tools to propose changes in the patient's pathway, or to identify needs for pathway redefinition.

Two pilot implementations demonstrate the benefits of CARE-PATHS in supporting healthcare professionals by reducing medical risks and making the relevant decisions:

- The CARE-PATHS pilot in Parma involves the domain of Cardiology/Cardiosurgery and Peripheral Vascular Surgery, and aims at implementing and testing the set of tools previously described in the emergency care setting.
- Valencia Pilot (La Fe Hospital) deals with the implementation of the CARE-PATHS solution in the domain of Pneumonology through its Home Hospitalisation Unit.

1.3. Noesis

NOESIS strategic objectives are to tackle the deficiencies and failures of medical decision making and to satisfy the need for effective information retrieval, thus improving the healthcare services provided to European citizens.

The selected clinical domain addressed by the project is Cardiology. In particular NOESIS will contribute to:

- Reduce the uncertainty in diagnosis of diseases, focusing on cardiovascular diseases;
- Support the process of diagnosis and treatment by reducing errors and minimising associated risks;

- Provide methods for establishing trust and confidence of users towards information sources.

This will be achieved by developing a computer-based application that enables the retrieval of up-to-date and valid medical information from heterogeneous, distributed sources. The NOESIS system combines:

- User-friendly Interfaces that enables the users to interact with the system and take advantage of the main functionalities that include:
  - o Information retrieval by simple queries. Search of information is beyond keyword matching enabling context and content based information retrieval;
  - o Information "feeding"; authorized user groups are able to:
    - insert with specific procedures, protocols, papers, articles, and other medical knowledge into the system;
    - make the appropriate characterization/annotation of that information, so that they will be categorised and retrieved according to their content-category.
- Profiling and Personalisation mechanisms;
- Resources integration and semantic interoperability;
- Knowledge management and retrieval;
- A Decision Support Framework capable of supporting the process of diagnosis.

Trying to reduce uncertainty in this complex domain of cardiovascular diseases, NOESIS assists health professionals in the diagnostic process allowing a smooth collaboration between established medical knowledge and personal judgment. Additionally, academic health professionals take advantage of the use of NOESIS, as a tool for training purposes of medical students for both handling diagnosis and treatment, introducing them to the way they should couple knowledge and make decisions.
The NOESIS solution will be tested and assessed by several user groups (within healthcare institutions) located in Italy, France, Cyprus and Greece.

2. Discussion and Conclusions

The comparison of these three projects has enabled the definition of a generic model for transforming shared and documented "Good Practices" into software entities; they can pro-actively advice users when they encounter difficult situations. This generic model of "Good Practice" Software supports:

- Interaction with existing Healthcare Patient Records,
- Ability to enforce rules and/or to propose advices,
- Ability to evaluate historical practices and performance to propose practice revisions.

We can abstract from this a more generic model called "Active Practice" Service. To support the definition, enactment and continuous revision of "Good Practices", this model is based on a generic scenario that can be split in 3 stages:

Table 1. Scenario for "Good Practices".

Phases	Activities
1. **Set up**	• Define Good Practices through the analysis of existing business processes and existing documentation (e.g. regulations, procedures definition, mission statement…) • Provide a gateway to existing Information Systems involved in the processes • Modelise Active Practice Templates through an analysis of past cases relevant to the Practice Definition
2. **Enactment**	While a practitioner is using his/her information systems, the Active Practice Service continually: • Monitors the case (and enriches a cases database) • Reminds the practitioner of key case info • Asks questions relevant to possible options for processing the case • Alerts the practitioner in case of "strong" deviation from the good practice • Proposes decisions
3. **Practices Evaluation**	• Deviations indicators are continually computed (cases *vs.* Active Practices) • Deviations are analysed at the level of Active Practice Template and proposals are made for Template revision • Deviations are analysed at the level of Practice Definition • Practitioners collaborate (chats, case discussion, opinion analysis, vote …) in the revision of Practices.

Transforming this scenario into a model led us to the definition of the "Active Practice" Service as described next page.

A first functionality would deal with analysing existing documentation in order to semi-automatically **generate Good Practice template**s. This could be twofold:

- A first analysis is needed on documents describing existing processes (care protocols, procedure manuals…) to get a Good Practice definition that could emphasise both formal aspects and semantics;
- From this Good Practice definition, interview reports with practitioners and excerpts from past cases, it is possible to go a step further, to model Practices, to describe security policies, and to define performance targets.

The **implementation of the Good Practice Template** among a healthcare organisation can be characterized by the following features:

- Good Practice Templates can be shared across the various services of a healthcare organisation;
- Each service handles access to its own existing information systems;
- When processing a case, each involved service must temporarily instantiate the relevant Good Practice Template into an in-service database.

Moreover, the management of co-operative practices induces the need for modeling processes by examples. In the context of distributed processes, this also implies that:

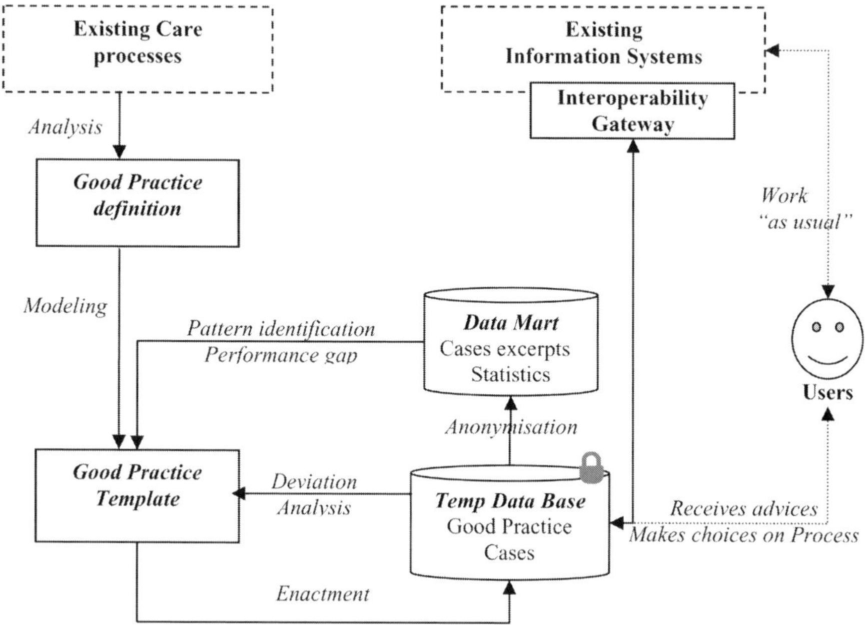

Figure 1. "Active Practice" Service architecture.

- The Case Management cycle would consist of 3 steps: "Monitoring a Case", "Deviation Analysis vs. Good Practice Template" and "Advising User"; this could rely on automation tools;
- The decision to exchange case data between users (and therefore healthcare institutions) is often left to users and cannot always be pre-defined. However data privacy remains an issue and it thus becomes mandatory to address security & privacy and data level rather than at service or case level.

Practices evaluation aims primarily at adjusting Good Practice Templates on the basis of identified patterns in past cases for improving performance and **revising Good Practices**. The steps needed to achieve this are the following:

1. To measure in a dynamic and secure way, the evolution of the care processes through networks which are created automatically by the interconnection of several Legacy systems
2. To extract, process in a protected and fair way the gathered data; then to store it to be able to exploit it in order to discover interesting patterns and thus to measure deviations
3. To analyse the selected patterns
4. To apply the results of these analyses in order to optimise the care processes.

This service then proposes to reduce risks related to care processes and help healthcare professionals to make the most relevant decisions by leveraging on the knowledge available about "Good Practices"; this reflects a willingness to enact good practices rather than to enforce them.

References

[1] IST-507863 PALLIANET – Decision Support and Knowledge driven Collaborative practices in Palliative Care, 2003, http://www.pallianet.eupm.net/.
[2] IST-1-507017 CARE-PATHS – An intelligent support environment to improve the quality of decision processes in health communities, 2003, http://www.carepaths.eupm.net/.
[3] IST-2002-507960 NOESIS – Platform for wide scale integration and visual representation of medical intelligence, 2003, http://www.noesis-eu.org/.

Medical and Care Compunetics 2
L. Bos et al. (Eds.)
IOS Press, 2005

Optimisation Issues of High Throughput Medical Data and Video Streaming Traffic in 3G Wireless Environments

R.S.H. ISTEPANIAN and N. PHILIP
Mobile Information and Network Technologies Research Centre, Kingston University, London Kingston upon Thames, KT1 2EE, UK
r.istepanian@kingston.ac.uk

Abstract. In this paper we describe some of the optimisation issues relevant to the requirements of high throughput of medical data and video streaming traffic in 3G wireless environments. In particular we present a challenging 3G mobile health care application that requires a demanding 3G medical data throughput. We also describe the 3G QoS requirement of m**O**bile **T**ele-**E**chography ultra-**L**ight r**O**bot system (OTELO that is designed to provide seamless 3G connectivity for real-time ultrasound medical video streams and diagnosis from a remote site (robotic and patient station) manipulated by an expert side (specialists) that is controlling the robotic scanning operation and presenting a real-time feedback diagnosis using 3G wireless communication links.

Keywords. 3G, wireless communications, mobile healthcare, telemedicine, robotics, tele-echobgaphy, frame rate control

1. Introduction

m-Health can be defined as 'mobile computing, medical sensor, and communications technologies for healthcare' [1]. This emerging concept represents the evolution of e-health systems from traditional desktop 'telemedicine' platforms to wireless and mobile configurations. Current and emerging developments in wireless communications integrated with developments in pervasive and wearable technologies will have a radical impact on future healthcare delivery systems. In this paper we present an advanced mobile healthcare application example (mobile robotic tele-echography system) that requires a demanding medical data and video streaming traffic in 3G wireless environments.

The advanced medical robotic system -OTELO (m**O**bile- **T**ele-**E**chography using an ultra-**L**ight r**O**bot) was a European IST funded project that develops a fully integrated end-to-end mobile tele-echography system for population groups that are not served locally, either temporarily or permanently, by medical ultrasound experts. It comprises a fully portable tele-operated robot allowing a specialist sonographer to perform a real-time robotised tele-echography to remote patients [2].

OTELO is a remotely controlled system designed to achieve reliable ultrasound imaging at an isolated site, distant from a specialist clinician [3]. Figure 1 shows the main operational blocks of the system. This Tele-echography system is composed of three main parts:

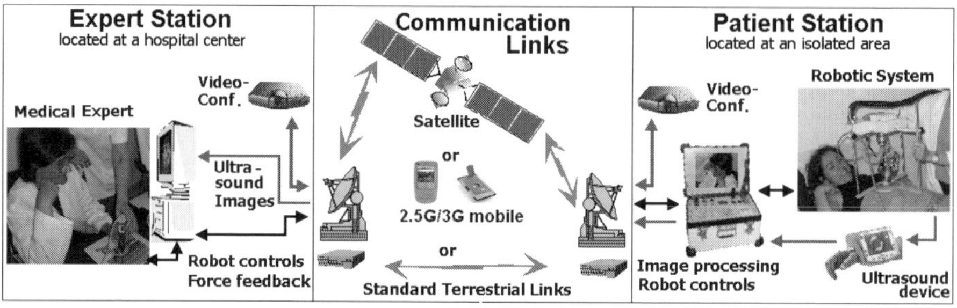

Figure 1. The OTELO Mobile Robotic System.

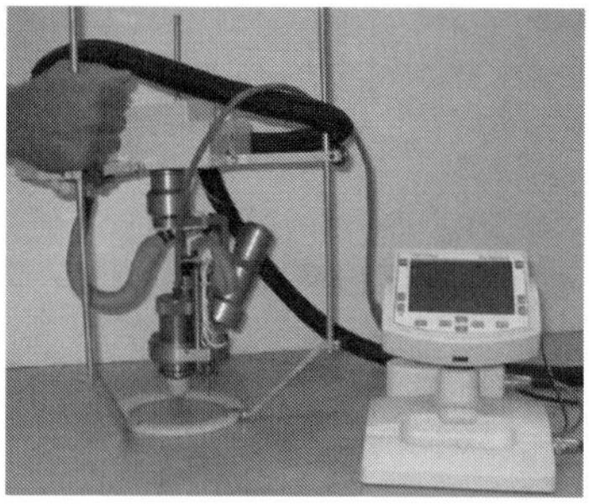

Figure 2. OTELO- The Mobile Robot system with the echograph Unit.

- An « expert » site where the medical expert interacts with a dedicated patented pseudo-haptic fictive probe instrumented to control the positioning of the remote robot and emulates an ultrasound probe that medical experts are used to handle, thus providing a better ergonomy.
- The communication media. We developed communication software based upon IP protocol to adapt to different communication (wired and wireless links).
- A « patient » site made up of the 6 degrees of freedom (Dof) light weight robotic system and its control unit (Fig. 2).

Reliable transmission of video over wireless links is becoming an increasingly important application requirement in mobile communications. However, supporting robust video communications over wireless networks is a significant problem, primarily because of two factors: low bandwidth and the time varying error characteristics of the transmission channel.

One of the main medical data type processed here is the ultrasound video stream. It is the most user of the available wireless bandwidth. Therefore we should implement some frame rate control that optimise the usage of the limited wireless bandwidth and in the same time guarantee the ultrasound video QoS.

This paper presents some of the optimisation issues relevant to the requirements of high throughput of medical data and video streaming traffic in 3G wireless environments. The functional modalities of the OTELO system over the 3G link is presented in the following part. Quality of Service (QoS) over UMTS for medical images is investigated in the third part. Fourth part concerns the optimised OTELO traffic issues.

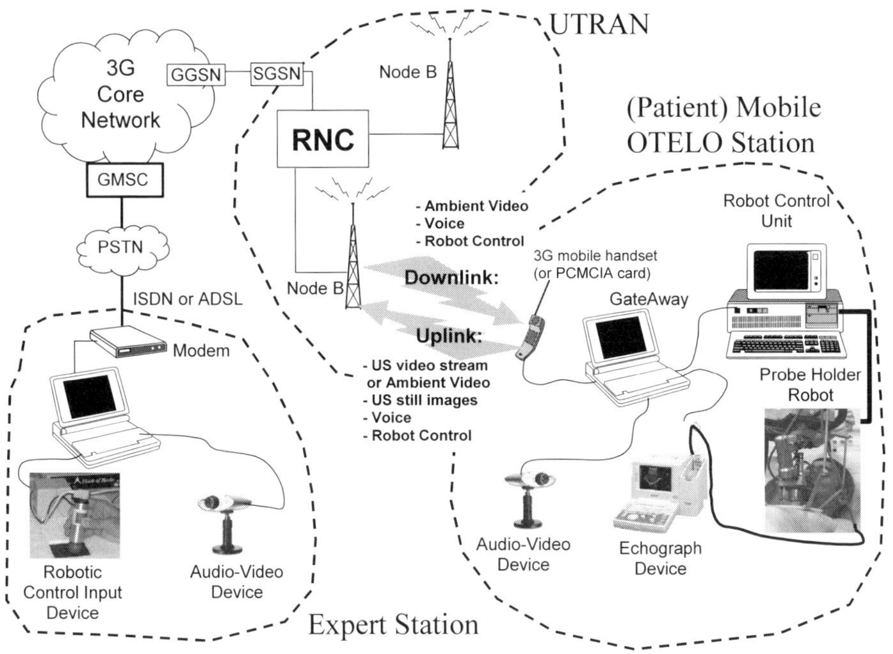

Figure 3. The UMTS OTELO connectivity scenario with a fixed expert station and a mobile patient station.

Table 1. OTELO medical data requirements and corresponding data rates.

	Ultrasound video stream	Ultrasound still images	Ambient video stream	Voice	Robot control data
Flow direction	Simplex: Patient to Expert	Simplex: Patient to Expert	Duplex	Duplex	duplex
Transport Protocol	RTP/UDP/IP	TCP/IP	RTP/ UDP/IP	RTP/UDP/IP	UDP/IP
Speed Requirement	Real-time	Non Real-time	Real-time	Real-time	Real-time
Payload data rate requirement over the air-interface (without protocol headers)	15 frames/s @ 210 kbit/s Uplink	1 frame/ 10s Uplink	15 to 1 frame/s symmetrically	16 kbit/s symmetrically	0.3 kbit/s symmetrically

2. OTELO Functional Modalities and Wireless Connectivity

OTELO can be considered as a multi medical data traffic with different classes of QoS requirements. These have to be transmitted simultaneously. Figure 3 shows the 3G connectivity of the OTELO system and the interface requirements with a typical UMTS network. The OTELO Expert Station may either link from the IP Multimedia Network or through the ISDN/ADSL or through UTRAN.

The detailed medical and non-medical OTELO data traffic are shown in Table 1. From this table it can be seen that the most traffic and bandwidth demanding OTELO traffic type is the medical video streaming traffic of the system.

Table 2. UMTS QoS classes and corresponding OTELO mappings.

1. Traffic class	Conversational class conversational RT	Streaming class streaming RT	Interactive class Interactive best effort	Background Background best effort
Fundamental characteristics	– Preserve time relation (variation) between information entities of the stream – Conversational pattern (stringent and low delay)	– Preserve time relation (variation) between information entities of the stream	– Request response pattern – Preserve payload content	– Destination is not expecting the data within a certain time – Preserve payload content
OTELO Medical and Operational Traffic	Robotic Control	Medical Ultrasound Video streaming and Ambient Teleconferene Traffic	Ultrasound Images	Other e-mail traffic

1) When the expert is searching for a specific organ (liver, kidney, etc.), high quality images may not be required: simple compression methods or lossy techniques can be applied. The lowest data rate acceptable to medical experts is 210kb/s with a frame update of 15 fps.
2) When the organ of interest is found and small displacements of the robot are appealed, it may be necessary to consider lossless compression techniques that would bring higher image quality to the expert. This lossless compression can be applied on the whole image or on an area of interest (A.O.I.). Form the medical perspective and in order to provide a real-time virtual interactivity between the remote consultant and the manipulated robot, the best round trip delay from the expert station between the robot commanded position and the received corresponding image should not exceed 300 ms.

3. 3G OTELO Quality of Service and Classes Mappings

Based on the functional modalities of the OTELO system and traffic classes of the system discussed above. The QoS classification of the OTELO traffic can be mapped to the three major traffic classes defined by the 3GPP UMTS QoS Classes. Table 2 illustrates the different QoS traffic classes with their corresponding OTELO mappings.

From this table, the robotic control data of the system can be clearly categorised within the 'Conversational Class' traffic because this traffic in the system is very sensitive to network time delay and tolerate only very small time delay variations, especially in this medical application. Ambient video and audio can be selected within the streaming class traffic and Ultrasound image are allocated within the interactive class traffic.

4. Optimisation Issues of OTELO Medical Video Wireless Traffic

It is well known that congestion is a common phenomenon in wireless communication that occurs when the offered load exceeds the designed limit, causing degradation in network performance (QoS) such as utilization. In addition to utilization, other symptoms of congestion in packet networks may include packet losses, higher delay and delay jitter [4]. To avoid the undesirable symptoms of congestion, control procedures are often employed to limit the amount of network load. Such control procedures are called rate control. It should be noted that different network technologies might implement rate control in different levels, such as hop-to-hop level or network level. Nevertheless, for inter-networks involving multiple networking technologies, it is common to rely on rate control performed by the end-hosts application layer.

Video applications generally have unique QoS requirements such as delay, packet loss and bandwidth metrics that differ from other data types. For wireless networks those metrics varies drastically over time, which is detrimental to video transmission. Therefore quality evaluation and monitoring is critical to maintain user satisfactions.

In particular medical video streaming need a special QoS traffic issues that need to be studied further. In the OTELO system the ultrasound images are acquired at the patient station at a resolution of 768 x 570. However, due to bandwidth restrictions, the chosen image size for real-time video transmission is 352 x 288. For the purpose of OTELO's ultrasound image streaming, expert evaluation has shown that the minimum requirements for an efficient diagnosis can be summarised as follows [6]:

1) The minimum frame rate of the received images should be 5fps.
2) The objective measure peak signal to noise ratio (PSNR) should be at least 36dB.
3) The delay of the received images should be less than 300 ms.

From Tables 1 and 2 above the five media streams are transmitted in such away that it is in admissible for one media to occupy the link and impede the transmission of others. For example the robot control data requires a relatively small portion of the bandwidth compared to the other four data type. For the ultrasound still images, although the file sizes of medical images are large compared to the other data type, the frequency of the image transmissions is much lower. Therefore we use TCP/IP congestion control. The video streaming data type is the subject of this section. As mentioned in Table 1, video streaming data type is transmitted over RTP/UDP/IP. UDP uses simple datagram with no congestion control. Therefore we use a congestion control technique in the application layer. Optimisation technique is used here to find the optimal frame rate that satisfies the QoS metrics mentioned above (utilization, packet losses, delay and delay jitter).

4.1. The Proposed Optimisation Technique

In this section we briefly introduce an optimization procedure to determine the optimal frame rate control required for the OTELO system 3G wireless functionality. It is well known that the frame rate control in 3G wireless networks is a multiobjective design problem. One approach to solve multiobjective design problems is to formulate the problem as a set of algebraic inequalities that must be satisfied for a successful design.

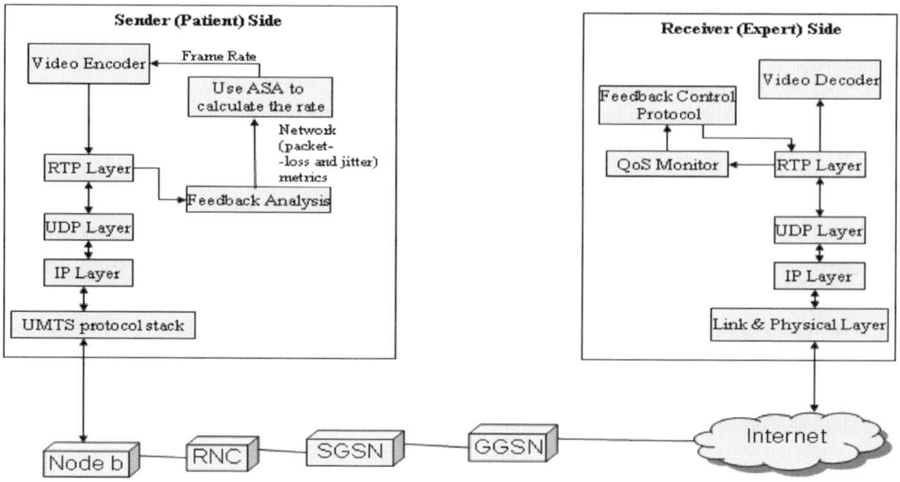

Figure 4. End-to-End System Architecture.

In this work we introduce Adaptive Simulated Annealing (ASA) Optimization technique and apply it for this multiobjective optimization problem. In particular we consider the packet loss and delay Jitter objectives function (Φ_i), therefore the algebraic inequality here are:

Packet loss $<= e_1$
Delay Jitter $<= e_2$

e_1, e_2 are the limits of these inequalities.

These can be combined as one equation that the optimization techniques will work on to find the optimum rate.

$$E(r) = \max \{\max \{((\Phi_i(r) - e_i) / \omega_i), 0\} : i = 1\&2\}$$

Φ is the objective function,
i is the number of QoS metrics elements,
r is the rate control value,
ω is the weightings.

Figure 4 shows a schematic diagram for the proposed rate control optimization architecture applied to OTELO system within UMTS network. The receiver (expert) side here monitors the QoS metrics at the RTP layer and sends these measurements via the RTCP receiver report (RR) protocol to the sender [5]. At the sender (patient) side, the relevant feedback information are analysed at the RTP layer and extract the packet loss, delay jitter, and feed them to the Optimization algorithm block to find the optimal rate. The encoder encodes the images according to this calculated rate.

The video streaming data type here is the highest bandwidth user by applying the rate control algorithm above we are optimizing the usage of the wireless bandwidth (utilization) in addition to satisfy the QoS metrics (which are the packet loss and the jitter).

Ongoing work is currently under way to analyse the performance of the system under different 3G network conditions and to verify the QoS metrics within this application.

The research work is analyzing the packet loss and delay jitter network QoS metrics. However as a future work the user QoS that is the ultrasound video stream PSNR issue will be considered.

5. Conclusions

Mobile health care 'm-health' is one of the emerging and most promising application domain for 3G and beyond 3G wireless systems. One of the major challenges for the larger deployment of such systems is the clear understanding of the medical data requirements and specific

In this paper we presented a multiobjective optimisation methodology to improve the QoS traffic requirements designed for medical video streaming data traffic for a mobile robotic tele-echography system. The 3G QoS of the system are also presented and their corresponding medical mappings are discussed. The ASA is presented as an optimisation solution to the relevant multiobjective optimisation problem. Ongoing work is currently underway to verify and validate the performance of this optimization technique in simulated 3G-based mobile tele-echography system.

References

[1] Istepanian, R.S.H., Jovanov, E. and Zhang, Y.T., 'm-health: Beyond Seamless Mobility for Global Wireless Healthcare Connectivity-Editorial', *IEEE Trans., Information Technology in Biomedicine,* Vol. 8, 4, pp.405–414, Dec. 2004.

[2] Garawi, S. A., Courreges, F., Istepanian, R S. H., Zisimopoulus, H., and Gosset, P., 'Performance Analysis of a Compact Robotic Tele-Echography E-Health System over Terrestrial and Mobile Communication Links', *Proceeding of the 5th. IEE International Conference on 3G Mobile Communication Technologies- 3G 2004*, London, 18–20, October, pp.118–122, 2004.

[3] Courreges, F., Istepanian, R.S.H. and Garawi, A.S., 'Wireless Challenges for Mobile Robotic Tele-Echography System, *Proceedings of the 2nd International Conference on Smart home and health Telematics-ICOST04*, Sept 2004, Singapore, In 'Toward a Human – Friendly Assistive Environment, Zhang, D. and Mokhtari M. (Eds.), IOS Press, pp.15–22, 2004.

[4] Jamalipour, A, 'The Wireless Mobile Internet: Architectures, Protocols, and Services', John Wiley & Sons, Ltd, ISBN: 0-470-84468-X, Chap. 9, Copyright 2003.

[5] IEFT 1889, "A Transport Protocol for Real-Time Applications (RTP)", July 2003.

[6] Cañero, C., Thomos, *N.,*Triantafyllidis, G., A., Litos, G. C. and Strintzis, *M., G.,* 'Mobile Tele-Echography: User Interface Design', *IEEE Transactions on Information Technology in Biomedicine*, Vol. 9, No. 1, March 2005.

Medical and Care Compunetics 2
L. Bos et al. (Eds.)
IOS Press, 2005

A New Algorithm for Content-Based Region Query in Databases with Medical Images

Dumitru Dan BURDESCU and Liana STANESCU
University of Craiova, Faculty of Automation, Computers and Electronics
burdescu@topedge.com, stanescu@software.ucv.ro

Abstract. This article presents an original method of implementation of the color set back-projection algorithm that is one of the most efficient method of automated detection of color regions from an image. The detected regions are then used in the content-based region query. The query is realized on one or more regions, having into consideration the color feature. The efficiency of the method was studied by means of a number of experiments effectuated with the help of a software system realized for this purpose, on a collection of medical images collected with an endoscope. The new method for the implementation of the algorithm is compared with the traditional one not only from the point of view of the execution time, but also from the point of view of the retrieval process quality.

Keywords. Image retrieval, content-based region query, medical images, color feature, color set back-projection algorithm, graph

Introduction

In present there are a variety of activity fields in which massive databases with grey level or color images were created. One of these domains is the medical field. For querying these imagistic collections, the traditional simple methods based on text are not sufficient. This is due to the fact that the information from images and in general from multimedia data, is not structured and in consequence the utilization of some attributes for describing its content is not possible. From this appears the big necessity of using alternative methods for retrieving with accuracy and rapidity the relevant information, from a massive imagistic collection, such that the user's query could be satisfied [1]. These techniques are known under the name of content-based visual information retrieval and they were centered in the attention of a lot of researchers, in the last years. In the medical field, images, and especially digital images, are produced and used for diagnostics and therapy in large amounts. In some medical areas, hundreds or even thousands of images are daily produced. A big part of them are color images, like the images collected with the endoscope's help, so to take into consideration the color characteristic in the content–based visual retrieval presents importance. There were proposed several methods based on the content, for accessing the medical images [2,3]. There are already some important systems, that can be integrated in the diagnosis process [4–6]. There are argued some important reasons that explain the need for supplementary methods for image retrieval:

- in the process of taking clinical decision, it may be very important to specify an image like query or some regions like query regions and to retrieve those images from the database that are most similar to the specified image query or region query, together with the afferent diagnoses.
- the education and the research activity can be improved by using the access visual methods.
- the visual characteristics allow not only the retrieving of the patients having the same disease, but also the cases where the visual similitude exists, but the diagnosis differs.

The content – based visual query may be realized either at the level of the entire image (content-based visual query), or based on the color regions existed in images (content-based region query) [7]. In a content-based region query, the images are compared on their regions. For realizing the content-based region query on a database with medical images, it is necessary an automated algorithm for detecting the color regions, significant for the diagnosis. It was chosen the color set back-projection algorithm, introduced initially by Swain and Ballard and then developed in the research projects at Columbia University, in the content-based visual retrieval domain [7]. This technique provides the automated extraction of regions and the representation of their color content. The extraction system for color regions has four steps [7,8]:

- The image transformation, quantization and filtering (the transformation from RGB to HSV color space and the quantization at 166 colors)
- Back-projection of binary color sets
- The labeling of regions
- The extraction of region features (the binary color set, the area, the centroid coordinates and the minimum bounding rectangle coordinates)

A Method for the Implementation of the Color Set Back-Projection Algorithm

In the first implementation of the color set back-projection algorithm (Method1), the image is read in a **.bmp** format. Each pixel from the initial image is transformed in HSV format and quantized. At the end of this processing there are obtained the global histogram and the color set of the image [8]. On the matrix that memorizes only the quantized colors from 0 to 165 it is applied a 5x5 median filter, which has the role of eliminating the isolated points [7]. Having the HSV quantized matrix it is possible to begin the process of regions extraction presented above. In the first implementation (Method1), it may be observed that this process is in fact a depth – first traversal, described in pseudo-cod in the following way:

```
procedure FindRegions (Image I, colorset C) is:
InitStack(S)
Visited = ∅
for *each node P in the I do
  if *color of P is in C then
     PUSH(P)
Visited ← Visited ∪ {P}
while not Empty(S) do
```

```
            CrtPoint <- POP()
      Visited ← Visited ∪ {CrtPoint}
      For *each unvisited neighbor S of
      CrtPoint do
            if *color of S is in C then
                  Visited ← Visited ∪ {S}
                  PUSH(S)
    * Output detected region
```

Proposition 1

The total running time of a call of the procedure FindRegions (Image I, colorset C) is $O(m^2*n^2)$, where "m" is the width and "n" is the height of image.

Proof

Recall that the number of pixels of image is m*n, where "m" is the width and "n" is the height of image. Observe next, that the first loop FOR of the algorithm is executed at most once for each pixel P in the image. Hence, the total time spent in this loop is O(n*m). The WHILE loop processes the stack S for each pixel which has the same color of its neighbor. The inner loop FOR processes the pixels of an unvisited neighbor. So, the total time spent in these loops is O(m*n), because are processed all pixels of image at most once. The result of the previous statements is that the total running time of this procedure is $O(m^2*n^2)$.

In the new original implementation of the algorithm (Method2), the image pixels were arranged into hexagons. The edge of a hexagon has a certain number of pixels (3, 4, 5). Only the pixels which correspond to the vertices of the hexagons with an established edge are taken into consideration. The image is viewed as a graph not as a pixel matrix. The vertices represent the pixels and the edges represent neighborhoods between pixels.

For each binary set is executed:

- the graph is inspected until it is found the first vertex having the color from the color set
- starting from this vertex, there are found all the adjacent vertices having the same color
- the process will continue in the same manner for each neighbor, until there are not found vertices having the same color
- it is verified if the detected region satisfies the imposed thresholds; in affirmative case, the region is labeled and introduced in the database

This process of regions extraction from a graph is in fact a breadth – first traversal, described in pseudo-cod in the following way

```
procedure construct_graph (Image I, Graph g, Edge edge) is:
   for * i->0,width/edge
     for * j->0;height/edge

        if (i mod 3==0)
                    *if(jmod2==0)
                                      g[i][j]=I[edge*i][edge*j+edge–1]
```

```
    *if(jmod2==1)
                g[i][j]=I[edge*i][edge*j+edge+2]

   if (i mod 3==1)
    * if(j mod 2==0)
                    g[i][j]=I[edge*i–1][edge*jedge]
    * if(j mod 2==1)
                   g[i][j]=I[edge*i–1][edge*j+edge*2]

   if (i mod 3==2)
          *if(j mod 2==0)
                   g[i][j]=I[edge*i–2][edge*j+edge–1]
          *if(j mod 2==1)
                    g[i][j]=I[edge*i2][edge*j+edge+2]

  //end for * j->0
  *output the graph g
//end for * i->0
 procedure FindRegions (Graph G, colorset C):
   InitQueue(Q)
   Visited = ∅
   for *each node P in the G do
     if *color of P is in C then
       PUSH(P)
       Visited ← Visited ∪ {P}
       while not Empty(q) do
         CrtPoint <- POP()
         Visited ← Visited ∪ {CrtPoint}
         for *each unvisited neighbor Q of
                                               CrtPoint do
               if *color of Q is in C then
                    Visited ← Visited ∪ {Q}
                   PUSH(Q)

   *output-detected region
```

Proposition 2

The total running time of a call of the procedure FindRegions (Graph G, colorset C) is $O(n^2)$, where "n" is the number of nodes of graph attached to an image.

Proof

Observe that the first FOR loop of the algorithm is executed at most once for each node of the graph. Hence, the total time spent in this loop is O(n). The WHILE loop processes the queue Q for each node which has the same color of its neighbor. The inner loop FOR processes the nodes of an unvisited neighbor. So, the total time spent in these loops is O(n), because are processed all nodes of graph at most once.

From previous statements results that the total running time of this procedure is $O(n^2)$.

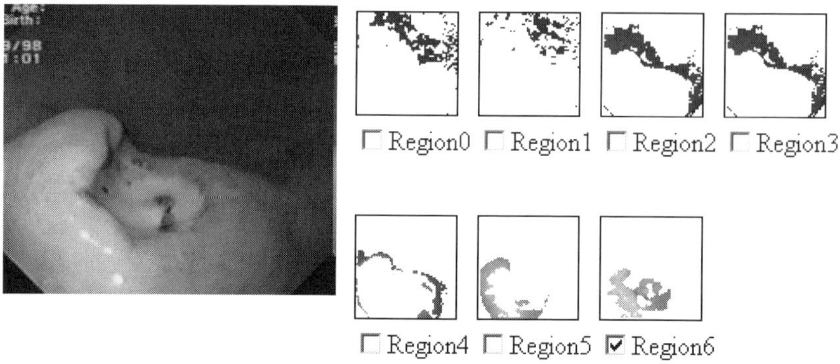

Figure 1. The image with detected color regions using Method2 and edge=3; Region6 (representing the sick area) marked for the content-based region query.

Taking into account that the color information of each region is stored as a color binary set, the color similitude between two regions may be computed either with the quadratic distance between color sets, or with Hamming distance between color sets. Here, there was used the quadratic distance between binary sets s_q and s_t that is given by the following equation [7]:

$$d_1 = \sum_{m_0=0}^{M-1} \sum_{m_1=0}^{M-1} (s_q[m_0] - s_t[m_0]) a_{m0,m1} (s_q[m_1] - s_t[m_1]) \quad (1)$$

Experiments and Results

For testing the efficiency of the new method and for comparing the two methods of implementation of the color set back-projection algorithm, there have been made some experiments over the medical images collection. For Method2 the hexagon edge can be equal to 3, respective 4. For each query, the images from the databases were inspected and relevance was assigned to them (1– relevant, 0 – irrelevant) and the retrieval effectiveness using recall and precision was recorded [7]. Below, there are presented the results of two such experiments.

Experiment 1:

In Fig. 1 there is the image for which there were detected the color regions using Method2 with edge=3. Region6 was chosen as query region, which appears as marked and emphasizes the sick area. The obtained results are presented in Fig. 2. It can be observed that the first five retrieved images are all relevant for this query. The graphic of the retrieving efficiency in the case of the two presented algorithms (Method1 and Method2 with edge =3) is shown in Fig. 3. The graphics corresponding to the two methods are superposed, which means that the results of this one region query are identical.

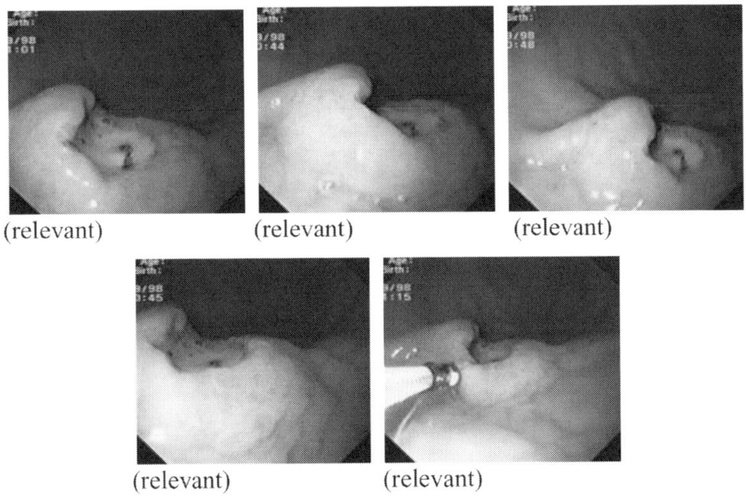

Figure 2. The retrieved images using Method2 and edge equal to 3, for the Region6 as query region.

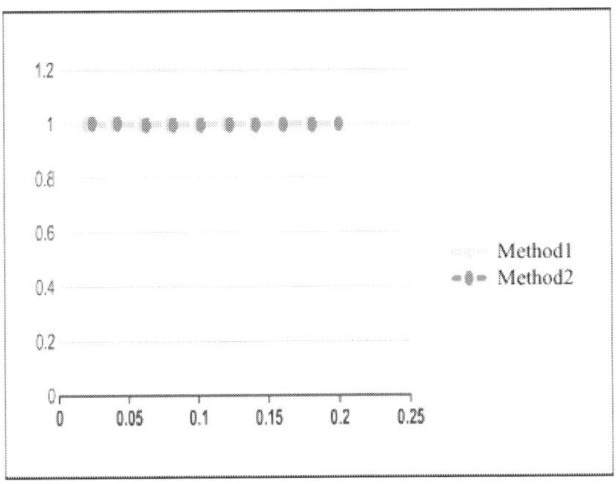

Figure 3. Experiment 1. The graphic of the retrieving efficiency for Method1 and Method2 with the hexagon edge equal to 3.

Experiment 2:

In Fig. 4 there is the image with detected color regions using Method2 with edge=3. Region8, Region9 and Region10, representing the sick area were chosen as query regions. The obtained results are presented in Fig. 5, where it can be seen that in the first five retrieved images there are four relevant images. The graphic of the retrieving efficiency in the case of the two presented algorithms (Method1 and Method2 with edge=3) is shown in Fig. 6. Identical results can be observed for the two methods.

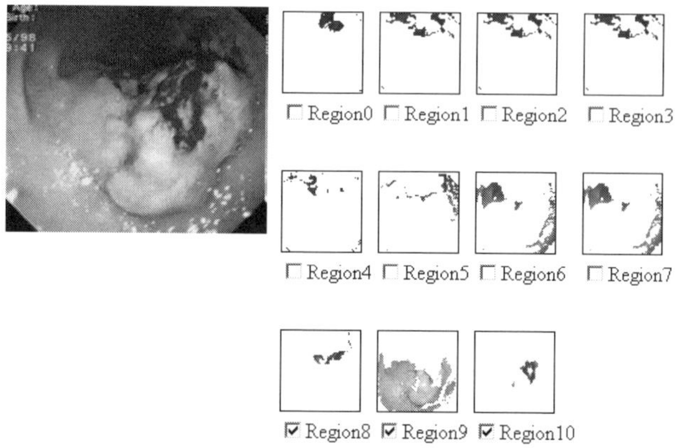

Figure 4. The image with detected color regions using Metod2 and edge=3; Region8, Region9, Region10 marked for the content-based region query.

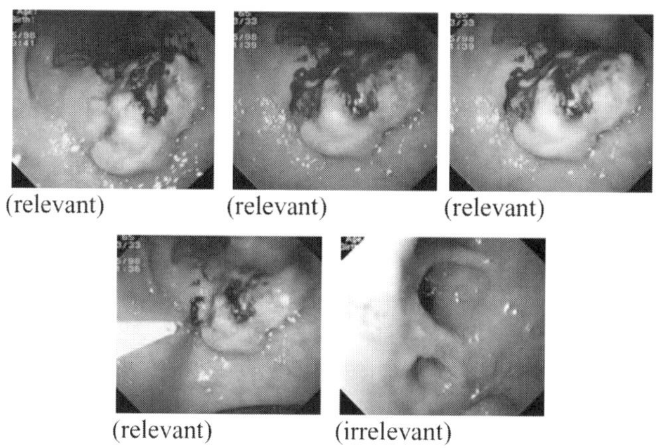

Figure 5. The retrieved images Method2 with hexagon edge equal to 3, for the Region8, Region9, Region10 as query regions.

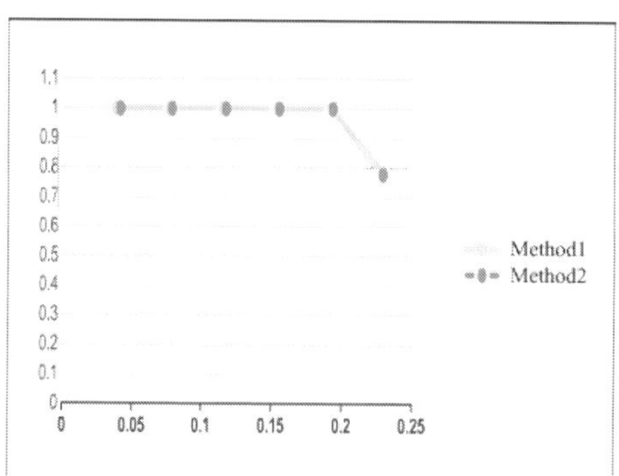

Figure 6. Experiment 2: The graphic of the retrieving efficiency for the two methods, with the hexagon edge equal to 3, for Method2.

Conclusion

This article presents an original method of implementation of the color set back-projection algorithm, algorithm that allows the automated detection of the color regions from a color medical image. The detected regions are then used in the content-based region query. The query can be realized on one or more regions, having into consideration the color feature. The efficiency of the two methods was studied by means of a number of experiments effectuated with the help of the Imtest system [9], on a collection of medical images collected with the help of an endoscope.

The very good results obtained in the effectuated experiments indicate the fact that each of the two implementations methods (Method1 and Method2) of the color set back-projection algorithm can be used in the processing of the content – based visual query. The experiments, some of which have been presented in this paper, show that the results obtained with the Method2 and edge=3 are closer in quality with those obtained with Method1.

The advantage of the second method (Method 2 with edge equal to 3) is given by the fact that for detecting the color regions it is not necessary the pixel-by-pixel image traversal, but only the pixels arranged in the vertices of a hexagon with edge equal to 3 pixels. If the processing time of the Method 1 is $O(m^2*n^2)$ (m is the width and n is the height of image), the processing time for the Method 2 presented here is $O(n^2)$ (n is the number of nodes of graph attached to an image) [10].

References

[1] Del Bimbo, A., 2001. Visual Information Retrieval. Morgan Kaufmann Publishers, San Francisco, USA.

[2] Müller, H. et al., 2004. Comparing feature sets for content-based medical information retrieval. SPIE Medical Imaging, San Diego, CA, USA.

[3] Müller, H. et al., 2004. A review of content-based image retrieval systems in medicine-clinical benefits and future directions. In International Journal of Medical Informatics, Vol. 73, pp. 1–23.

[4] Lehmann, TM et al., 2004. IRMA – Content-based Image Retrieval in Medical Applications. In Proceedings of the 14th World Congress on Medical Informatics (Medinfo 2004). IOS Press, Amsterdam, pp. 842–848.

[5] Lehmann, TM., et al., 2004. The IRMA Reference Database and Its Use for Content-Based Image Retrieval in Medical Applications In: Ammenwerth E, Gaus W, Haux R, Lovis C, Pfeiffer KP, Tilg B, Wichmann HE (Hrsg): GMDS 2004 – Kooperative Versorgung – Vernetzte Forschung – Ubiquitäre Information. Verlag videel OHG, Niebüll, 251–253.

[6] Shyu, C. et al., 1999. ASSERT, A physician-in-the-loop content-based image retrieval system for HRCT image databases. In Computer Vision and Image Understanding, Vol. 75, Nos. 1/2, pp. 111–132.

[7] Smith, J.R., 1997. Integrated Spatial and Feature Image Systems: Retrieval, Compression and Analysis. Ph.D. thesis Graduate School of Arts and Sciences, Columbia University.

[8] Stanescu L., Cojocareanu C., 2000 The Color Set Back-Projection Method for Color Image Retrieval, Sintes 10, Craiova.

[9] Stanescu, L. and D.Burdescu, 2003. IMTEST-Software System For he Content-based Visual Retrieval Study.In: 14th International Conferece On Control Systems And Computer Science. Bucuresti.

[10] Burdescu, D.D., 1998. Analiza complexitatii algoritmilor. Ed. Albastra Cluj-Napoca.

Medical and Care Compunetics 2
L. Bos et al. (Eds.)
IOS Press, 2005

Economic Impact of Telemedicine: A Survey

Jasjit S. SURI[a], *PhD., MBA, Fellow AIMBE, Sr. IEEE Member*, MAAPM,
Alan DOWLING[a], *PhD.*, Swamy LAXMINARAYAN[b], *ScD., Fellow AIMBE,*
and Sameer SINGH[c], *PhD*

[a] *Weatherhead School of Management, Case Western Reserve University, Cleveland, OH, USA*

[b] *Rural Healthcare/Biomedical Engineering Dept., State University of Idaho, Pocatello, ID, USA*

[c] *Department of Computer Sciences, University of Exeter, Exeter, UK*

Abstract. The economic evaluation of telemedicine has faced difficulties, both in terms of the effectiveness and cost-benefit analyses. The main challenges that lie ahead for economic assessment are: (a) technological changes; (b) sustainability of applications; (c) availability of outcomes and other patient data; (d) generalisability of evaluation results. These challenges have lead to an unsatisfactory modeling of cost analysis of teleradiology systems versus non-teleradiology (visiting radiology services) applications.

This paper presents the analysis on the impact of telemedicine on health care. It particularly emphasizes a model for teleradiology cost systems. We study and compare cost analysis of teleradiology system versus non-teleradiology systems. Finally, a model is presented which is made viable for computing the number of patients needed to demonstrate the viability of the telemedicine systems.

We conclude the following: (a) that large number of patients is needed to validate the economic impact of telemedicine services; (b) cultural change in USA will bring most prominent effect in improving health care thereby bringing health care costs down. This when combined with improving cost effective technology like telemedicine services will bring the overall health care costs down.

1. Introduction

Telemedicine (TM) is a field of engineering in medicine where we use information and communication technology to provide healthcare services to people who are at a distance from the provider. It involves the interaction of a variety of information technologies and health services. Today, when the visiting nurse calls on a homebound patient, she uses the phone. The nurse will do the same kinds of exams she would have done in person: take the patient's blood pressure, listen to the heart and lungs, record body temperature, take other vital signs and give the patient a visual once-over. But the nurse could be hundred's or even thousands of miles away. A virtual visit can now be done with *computerized devices* and a standard *phone line*. With the blend of telephone and television, computer connections and the internet, the idea of medicine at a distance has steadily matured. While much of the work remains in experimental stage, the future vision has clarified enough for federal agencies to form the joint working group on telemedicine. Members include departments of defense, agriculture, commerce, health and human services, justice and veteran affairs, the office of management and budget, the Appalachian Regional Commission and the NASA.

As technology advances rapidly it has become important to demand for value for money in allocation of healthcare resources. The healthcare providers are increasing pressure on evaluators to find out if telemedicine is economic or not? They need an answer to the question: "should healthcare providers invest in TMS (Telemedicine Systems)?" Cost-benefit understanding is thus important for evaluators, health care providers, engineers who play a role in TMS design. It can be difficult to establish on observable and empirical link between telemedicine and change in patient outcome. The availability of administrative and other data for conventional services may be limited. In addition, differences in outcomes between the telemedicine and conventional options may be modest, and the power of the studies may be low. Telemedicine system is also an information and communication technology that facilitates rapid and accurate diagnosis by remote specialists, thus reducing risks of harmful events occurring. By using telemedicine links for establishing diagnoses in non-urgent cases, wasteful journeys to tertiary centers may be avoided for say to pregnant women and families with young children.

Wooton et al. [5] writes that telemedicine must be implemented with a clear idea of why it is being used. What should be the goal: given the task, fit the new technology OR take the task and adapt to the practice in to the new technology framework. The more you utilize the equipment, more is the cost of the telemedicine. Much depends, however, on variable costs, especially those associated with the personnel required to produce the service and with the time used for telecommunication. An example is PACS, where utilization must be very high to make investment in the system worthwhile. Another example is the *video conferencing* where use of the equipment for many types of consultations across different specialties may increase efficiency, provided the institution can adjust. If the patients are benefiting, healthcare professionals are benefiting so are the mangers in the industry, then the telemedicine technology is acceptable.

The economic evaluation of telemedicine has faced difficulties, both in terms of the effectiveness and *cost-benefit* analyses. The main challenges that lie ahead for economic assessment are: (a) technological changes; (b) sustainability of applications; (c) availability of outcomes and other patient data; (d) generalisability of evaluation results. These challenges have lead to an unsatisfactory modeling of cost analysis of teleradiology systems versus non-teleradiology (visiting radiology services) applications.

This paper thus presents the analysis on the impact of telemedicine on health care. It particularly emphasizes a model for teleradiology cost systems. We study and compare cost analysis of teleradiology system versus non-teleradiology systems. Finally, a mathematical model is presented that has made viable for computing the number of patients needed to demonstrate the viability of the telemedicine systems. We rationalize why the overall costs of health care is increasing even though telemedicine has become so advance and technology to treat patients has been improving. Should we blame to technology or to the costs of telemedicine services or can cultural change play a role in bringing the overall costs down? We will address some of these issues in this paper.

The layout of this paper is as under: Section 2 presents the challenges in telemedicine. Section 3 presents the economic impact of telemedicine. Section 4 presents the digital radiology systems. The evaluation of the telemedicine system is presented in Section 5. Finally, the conclusions are presented in Section 6.

2. Challenges in Telemedicine

This section presents the reasons as to why it is difficult to evaluate the telemedicine systems.

- *Modularity of Equipment:* Telemedicine technologies continue to evolve rapidly. Reid et al. [3] points out that the lifespan of most microprocessor-based technologies is no greater than three years. The product themselves may last longer, but in that short time they become obsolete. Changing equipment and data transmission technology adds difficulty in economic appraisal: successive versions of equipment have different, typically decreasing, prices. For example, equipment prices for a teleradiology application decreased from $A520K to $A150K over the period of 3 years [4]. In future, internet and radio technologies will provide realistic alternatives to the current information technology networks. Continuing improvements in technology have important implications for those seeking to introduce and operate telemedicine. It is questionable if acquisition of new equipment reduces costs. It is also questionable if delay in replacement of working well systems reduces costs. There may also be changes to non-telemedicine services that make telemedicine a less attractive.
- *Resistance to Change*: The physicians, technical staff and patients are the key components of telemedicine. Surprisingly patients are many times the least resistant to the telemedicine system. Self-consciousness of being on camera and on video is concern for some physicians, staff, and patients. Thus, it poses a challenge to TMS design.
- *No Solid Model for Telemedicine Cost Analysis*: Due to the lack of credible data sets, it has not been possible to access the economic impact of telemedicine. There has been no good model to analyze the economic impact of the teleradiology or other telemedicine systems. We will discuss this in Section 4 ahead.
- *Licensing Issue*: The question is: "Does a physician have to be licensed to practice medicine in a state in which he/she provides a remote interactive video consultancy?" The state laws for license to practice medicine are different for each US state. There are licensing fees, expenses and time in meeting continuing education requirements, and time in keeping informed of the changes that occur in each state's requirements. Some states have addressed telemedicine issues that relate to licensing in a ways that are well-defined and provide for a positive environment for telemedicine, such as Texas, but many others have ill defined definitions or have not addressed the issue. (see [22], page 88). The possibility of national legislation governing telemedicine has been proposed but as yet has not been successful.
- *Institutional Credentialing Telemedicine Practitioner*: The issue of institutional credentialing of each practitioner in order to grant privileges to practice medicine is a concern. This process is timing consuming, and usually involves obligations with the institution that someone at a distance could not fulfill, and requires staff membership fees.
- *Formats of the Telemedicine/Confidentiality/Privacy*: All information formats; patient identifiable images, text, video are protected by confidentiality laws and require security. In order to protect the health information that is or

will be in electronic form three areas need to be addressed. Namely, (i) updating laws and institution's policies to incorporate telemedicine situations, (ii) in service of health care providers to safeguard the information in special circumstances of telemedicine, and (iii) implementation of safeguarding technologies that prevent unauthorized access. This includes but is not limited to firewalls that safeguard access to networks, encryption to encode the data so it can only be read by one with the decoder, and auditing programs of what data was accessed in the system and by whom. Encryption does protect privacy, but it drives the costs up.

- *Malpractice Liability for Telemedicine*: Malpractice liability is a major issue and like licensure is governed by each state's laws and the accepted standard of care practiced in a locale. As practice standards continue to develop nationally by specialty, this issue may be resolved. There is very limited case *law in telemedicine issues*, so it is still unknown how the courts and juries will view telemedicine parties' responsibilities.
- *Lack of State Telecommunication Laws*: Federal and state telecommunications policy greatly effects telemedicine. The Federal Communications Bill of 1996 which is the major revision of the Communications Act of 1934 allows for long-distance telephone companies, cable companies and others to compete with local telephone companies and provides for universal communication service at affordable rates for all areas of the country. This will help in the rural and previously isolated areas. Several federal programs and agencies are working to develop national telemedicine standards in infrastructure such as the High Performance Computing and Communication (HPCC) program, which promotes research, advanced technology, such as virtual reality tools in surgery, and networks. State telecommunications laws are lacking in all but about 10 states.
- *Reimbursement Telemedicine Services:* Reimbursement is a major issue. Medicare, Medicaid and most insurance carriers have reimbursed teleradiology. This is because face-to-face encounter is not required for the interpretation of radiography as is required in other patient care consultations. Some payers are beginning to pay for consultations by interactive video and some *store-and-forward* telepsychiatry, tele-home health, telepathology and teledermatology. But few payers have national policies governing telemedicine. It is estimated that Medicare is years away from establishing a telemedicine reimbursement policy. (See [21], pg. 46). It is the managed care programs that are providing much of the financial impetus to develop telemedicine services. This is because systems improve the quality of care or at least not diminish its quality of care and deliver it in less costly manner will win the managed care contracts. Medicare does not pay for all telemedicine applications. The main problem is the lack of data showing that patients benefit from these telemedicine technologies. There are also questions about whether these technologies will ultimately save money. This is exactly this paper is all about.
- *Bandwidth Capability of Transmission in Telemedicine Framework*: The bandwidth capability of the telemedicine system determines the constraints of the system. The greater bandwidth produces higher costs but provides greater capacity for real-time images, video, and higher quality resolution. The qualities of transmission issues of importance to medicine are sound fidelity, image resolution (spatial or contract), range of motion depicted, and transmission

speed. (See [22], pg. 66). If the Internet 2 is further developed and made available to other participants besides universities and government agencies, Internet 2 could be telemedicine's answer to the need for high-speed transmission of high quality video. (See [23], pg. 18).

Having discussed some of the major challenges, we now discuss about a telemedicine system such as: Digital Radiology Systems (DRS) and understand why the costs are high. We will also discuss who are the major players who interact in DRS and what kind of benefits they receive?

3. Digital Radiology Systems: Why Costs are High?

An economic analysis must take into consideration both *costs and outcomes* and must compare the project with what would have happened in its absence. Van Gennip et al. [19] and Crowe et al. [20] have commented on the lack of uniformity in a number of cost-benefit studies of PACS and have demonstrated the need for uniform, well defined criteria for the calculation of costs and benefits.

Figure 1 below shows the framework which helps in understanding the cost structure for the "digital radiology systems". The second name of this is PACS (Picture Achieve and Communication System). We first discuss the direct impact of DRS, followed by the rational for its high cost.

3.1. Benefits of D-R-S to Hospitals, Patients and Providers

Figure 1 below shows the three areas where the benefits of PACS have reached. It can be via: (a) hospitals; (b) patients and (c) provider. To a hospital, PACS brings more speed, which in turn brings higher productivity and which leads to more income. To a patient, PACS reduces the service time that brings the examination time shorter. Thus physicians spend less time for service, which means low attendance cost. This brings more number of patients at hospitals and hence more revenue. The last is the benefit to the health care provider. It reduces the length of stay. This further brings gain in productivity and uses low resources that bring more earnings.

3.2. Cost Analysis of D-R-S

Figure 2 below shows the cost analysis of the DRS system. It has six inputs to the ellipse named as "DRS". These are: (i) technology changes; (ii) capital costs; (iii) tangible costs; (iv) health care policy costs; (v) cost for hospital staff and (vi) organization (administrative changes). The output of DRS system is shown in figure A, B and C given as: (A) storage system services; (B) three-dimensional image analysis services; and (C) transmission services. Also shown in the figure are seven types of tangible costs: (a) staff requirements; (b) training requirements; (c) productivity; (d) hospital infrastructure; (e) diagnostic accuracy; (f) file integrity and (g) emergency services. The important thing to note here is what kind of technology-based output the system provides and how dynamic it is. *Storage services* are one of the output which changes very frequently. *Image analysis services* are very dedicated outputs which are based on the image processing expertise. This requires design of the CAD system. These CAD design systems are very valuable tools necessary for detection of cancers in the image

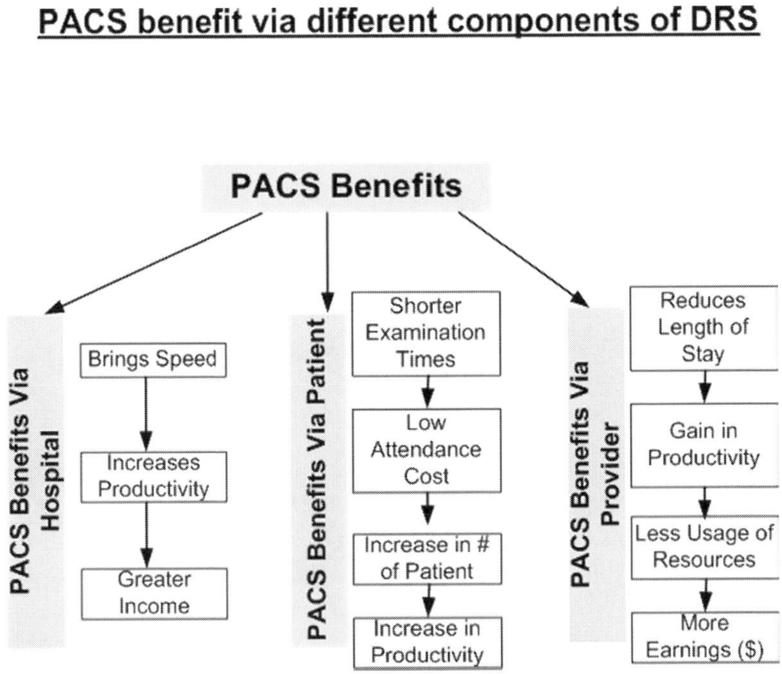

Figure 1. The figure demonstrates how the PACS benefit the three streams of healthcare system. They are: (a) Hospitals; (b) Patients; and (c) Health Care Providers.

volumes produced by medical imaging modalities like MR, CT, X-ray, PET and Ultrasound. We will discuss the embedding design concept where PACS are becoming more diagnostic based system designs. This raises the costs of telemedicine system even higher and therefore there is a motivation for cost reduction. This is going to be the future of telemedicine design. The last set of services is *transmission services*. The technology used by PACS uses the transmission services which is also very heavily technology-based and changes very rapidly (modularity effect).

The costs of operating an existing film library are often either in the overall hospital budget or are hidden in personnel time searching for "lost films" Thus there is a need for more precision in determining the costs of existing system. The next section presents an exemplary evaluation system discussing different kinds of cost/benefit analysis.

4. Evaluation of Telemedicine Systems?

4.1. Evaluation Algorithm

Evaluation of telemedicine systems is the very essential for cost-benefit analysis. The Fig. 3 shows the new algorithm developed by *Suri, Dowling and Laxminarayan*. The heart of the "evaluation algorithm" is the evaluation process and the feedback loop. Given, initially are the two sources: telemedicine system (TMS) and the telemedicine gold standard (TMGS) along with the assigned evaluator. The evaluation process re-

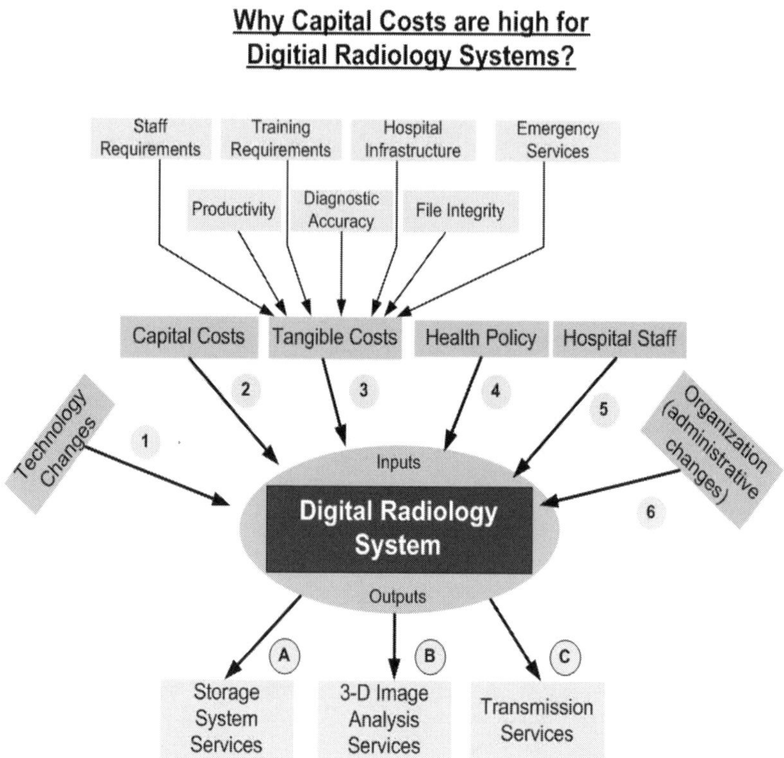

Figure 2. The figure demonstrates why the Digital Radiology System (DSR) has more cost. The output of the system has three deliverables: (A) Storage System Services; (B) 3-D Analysis Services and (C) Transmission Services.

ceives three inputs and returns one output, the scale (see block "Evaluation Scale"). This scale is used as an

Evaluation criteria. The algorithm will then check for acceptance. If the TMS is okay, the process accepts the TMS. If the algorithm finds that the scale is not in range, then it makes two initial choices: either update the "evaluator" or update the "Telemedicine System". These are called the feedback loops. The TMS in itself is very complex (say for example, Diagnostic Radiology System) is an example of TMS as shown in Fig. 2 (DRS).

The *novelty of the telemedicine evaluation system* lies in its iterative methodology to automatically bring corrections. It will check for all the components and frameworks for the TMS system and sees how far it is from the gold standard. The second *new feature* of the "evaluation system" lies in its *scale computation*. The scale is a decision criterion for acceptance or rejection. So the system quantifies in terms of numbers and hence there cannot be any fuzzy criteria. If the convergence does not happen, then in such cases one needs to study the gold standard.

4.2. Break-Even Analysis: Teleradiology Costs Vs. Visiting Services

One of the very important aspects for studying the economic impact of telemedicine is to develop a model to compare the costs between two alternatives: teleradiology and

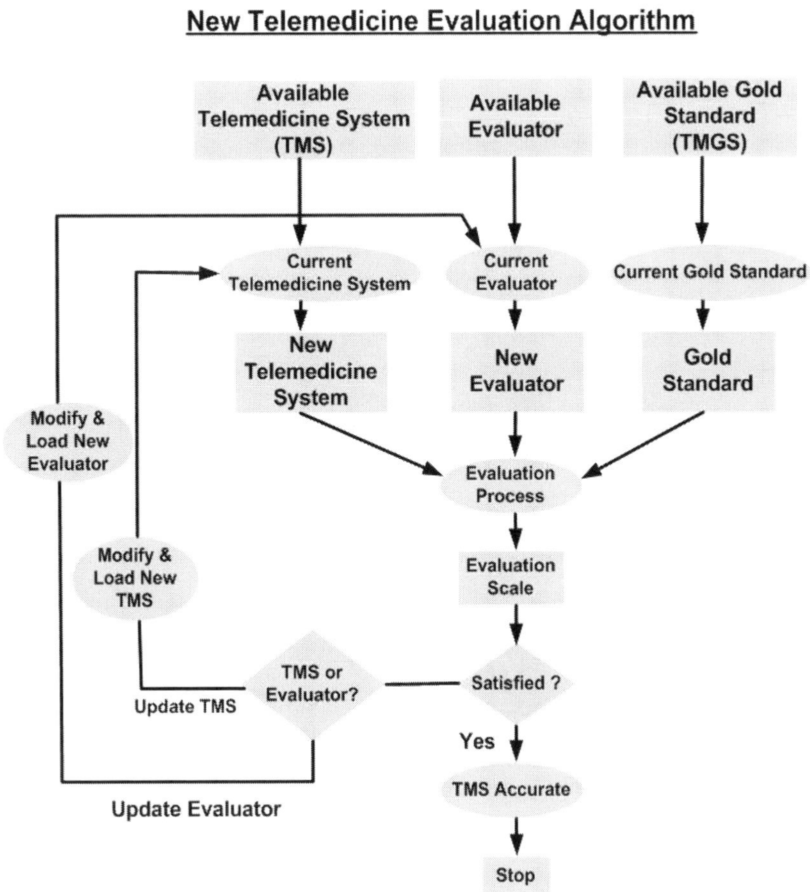

Figure 3. New Telemedicine Evaluation Algorithm. It has three inputs: TMS, TMGS and the evaluator. The main engine is the evaluation process. If the evaluation scale is not in range, the two feedback loops make the decision process either to update TMS or Evaluator.

non-teleradiology (conventional or visiting radiology services). Non-teleradiology costs are also called as visiting services costs, since a visiting radiologist is used for this purpose. Teleradiology cost consists of: Sparc Stations, Sun Stations, Disk Space, Communication Software, scanners for X-ray films and some printers like HP Scanjets. This also includes ISDN routers (like Cisco 2500) (see Fig. 4, marked by letter A). (b) The second is the visiting services cost (cost due to visiting radiologists) (see Fig. 4, marked by letter B). In the visiting radiologist service, a senior radiologist from the central hospital travels once a week (say for example) to the rural hospital to report the previous week's examination. Traveling accounts to about 50% of the time. If there is no availability of teleradiology services then, some of the patients will have to travel to the rural hospital as emergency transfers. The emergency transfer rate is assumed to be 5% of all the patients who were radiographed at the rural hospital. Since rural hospital has only analogue X-ray equipment, thus the film developing expenses had to be taken into account. The travel costs for the visiting radiologist are assumed to be fixed.

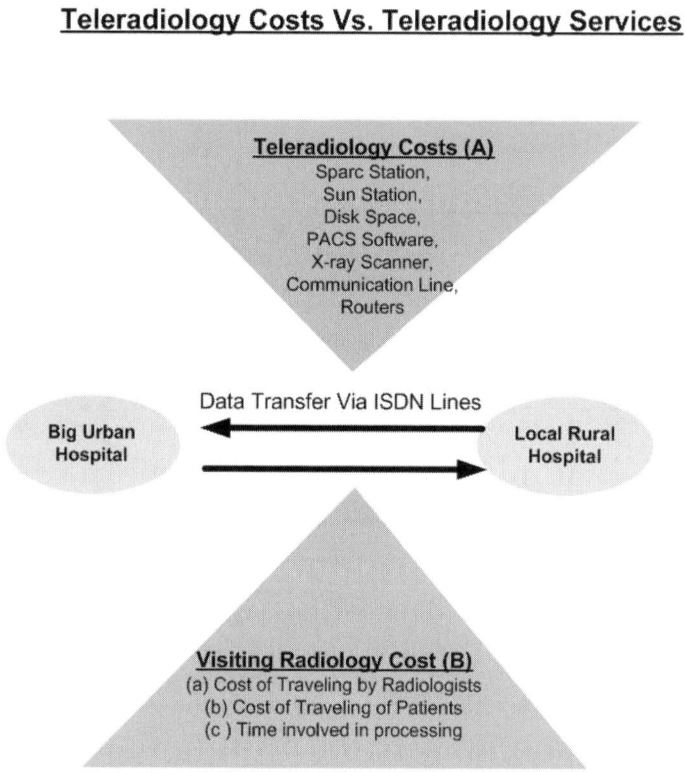

Figure 4. Teleradiology Costs Vs. Teleradiology Services.

As pointed out before, one can find out how the cost behavior changes with the number of patients in the database. This can be seen in Fig. 5. It shows the cost per patient for both teleradiology and the visiting radiologist service. With small number of patients there are large cost differences between the two alternatives. With higher number of patients, the lower cost per patient favors teleradiology. The threshold value can be computed by running the breakeven analysis.

4.3. Teleradiology Costs

Teleradiology costs consist of "fixed" and "variable" costs. This can be given as:

Fixed Costs = Equipment Cost (E) + Maintenance Cost (M) + Line Rental Cost (R) (Equation 1)

Variable Costs consist of the following:

Variable Cost =

Cost spent using communication line L1 * time spent in hospital H1 +
Cost spent using communication line L2 * time spent in hospital H2 +
Wage of technician * hours spent by technician +
Wage of radiologist * hours spent by radiology) (Equation 2a)

In symbols:

Variable Costs = $(L1 * t1 + L2 * t2 + T * h1 + R * h2)$ (Equation 2b)

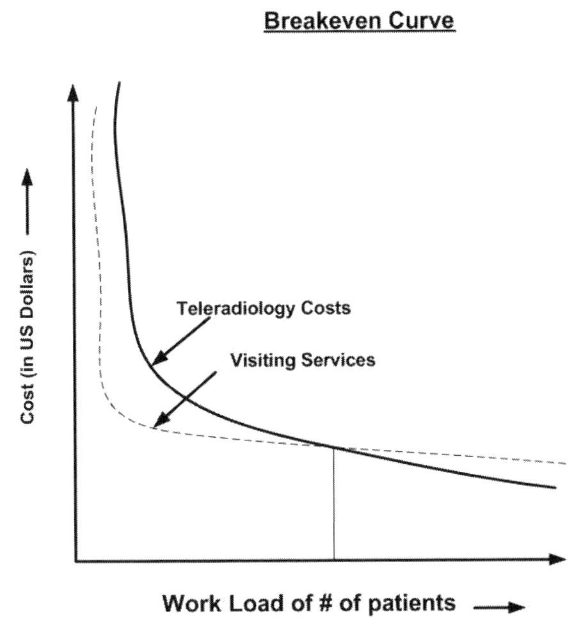

Figure 5. Breakeven Curve between Teleradiology Costs and Services.

Thus total cost is computed by adding Equation 1 and Equation 2b and is given as:
Thus total costs = E(equip) + M + R(line) + (L1 * t1 + L2 * t2 + T * h1 + R * h2)
(Equation 3)

4.4. Cost of Visiting Radiology Services

Variable Radiology Services costs consists of fixed and variable costs.
Fixed Costs = Travel Costs (T) + Allowance Cost + Rest
= Travel Cost (T) + A +
(Hourly wage of Visiting Radiologist * Working Hours/year) +
(Film Processing Cost * Number of X-ray Films) +
(Emergency Transfer Cost * Number of emergency Transfers/year)
Total Visiting Radiology Services Cost = T + A + (Rcost + Pf + E) (Equation 4)

4.5. Breakeven Analysis: Computing the # of Patients

Total Cost of Teleradiology = Total Cost of Radiology Services
(Non-Teleradiology Cost)
Substituting Equation 3 and Equation 4, we get:
E (equip) + M + R (line) + (L1 * t1 + L2 * t2 + T * h1 + R * h2) =
T + A + (Rcost + Pf + E)

This can be written as:
F (tele) + V (tele) * x = F (visiting) + V (visiting) * x
The total number of patients (x) = [F (tele) – F (visit)] / [V (visit) – V (tele)]
(Equation 5)

Thus the total number of patients is computed as the ratio of difference of fixed costs between teleradiology and visiting services to difference of variable cost of visiting services and teleradiology.

If the fixed costs of teleradiology systems is large, this means F (tele) >> F (visit). Under this condition, the number of patients for establishing the effectiveness of telemedicine systems (TMS) would be large. If the difference between the fixed costs of TMS and visiting services is small, it means less number of patients will be needed for break even. This could also mean that we can derive the benefit of TMS if more patients are treated using TMS.

It is interesting to see that the denominator has two components (see Equation 5): Variable costs due to visiting services, V (visit), and variable cost due to teleradiology systems, V (tele). Usually, the visiting costs for radiologists is dependent upon number of hours used by visiting radiologists, his hourly wages, the number of emergency transfers per year and costs for processing the films times the number of films. The hourly wages of visiting radiologists is partially dependent upon the city he/she lives in. The wages for visiting radiologists in New York and California are more expensive compared to the wages of visiting radiologist in Cleveland and Idaho. On the contrary, the visiting radiology service depends upon the wages of the technician (see Equation 2a and Equation 2b). Since wages of the technician (in variable cost of teleradiology) << wages of the physician (in variable cost of visiting radiology services), the variable cost of visiting radiology services is much more than the variable cost of the teleradiology. As a result, the denominator is positive. The more the number of patients seen by the visiting radiology services, the larger the difference between V (visiting) – V (teleradiology). Since we are interested in establishing more number of patients for validating TMS, we want denominator to be low. This can only happen if the variable cost for visiting radiology services is high, i.e., V (visiting) is high. If we try to make V (visiting) high, we would have to give more wages to the visiting radiologists or let them work more number of hours (see Equation 4). They have a limit on the number of hours they can give (since they are employed elsewhere and the main organization will loose money if they try to be away from their work). *Thus there is a tradeoff between the wages of the visiting radiology services Vs. number of patients.*

5. How to Design Successful Telemedicine Systems?

As seen in the previous sections that there is a tradeoff between the number of patients needed to establish the validity of the telemedicine systems and the wages of the visiting radiologists in non-teleradiology systems. This is a very interesting relationship. Though, these factors are one side of the equations, but lot of financial analysts fails to understand the issues related for the successful design of the TMS. One reason being they either do not have knowledge about the inter-relationships between different components of telemedicine or they tend to ignore the engineering aspects of telemedicine. Since the TMS design is engineering in medicine application, there are lot engineering issues which need to be discussed for successful TM systems design. Not only this, but the relationships between patients, hospitals and engineering design has its own importance for superior quality of TM designs. We thus need to discuss in this section, what are the key factors that can help reduce bringing the cost of telemedicine down. These are also the reasons for finding out why the evaluation of the TMS fails.

- *De-acceleration of the funding*: When ever the funding for the TMS development stops or there is a de-acceleration, the evaluation of the TM systems cannot be done. Thus there are no proper methods for continuous evaluation of the TM systems. Since the TM systems are collaboration between engineering framework, hospital administrative frameworks, and the medicine frameworks, the funding cuts can jeopardize the evaluation process.
- *Formation of Cooperative Groups To Avoid TMS Failure*: One way to avoid failures is to form cooperative groups. These groups can lead into discussions about TM systems and thus sharing knowledge and information which can help the understanding of all the telemedicine frameworks.
- *Better Understanding of Engineering Perspective of TM systems*: By understanding the engineering perspective of the TM systems, there, is less chance of failure of the TMS.
- *Better Understanding of the Medical Perspectives:* Since TMS is a technology service to the medical hospitals, better understanding of the medical perspective will avoid the chances of the failure of the telemedicine systems.
- *Better Understanding of different Medical Imaging Modalities:* This is one of the most important issues which seem to be the spearhead of advancement in imaging. People in telemedicine area very interested in using different modalities like MRI, CT, X-rays, Ultrasound, Elastography and fusion of these for diagnostic information but they totally do not understand the concepts of how to embed this diagnostic information. This will be a challenge of the future and some advance development groups are working on it (*discussion with Dr. Swamy Laxminarayan, Idaho State University, Pocatello*).
- *Update to the Hospital-Based Customers:* Since TM systems are designed by engineering people and the customers are hospitals, they need to be updated as soon as there is an update by the engineering group on the TMS group. This also includes having a proper relationship (see Fig. 4).
- *Building a Standard for all Institutions:* Since there are too many institutions involved in building the telemedicine system and there is no one standard, it is hard to cope up with changes. There is no standard at this time. We have not set up a standard because the image processing stage is dynamically changing (see 7 books by Suri et al. [26–29]).
- *Confinement of Telemedicine System:* Many relevant telemedicine applications are confined to specific geographic regions with a space population and thus, large sample sizes that are needed for statistical reasons are hard to obtain.
- *Improving the Direct HealthCare to Providers:* Another way, we can improve the telemedicine evaluation system would be by improving the direct access to other healthcare providers.
- *Patient Satisfaction:* By improving patient satisfaction by actively participating in a synchronous tele-consultation.

The other factors which affect the telemedicine evaluation are: (a) local physician vs. distant expert physician; (b) patient selection; (c) diagnostic category; (d) building the gold standard and (e) sample size.

If telemedicine is developed into user friendly systems for practitioners and patients and provides quality health care at an economical rate telemedicine will become common place in U.S. and many other countries.

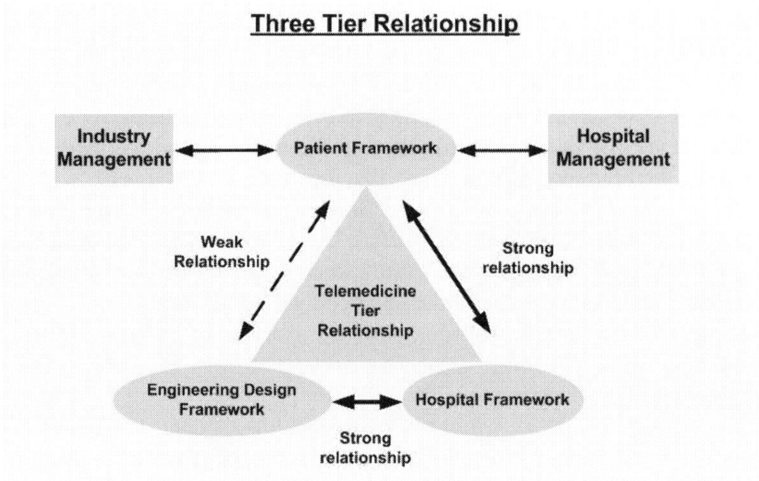

Figure 6. Three Tier Relationship Development.

6. Conclusions

We saw in earlier sections the importance of TM systems, challenges in TM system design and who are the major players in PACS designs, cost analysis of TMS designs and the major design challenges. During all the discussions in our previous sections, we also found that technology changes rapidly, it improves and becomes cost effective over time, but still the health care costs are high and the blame starts to come on the TM systems designs that they are too expensive to operate. Is it really true? We will examine here the main reasons for escalating health care costs in USA. In second part of our conclusion section, we briefly talk about the clinical trials for telemedicine systems.

6.1. Should Telemedicine be Blamed for High Costs?

Physicians are every thing in the telemedicine process when it comes to evaluation. They should feel comfortable about using it. The more they bring TMS to daily usage; they can make patients comfortable to use it. The patients on the other hand should not be surprised with sudden new technology when it comes out. They should be gradually informing as physicians in their learning stages of this new technology. Physicians should be open to new technology, the way they are open to new drugs. Drug representatives from Pharmaceuticals companies take special preparations to train physicians about new drugs. They go from hospital-to-hospital to train physicians and are being used to propagate this information. Free samples of drugs are distributed to physicians in hospitals to make physicians comfortable. In a similar way, the TMS design companies can train physicians about their system. Now unlike drugs, TMS are expensive and they cannot be distributed easily. One method would be to setup a "Virtual TMS" at industries, where physicians can be invited to learn the usage of TMS. Now this can be expensive ordeal for physicians, because they have to spend time traveling to TMS design sites and stay 1–2 days in learning the TM systems. Physician's time is very expensive. Three days of their time means 75 patients. Even if the hospital generates an average of $100 to $500 per patient, they make $7500 to $38,000, which is much more than the return on telemedicine.

What strategy can hospital adapt? They should keep physician time engaged with patients. One alternative for TMS companies is to integrate their training program with imaging machines. This means when big giants like Philips, Siemens, and GE must have package deals for radiologists, where they not only train them on how to operate on medical imaging scanners, but also teach them about TM system designs. This is win-win for all. By integration and alliance, the cost can be distributed among TMS, physician/hospitals and diagnostic imaging companies. Thus, diagnostic imaging companies share the cost between the other two.

We cannot blame technology for high health care costs. The people who are 85 years or older are living longer but in troubled state of minds. They do get the benefit of technology, but they are two issues: (a) First, old age people are more depressed than younger people. They are single due to 50% divorce rate. They are not happy over long time. The non-happiness brings stress at homes and this causes cancer in old age people. (b) second, the issue of delayed health care escalates the costs of living. We need a cultural change in USA so that old age people are happier. Thus the technology alone cannot be blamed for high costs, rather a cultural change is needed.

Figure 7 shows the cultural effect on the cost of the healthcare. Figure 7a shows the graph of "illness", "unhappiness" and "total cost" during the life span of a person. As the "illness" increases with age, the health care costs increase. Similarly, as the "unhappiness" increases (for some people) over age, the cost of illness increases. In Fig. 7b, we see that over time, the cost of the technology falls down (line a). This is due to better system design, cheap electronics etc. Since the "illness" is high over time (line b1), the total cost is given by the sum of "technology cost" and "illness cost", which is very high (line a+b1). In Fig. 7c, due to the cultural effect, the "illness cost" will decrease (as shown in the diagram) (line b2), thus the overall cost will also decrease (see Fig. 7c), i.e., (a+b2) < (a+b1). So, the assumption that technology is not bringing the overall cost down is not valid all the time. No doubt that the technology brings the cost down over time, but a stronger component is the "cultural effect", which can bring the overall health care costs down, i.e., if b2 <<< b1, then (a+b2) <<< (a+b1).

6.2. Role of Trials in Telemedicine

We saw that economic impacts of telemedicine are in question. It is necessary for patients, doctors or the health service? Randomized trials of telemedicine were first performed two decades ago, but some recent studies seem to have been drive by *technology push* rather than *clinical pull* (see Dunn et al. [21]). These studies give inadequate attention to three fundamental aspects of any given trial: (a) defining what is done (such as speed at which is done); (b) to whom is it done for (such as doctors, patients); and (c) and what is measured (such as patient satisfaction, compliance and outcomes).

Trials of telemedicine need to be conducted on representative cases and subjects to ensure that results can be generalized. The control intervention must be the best that can be achieved without telemedicine, as otherwise it is hard to credit any benefit to telemedicine itself. Since telemedicine is simply another kind of medical technology,

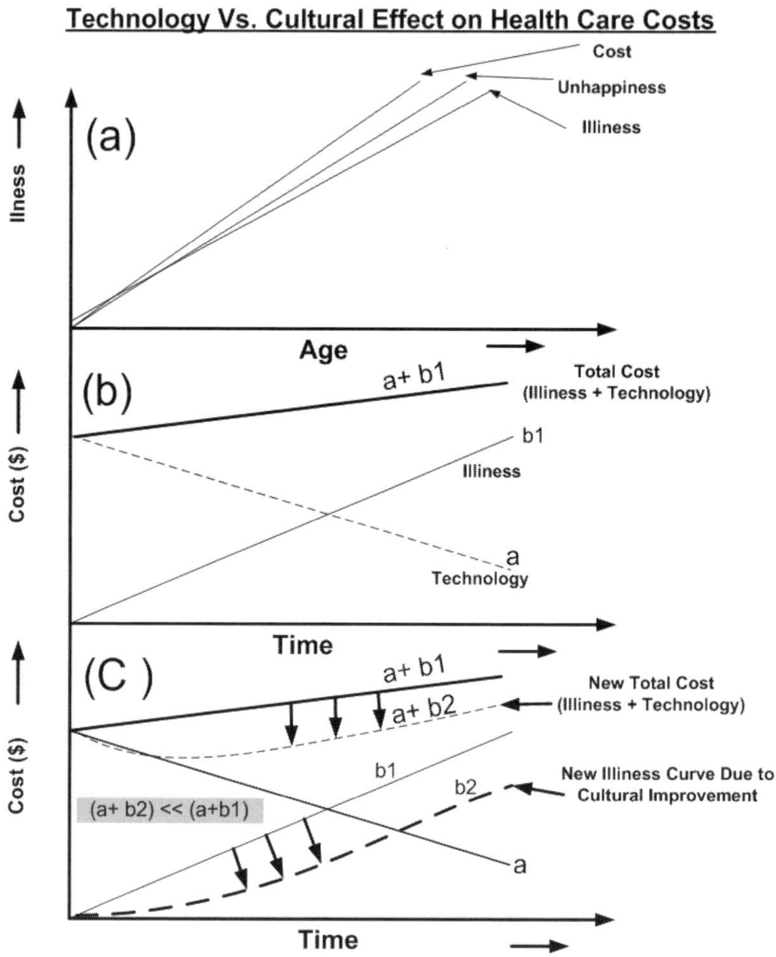

Figure 7. Effect of Culture Change on Health Care Costs.

the same principles of rigorous evaluation of costs and benefits apply. However, investigators may need to strive harder to maintain their clinical perspective and scientific rigor, since these trials often driven by high technology and sponsored by those who provide it.

Acknowledgements

I would like to thank Professor Alan Dowling for giving the guidance in development of this report. I also would like to thank Professor Swamy Laxminarayan for his constant guidance in several other Telemedicine projects and grants. I would also like to thank participants of IT Health Care class. Thanks are also due to the discussion CASE board participants, where time-to-time relevant articles were posted to enhance my knowledge in IT health care.

References

[1] *Begmo, T. S.*, An Economic Analysis of Teleradiology versus a visiting radiologist service, *Journal of Telemedicine and Telecare*, Vol. 5, pp. 136–142, 1996 (Request Received. Transaction Number:115857, CWRU request).

[2] *McIntosh E., Cairns, J.*, A framework for the economic evaluation of telemedicine, *Journal of Telemedicine and Telecare*, Vol. 3, pp. 132–139, 1997 (*Request Received. Transaction Number:115858).*

[3] *Hailey, D. Jacobs, P., Simpson, J. et al., An assessment framework for telemedicine applications*, *Journal of Telemedicine and Telecare*, Vo. 5, pp. 162–170, 1999 (*Request Received. Transaction Number:115859*).

[4] *Patterson V, Hoque F, Vassallo D, Farquharson Roberts M, Swinfen P, Swinfen R.* Store-and-forward teleneurology in developing countries. *Journal of Telemedicine & Telecare.* 2001; 7, No. 5, 52–3 *(available on line).*

[5] *Minion DJ, Sprang R, Endean ED.* A review of telemedicine in vascular surgery. *Minerva Chirurgica.* 2002; 57:237–44 *(not available on line).*

[6] *Marescaux J, Rubino F.* Telesurgery, telementoring, virtual surgery, and telerobotics. *Current Urology Reports.* 2003; 4:109–13.

[7] *Settakorn J, Kuakpaetoon T, Leong FJ, Thamprasert K, Ichijima K.* Store-and-forward diagnostic telepathology of small biopsies by e-mail attachment: a feasibility pilot study with a view for future application in Thailand diagnostic pathology services. *Telemedicine Journal & E-Health.* 2002; 8:333–41 *(not available on line, Possible via Ohio Link).*

[8] *Marescaux J, Soler L, Mutter D, et al.* Virtual university applied to telesurgery: from tele education to telemanipulation. *Studies in Health Technology & Informatics,* 2000; 70:195–201.

[9] *Micali S, Virgili G, Vannozzi E, et al.* Feasibility of telementoring between Baltimore (USA) and Rome (Italy): the first five cases. *Journal of Endourology.* 2000; 14:493–6.

[10] *Moore RG, Adams JB, Partin AW, Docimo SG, Kavoussi LR.* Telementoring of laparoscopic procedures: initial clinical experience. *Surgical Endoscopy*. 1996; 10:107–10.

[11] *Rosser JC, Wood M, Payne JH, et al.* Telementoring. A practical option in surgical training. *Surgical Endoscopy*. 1997; 11:852–5 *(Not available online, but present in Alan Library).*

[12] *Smith RS.* Telemedicine and trauma care. *Southern Medical Journal.* 2001; 94:825–9 *(Present in Allan Medical Library).*

[13] *Briggs, A., Schulpher, M. Buxton, M,* Uncertainity in the economic evaluation of health care technologies: the role of sensitivity analysis, *Health Economics*, Vol.3, pp. 95–104, 1994 (Request Received. Transaction Number:116223).

[14] *Bryan, S., Keen J., Muris, N. et al.*, Issues in the evaluation of picture archiving and communication systems, *Health Policy,* Vol. 33, pp. 31–42, 1995 (Request Received. Transaction Number:116224).

[15] *O'Brien, B., Gafni, A.*, When do the dollars make sense? Towards a conceptual framework for contingent valuations studies in health care, *Medical Decision Making*, Vol. 16, pp. 288–299, 1996.

[16] *Mcclean, J. R.*, Telemedicine and the nurse: the benefit or burden of new technology, *Journal of Telemedicine and Telecare*, Vol. 2, Supplement 1, pp. 54–55, 1996.

[17] *Darkins, A., Dearden, C. H., Rocke, L. G., Martin, J. B., Sison, L., Wootoon, R.*, An evaluation of telemedical support for a minor treatment center, *Journal of Telemedicine and Telecare*, Vol. 2, pp. 93–99, 1996 (R*equest Received. Transaction Number:116226).*

[18] *Tachkra, S. Freij, R., Mullett, S., Sivakumar, A.*, A Teleradiology or telconsulation for emergency nurse practitioners*? Journal Telemedicine and Telecare*, Vol. 2, pp. 56–58, 1996 (R*equest Received. Transaction Number: 116227).*

[19] *Van Grnnip, EMSJ, Ottes, F. P., et al.*, Why do cost-benefit studies of PACS disagree? *SPIE Medical Imaging,* IV, 1990, Vol. 1234.

[20] *Crowe, B. L., Hailey, D. M. and Carter, R.*, Assessment of Costs and Benefits in the introduction of digital radiography systems, *International Journal of Biomedical Computing*, Vol. 30, pp. 17–25, 1992.

[21] *Dunn, E. V., Conarth, D. W., Bloot, W. G., Transquanda, B.*, An evaluation of four telemedicine system for primary care, *Health Service Research,* Vol. 1, pp. 19–25, 1977.

[22] Emory University's Virtual Reality in Medicine. (URL: http://www.gen.emory.edu/medweb/medweb.vrmed.html).

[23] Ferrini, Leslie. *Advance for Administrators in Radiology,* the State of Connectivity, November, 1997, 66–69.

[24] *Grimes, G. J.*, Remote Microscopy for hi-res and real-time interactive pathology, *Advanced Imaging*, Vol. 12, No. 7, pp. 12–16, 1998 *(*Transaction Number:118954).

[25] *Taylor, P.*, A survey of Research in Telemedicine, Part-II, *Journal of Telemedicine and Telecare, Vol. 4, 1998.*

[26] *Suri, J. S.,* Advanced Algorithmic Approaches to Image Segmentation: An application in Cardiology, Neurology, Pathology and Mammography, *Springer-Verlag*, 2001.
[27] *Suri, J. S.,* PDE and Level Sets: State of the art segmentation techniques for static and motion imagery, *Kluwer Publishers*, 2002.
[28] *Suri, J. S.,* Angiography and Plaque Imaging, *CRC Press*, 2003.
[29] *Suri, J. S.,* Hand Book of Medical Imaging: Segmentation and Registration Models, *Acadmeic Publishers*, 2004 (*to appear in June in 3 Volumes*).

Appendix

Sample Questions for Evaluation of Telemedicine

Understanding the main objectives of a telemedicine project should provide an indication of where costs may be incurred and where benefits may be achieved, and thus aids in the identification of key questions for the evaluation. The cost-consequences approach discussed above can be more formally identified using a set of key questions.

1. Evaluation time: Here the question arises as to when should the TM evaluation be done?
2. Choosing an evaluator: This involves who would be doing the evaluation.
3. Effect of TM on cost: will the TM bring more cost?
4. Effect of TM on human resources: Will it increase or decrease?
5. Treatment cost: will it increase or decrease?
6. Outcome on patients: will it increase or decrease?
7. Non-health outcomes: should non-health outcomes be included in evaluation?
8. Referral patterns: will this pattern change due to TM?
9. Activity levels: will the activity levels change upon implementation? If so, how will differing levels of throughtput affect the cost-effectiveness of the programme?

Medical and Care Compunetics 2
L. Bos et al. (Eds.)
IOS Press, 2005

ICT, e-Health & Managing Healthcare – Exploring the Issues & Challenges in Indian Railway Medical Services

Dr. Santanu SANYAL M.B.B.S (Cal), M.H.A (TISS)
Central Hospital, South Eastern Railway,
11 Garden Reach Road, Kolkata-700043, India
Email:sanishita@vsnl.net

Abstract. This paper attempts to detail the evolution of a system synergy for more than 3 decades where the health services researchers; clinicians and others have been investigating the use of advanced information and communications technologies (ICT) to improve Indian health care. At the core of all these efforts lies a successful system synergy or a marriage between medicine and ICT and combination of innovative and mainstream technologies. The system is being developed in the context of the medical standards and practices in India, addressing issues, challenges and problems specific to Indian health care scenario where its 1 billion populations are predominantly rural and distributed in distant geographical locations. The health and medical facilities presently available in the non-urban parts of the country is inadequate and there are wide disparities in terms of health care infrastructure, facility, manpower and funds between rural and urban communities, and between different states and even districts within states. This calls for innovative methods of utilization of science and technology for the benefit of our society and ICT and medicine assumes a greater significance to revolutionise the health care system in India.

Keywords. ICT, e-Health, telemedicine, HIMS, IRMS

Introduction

Continual changes in the Indian healthcare scenario now dictates the viability of a hospital but some hospital still resist and even fear change. The Indian Railway Medical Services (IRMS) understood the need for switching over to a computer based Hospital Information Management System (HIMS) way back in 1990 when this new HIMS facility was conceptualized to create environment conducive for comprehensive computer coverage of most of the hospital functions.

With the help from the Centre for Railway Information System (CRIS) it initiated a pilot project at the Southern Railway and subsequently in South Eastern Railway, Kolkata, Northern Railway, New Delhi and Central Railway, Mumbai. After a decade it reveals that the system failed to cope up with the rapid strides of changing ICT world. Reviewing planning failures that prohibited getting the desired results under the current changing scenario and overcoming these obstacles with the current growth of the Information and Communication Technologies (ICT) and offer a practical solution was the basis of this study.

1. Objectives

1. To understand the key health issues in the current perspective and synergy of ICT, Medical Science & Technology in an upcoming horizon.
2. To understand the ICT capability and core competence of the Indian Railways Medical Services (IRMS).
3. To understand the difficulty that is being faced in current perspective and the viable challenges, issues, opportunities in the current perspective and to understand the possible drivers of the future and catalysts for growth in Indian Railway healthcare scenario.

2. Methodology

This is a mixed study both quantitative and qualitative with the sole aim to understand and add value to the existing services if any and the methodology obtained are:

1. Collection and compilation of primary data on HIMS centre to be made available through surveys and structure questionnaire keeping in mind the four essential processes that can foster lasting change within an organization.
2. Collection and compilation of secondary data of the HIMS centre available from the files, registers etc.
3. Semiformal interviews with the experts, staff and administration, repeated brainstorming over the issue.
4. Review of literature & Internet surfing.

3. Indian Healthcare: An Overview

Constitution of India dictates that healthcare provision to ill person is a state responsibility but various reasons inherent in our socio-economic milieu inhibits this ideal and the growth expected in the Indian health care delivery system. As a result it has failed to grow and develop as neither to our expectation nor to the needs of the people of India. A large number of people had to spend from their pocket towards own and family health care of the individual.

The "out of pocket" expenses on health have been estimated to the extent of 83% of total expenditure on health. This is probably the highest expenditure on health care in the world and has been identified as one of the main reasons for remaining the below poverty line (BPL) due to the inherent 'double trouble' i.e. health care expenses on one hand and being away from the daily wages during the ailment.

Present healthcare spending: India spends about 86,000 crores in health care i.e. 5.2% of its GDP where Government share is meager 0.9%. The other contributors are from Employers (15%), Private Insurance (2%) and from direct out of pocket spending (83%). Out of 17,200 crores of the Government spending the distribution of expenditure in Primary Care is 2064 Crores (12%) and vertical Health Programmes get 4472 Crores (26%) but in Secondary and in Tertiary Care it is whopping 10664 Crores (62%).

With this health expenditure for 5 decades, we could create 128 tertiary Medical College Hospitals, 5600 district hospitals, 2400 Community Centers, 23000 Primary Centers and 132000 sub centers Now the emphasis is more on

1. Acute to chronic illness and life style diseases.
2. Curative to preventive and restorative to comprehensive medicine.
3. Inpatients care to outpatient care, daycare and home care.
4. Isolation function to area wise function or regional function
5. Individual to community orientation.

Indian Health Sector few facts:

1. India today has more than 1 billion population and there is finite limit of elasticity in providing health care in terms of infrastructure, facility, the manpower and the funds.
2. Wide disparities still persist between different income groups, between rural and urban communities, and between different states and even districts within States where the population is predominantly rural and distributed in distant geographical locations apart from the high-density urban areas.
3. Epidemiological transition is viewed in the form of population growth pattern with increasing awareness and expectation of the patient from the health providers.
4. To provide the basic minimum health care has been one of the priorities of the Health administration all along but high cost of curative health care and lack of investment for health care in rural areas is creating inadequate, inequitable distribution of medical facilities in rural and inaccessible areas.
5. Problem of retaining doctors in rural areas and the specialist doctors cannot be retained at rural areas as they will be professionally isolated and become obsolete and even monetary incentives also cannot prevent it. A recent survey by the Indian Medical Society revealed the facts that 75% of qualified consulting doctors practice in urban centers and 23% in semi urban areas and only 2% from rural areas whereas majority of the patients come from rural areas. The number of Neurosurgeons in Chennai city alone far exceeds those in the entire North Eastern Region.

4. Synergy of ICT & Medical Science

In India, the growth of ICT in last 15 years has been in leaps and bounds. Medical Science & Technology has also viewed a significant growth in the last decade. The arena of globalisation and consumerism catalysed a marriage between the parallel growths. The resultant synergy helped upwardly mobile success and a growing phenomenon is viewed in the current and in the upcoming horizon where this bondage between ICT and Medical Sciences is inseparable.

The Government (both State and Central), The Railways and the Municipalities in India are by far the largest healthcare providers in the country and I think they are all currently asking a very similar questions. Management of many hospitals is seriously introspecting that what phase they are currently in and what needs to be done to have a level playing field. Other Hospitals still give the ICT and HIMS lower priority that it deserves. The above scenario describes what is generally happening today in the Indian healthcare industry. Inspite of the presence of top class professionals in the form of doctors and IT people this sector was considered an unorganised sector in recent past.

With the corporate sector getting into the act and opening up of insurance sector can stimulate and streamline the healthcare scenario. It is already perceived in India that there is a paradigm shift in Healthcare reality where the market concept is bringing in more consumer friendly atmosphere. The key factor for survival now will be based on the following parameter:

- Competitive healthcare strategies in a 24x7 atmosphere.
- Consumer friendly care.
- Service quality not quantity.
- Speed with which the same is provided.
- Satisfaction of the customer.
- Web based e-Health adaptability and
- Healthcare professionals need to switch from traditional framework and
- Provide more patient involvement in the decision-making.
- Bring in transparency in the operational procedures.

5. IRMS-An Overview: Indian Railways the 'Lifeline of the Nation'

- 62023 route kilometers.
- 44000 coaching vehicles, 7700 locomotives and 0.216 million wagons.
- 6850 block stations.
- 43 workshops and production units.
- 52 crores spent on staff/day.
- 99 cr. revenue expenditure/day.
- 1.511 million work force and 7.12 million beneficiaries.

The IRMS is now one of the biggest comprehensive multidisciplinary multispeciality health care delivery providers in India and caters to the medical need of its 7.12 million beneficiaries through its three-tier system spread in 124 hospitals and 591 Health Units with 13758 beds, 2552 doctors and 52088 paramedical staff.

The service outcome is an annual load of 30.3 million OPD cases, 36797 admissions and over 32329 major operations.

Table 1. IRMS beneficiary categories.

Category	Number in million	No. of Dependants	Total
Serving employees	1.51	4	6.04 million.
RELHS	0.29	3	0.87 million.
RECHS	0.09	2	0.18 million.
Non Railway case	0.03	1	0.03 million.
Total beneficiaries	1.92	3.7	7.12 million.

Category of beneficiaries in IRMS

Table 2. Health expenditure distribution in IRMS.

FY	Ordinary working expenses	Expenditure on medical treatment	Percentage
2000-01	34142 crores	439 crores	1.28%
2001-02	36164 crores	459 crores	1.26%
2002-03	38967 crores	498 crores	1.27%
2003-04	39783 crores	532 crores	1.33%
2004-05	40381 crores	660 crores	1.63%

Health expenditures in IRMS

Table 3. Healthcare expenditure in IRMS.

FY	IRMS Expenditure	Beneficiary	Exp/Person/year
2000-01	439 crores	6.93 million	633.47
2001-02	459 crores	6.98 million	657.59
2002-03	498 crores	7.03 million	708.39
2003-04	532 crores	7.12 million	747.19
2004-05	660 crores	7.23 million	912.86

Financial implications in IRMS Healthcare per person/year

Table 4. Comparative Health Indices in IRMS.

	India	Kerala	Sri Lanka	IRMS
IMR/1000/year	68	14.0	15.4	13.76
MMR/lakh/year	407	87.0	59.6	27.0
CBR/1000/year	26.1	18.2	17.3	9.82
CDR/1000/MYP	8.70	3.12	5.70	1.35

Heath Indices in IRMS

6. Difficulties Faced in Current Perspective

The private healthcare market in India with its estimated growth potential to double by 2010 is now in a state of dizziness. Growing public awareness, rapid technological advances, likely impact of global health insurance players, growing concept on hospital accreditations and corporatisation of Indian Healthcare is rapidly altering the patterns of healthcare.

Profits have now become the key in hospitals function just like any other service industry and the thrust on profits promises to revolutionise healthcare delivery like never before. Never before has hospital administration assumed so much importance in the private healthcare sector.

7. Drivers of Change in IRMS Health Care

- Rise of sophisticated consumers in a 24x7 society with growing public awareness, increasing expectations, increasing public and social accountability courtesy ICT age.
- Presence of big players in the arena due to liberalised policies of the Government creating lack of level playing ground for genuine competition and changing boundaries between hospital and home care with increased emphasis on cost containment.

Today we have the most difficult customer to serve, where expectation are high, situation is tense, services under constant scrutiny. The journey from chaos to clarity has begun with professional healthcare management and a marked change in hospital management has been noticed with the shift from empirical to professional administration and now the hospital administration is no longer a monopoly of doctors who shuttled between clinical care and administration, or who settled down for administration after two decades of experience. In India now the hospital administration is a full-time vocation handled by professional managers.

8. Catalyst for the Growth

1. Incentives for investment for the improvement in infrastructure like sanitation, potable water supply and education.
2. Health Care Quality Standards are a must and can be laid down by the Government or by the Industry or a combination of both. This will give credibility to the public for usage.
3. Health Insurance can be the biggest driver for Healthcare in India which now covers only 4 million lives as compared to 80% coverage In USA.
4. Telemedicine is one of the biggest factors to open up and can make a lot of difference in bringing quality health care to rural India.
5. Corporate hospitals have started medical tourism in India has taken the lead.

9. Conclusions

Indian Healthcare in general and Indian Railways Medical Services in particular is viewing a silent yet paradigm shift. While equity of access and quality care are the benchmarks of good hospital administration, in India both of them comes at a price. In our country quality of cure is available to the consumer who can pay, and hence there is some over-use of services in the private sector. While most of the administrative changes occurring had given a thrust to healthcare industry, there needs to some changes in over-use of services. Perhaps the opening up of insurance would do the trick. In relation to above IRMS is providing outstanding health care delivery system to its serving employees and family members at extremely low cost. The scope of treatment is comprehensive health care delivery comprising of curative care in primary, secondary, tertiary level and in some super specialties. In addition the preventive, promotive and rehabilitative health care is also getting the due care. The service provided is also. IRMS is now gearing up to take this challenge for the future to provide quality heath care more effectively and efficiently with the increasing use of ICT.

References

[1] SEARO Country Health Profile, WHO: (2004).
[2] Technical Working Group for Telemedicine Standardization; *Recommended Guidelines and Standards for Practice of Telemedicine in India* (New Delhi: Department of Information Technology, Ministry of Communications and Information Technology, (2003).
[3] Indian Railway Medical Manual, Revised edition (2000).

EC e-Health Projects Symposium

Medical and Care Compunetics 2
L. Bos et al. (Eds.)
IOS Press, 2005

Intracorporeal Videoprobe (IVP)

A. ARENA [f], M. BOULOUGOURA [c], H.S. CHOWDREY [d], P. DARIO [f], C. HARENDT [a], K.-M. IRION [b], V. KODOGIANNIS [c], B. LENAERTS [e], A. MENCIASSI [f], R. PUERS [e], C. SCHERJON [a] and D. TURGIS [e]

[a] *Institut für Mikroelektronik Stuttgart, Allmandring 30a, 70569 Stuttgart, Germany*
[b] *Karl Storz GmbH & Co KG, Mittelstr. 8, D-78532 Tuttlingen, Germany*
[c] *University of Westminster, School of Computer Science, London HA1 3TP, UK*
[d] *School of Biosciences, University of Westminster, 115 New Cavendish Street, London W1M 6UW, UK*
[e] *Departement Elektrotechnik, ESAT - MICAS, Kasteelpark Arenberg 10, B-3001 Heverlee, Belgium*
[f] *Scuola Superiore Sant'Anna - CRIM Lab, Polo Sant'Anna Caldera, Scuola Superiore Sant'Anna, Viale Rinaldo Piaggio 34 - 56025 - Pontedera (Pisa) - Italy*

Abstract. The objective of the work in the EC project IVP is the development and evaluation of two prototypes of video systems:

– a small wired videoprobe with a CMOS image sensor

and

– an autonomous video-capsule with a telemetric link for image data transfer to an external PC-based system.

Introduction

Visualisation of the status of organs health is one major task in medical diagnosis and therapy. Endoscopy and minimal invasive surgery are techniques for this purpose in medical applications. Recent developments in microelectronics allow the fabrication of advanced and highly integrated image sensors and improved solutions for miniaturisation and wireless data transmission.

In endoscopy important aspects are the demand for smaller devices and the wish to integrate high quality, but low cost visualisation techniques [1]. Moreover the problems and cost of sterilisation raised the wish to fabricate disposable endoscope heads.

While the majority of endoscopes uses optical lens systems (rigid endoscopes) or fiber bundles (flexible endoscopes) to transmit the images to a camera, video-endoscopes have the camera directly at the tip. Thus such an endoscope head is a microsystem with image sensor chip, optics and illumination and electrical wiring. Image data are transmitted via cables, which also provide the power for the system. The wired videoprobe IVP1 is described in the first part of the paper.

Autonomous videoprobes on the other hand, use wireless data transmission and need an internal the power supply. The most prominent development of such an autonomous video-capsule is the M2A system of Given Imaging [2] a battery powered system with a CMOS image sensor. Other developments in this field describe external powering systems [3] or even work with CCDs (Charge Coupled Devices) and external

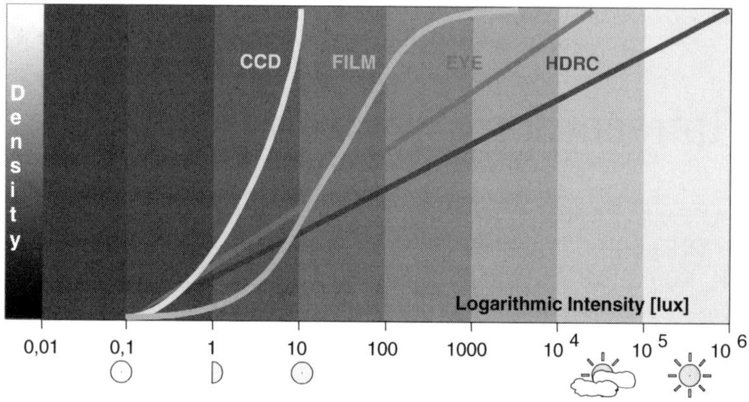

Figure 1. Response for different illumination conditions.

guidance systems [4]. The IVP2 system approach is described in the second part of the paper.

The main applications for these wireless videoprobes are the diagnosis of the gastro-intestinal tract, but depending on the performance of the system special applications (temporary implant, special diagnosis, etc) are feasible.

In the field of image sensor technology the CCD has been the main stream technology since more than 20 years, but CMOS image sensors gained increasingly market shares recently. CMOS (Complemetary-Metal-Oxide-Semiconductor) tech-nology is the basis of modern microelectronics. With advanced CMOS technologies (in submicron dimensions) sensor pixel sizes of a few microns are feasible. Therefore image sensors with good resolution and performance could be fabricated for a reasonable price. A further advantage of this technology is the possibility to integrate additional functions.

The High-Dynamic-Range-Camera (HDRC®) [5] is a special type of CMOS image sensor with a logarithmic response of the pixel.

Figure 1 shows the response versus illumination for different image detection systems. The sensitivity of the human eye is similar to a logarithmic responding of the sensor. As indicated in the Fig. 1 the HDRC sensors [6] cover a wide range of illuminations (dynamic range over 120dB). Thus no mechanical shutter is necessary to avoid saturation. There is no loss of information even for very bright spots or in high contrast scenes. The sensor shows colour constancy for all displayable illumination conditions, which is very important for medical applications, where the colour information essential.

1. The Wired Videoprobe IVP1

The major objective during the development of the **IVP1 image sensor** was the size of both the image area and the overall chip. Thus additional to the general objectives three issues had to be addressed:

- The minimisation of the pixel size to allow an acceptable dimensions for this sensor.

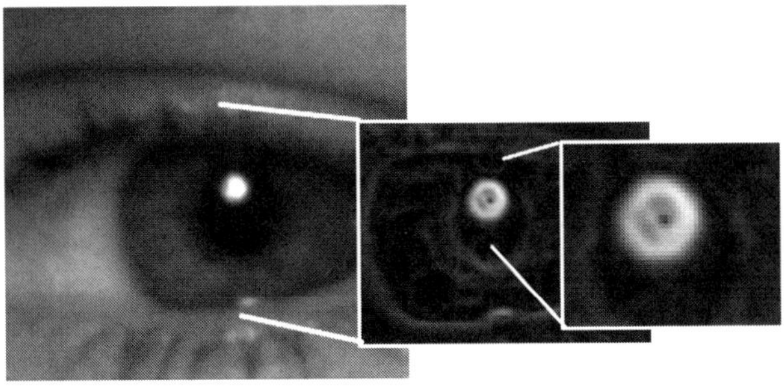

Figure 2. Colour image obtained with IVP1 image sensor. The enlarged images show details revealed after edge detection.

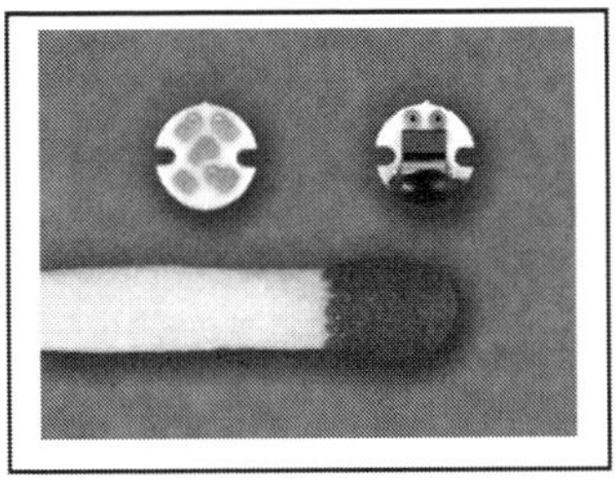

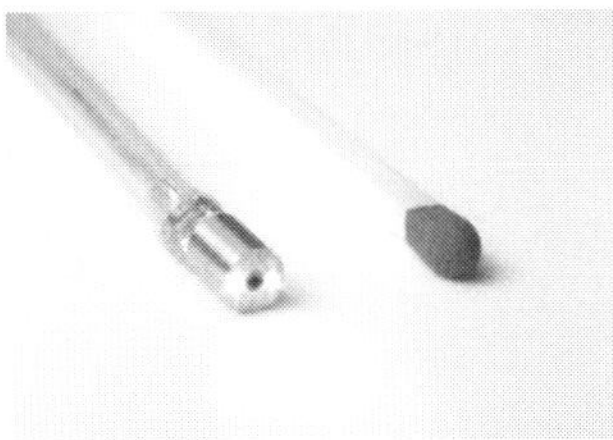

Figure 3. Ceramic board with IVP1 image sensor and pad connectors (left), IVP1 videoprobe head with optics and illumination (right).

- The reduction of the number of pad connections, because bonding pads with its area and the required sizes for pad circuitry cover a significant area of the chip. Additionally each bond requires also size on the package.
- The testability off the device to allow complete evaluation and verification of the first devices.

The resulting sensor has an image field of 200 x 180 pixels with a pixel size of 4,6 μm. The overall chip size is 1,7 x 1,3 mm^2 and the device has 4 connections. The chip is originally equipped with 43 pads, which are used for the complete digital test. The majority of these pads are cut-off before the final mounting of the chip.

The image sensor is coated with colour filters (red, green, blue). Figure 2 shows a colour image of a human eye obtained with an IVP1 image sensor. Although the bright reflection in the centre seems to be saturated, more details are visible in the enlarged images, which have been processed with an edge-detection software. The details are the shape of the spot light used for the illumination during the shot.

For the fabrication of the **IVP1 prototype** the chip is mounted on a circular (Ø 3mm) ceramics (see Fig. 3), where it is connected to the cables. Two openings in the circuit board are used to fix the optical fibres for the illumination: A metal cap with the optics completes the distal end of the endoscope. The analogue image data are transferred via the cables to a PC, where the image data are processed and subsequently displayed.

The prototype IVP1 has no internal **steering mechanisms** to produce tilting movements. For the first version of the video probe an external rigid pipe has been

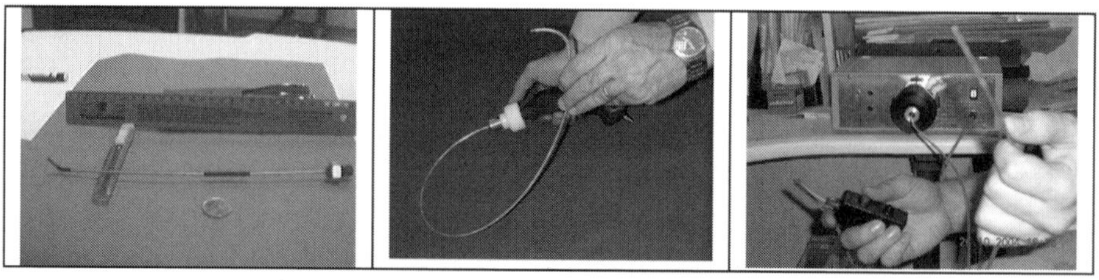

Figure 4. IVP1 steering: the movable tip (l), steering with a handle (m), motor driven system (r).

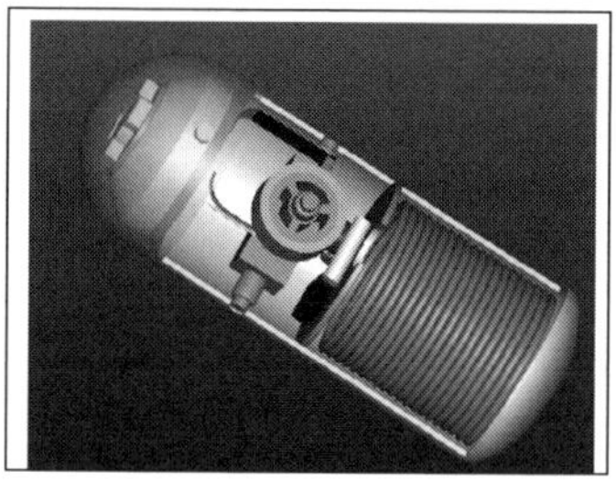

Figure 5. Scheme of the capsule.

used, in order to generate an axial rotation movement into the capsule; a joint with one degree of freedom will be included in order to produce the bending movement. The pipe must be hollow for electrical wires and optical fibers connection. The external diameter of the pipe is about 3 mm. We can easily obtain movements of the tip of +/– 90 degrees.

A second prototype with a more flexible connection (rubbery multilumen tube) between the steerable tip (which includes the camera and the optical fibre) and an ergonomic handle, which allows the actuation of the steering mechanism, has been developed. In particular the diameter of the tube is 3.5 mm, moreover, in order to have a better steering angle, the distal part of the tube has a different hardness as regard with the rest of the tube itself. The steering of the tip is obtained thanks to two push-pull cables connected to the tip and actuated manually or by a motor positioned in the handle. The systems are shown in Fig. 4.

For the manually actuated version, a sort of wheel can be screwed on a threaded shaft where the proximal end of the hollow pipe is fixed. As regards the motorized version, a geared motor is used to pull the push pull cables (Fig. 4 c).

2. The IVP2 Capsule

The autonomous IVP2 system (Fig. 5) contains a CMOS image sensor with camera, optics and illumination, a transceiver, a system control with image data compression unit and a power supply. The optical part is located on a tiltable plate, which is driven by a wobble motor.

The **IVP2 image sensor** for the IVP2 capsule is a HDRC image sensor with a resolution of 768 x 496 pixels. The sensor has a sensitivity of 120 (digits/decade). Its dynamic range is 150dB and the minimal detectable illumination is 0.005lux. Frames

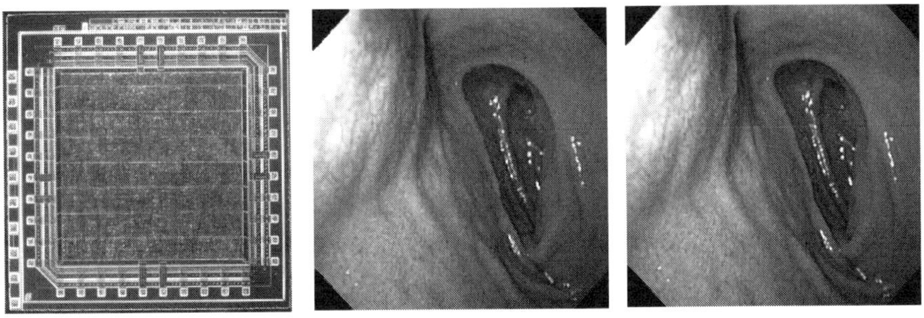

Figure 6. a) chip picture, b) original picture, c) compression by 20.

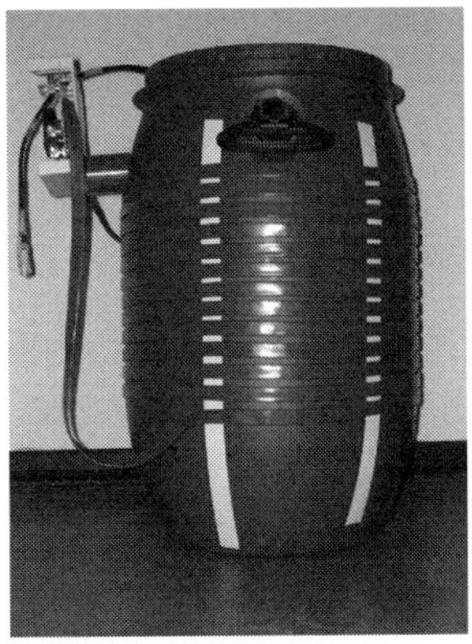

Figure 7. External coil with class E driver.

are generated at 14 MHz. The has a pixel pitch of 7,4 μm. It has an integrated A/D converter. Similar to the IVP1 sensor organic colour filters are used.

This image resolution and frame rate in capsule endoscopy lead to a bottleneck problem: the data rate allowed by data transmission is too low to reach both high image resolution and high frame rate. The HDRC image sensor operated at 10 images per second will produce about 30 106 bits. On the other hand data transmitters available for capsule endoscopy can transmit between one and two megabits per second.

The solution proposed is an **image compression** dedicated for endoscopic images that meets both high compression ratio, and low power consumption. Such a result is made possible by the endoscopic image characteristics: there are mainly smooth and small changes in the image. [7]

A technique, which uses the prediction of pixels by its predecessors to reduce image size has been tested and implemented on a dedicated ASIC of 2x2 mm (Fig. 6a) with a power consumption of 10mW. The comparison between an image (Fig. 6b) and the same image compressed by a factor 20 (Fig. 6c) let see the small degradation of the image quality.

The feasibility of an inductive link meeting all the power specifications imposed by capsule endoscopy is shown in previous work [8]. The **power link prototype** consists of one external coil and three internal coils, both parts equipped with their respective driver or receiver electronics.

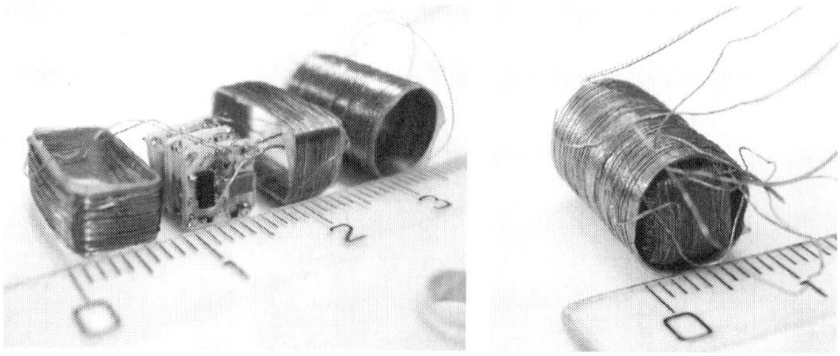

Figure 8. (a) Three orthogonal coils and receiver electronics integrated on a stack of thick-film substrates. (b) Electronics and coils assembled for integration in capsule.

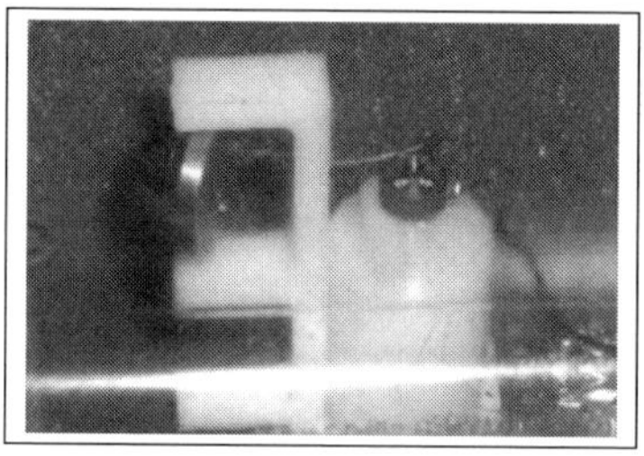

Figure 9. Wobble motor for the tilting movement of the camera head.

In Fig. 8 the receiver part is depicted. It consists of three orthogonal coils and a stack of thick-film substrates fixating and interconnecting the receiver electronic components (Fig. 8(a)). The three coils can be slid into one another to form a compact cylinder with the electronics inside (Fig. 8(b)). Because of their orthogonallity, there is always at least one coil capable of extracting power out of the external magnetic field, no matter the orientation of the capsule.

Two stable DC voltages are delivered by the link output to the rest of the capsule electronics: one at 3.6 V and one at 2.5 V. The worst-case power efficiency was measured to be 1.5 % for this prototype.

The basic concept is to use a frontal view system with a vision angle upper to 120 degrees and a **tilting mechanism** able to steer the vision system (optics, illumination and image sensor) between about ± 30 degrees in one plane. By exploiting this technique, the device will perform an optimal view between ± 90 degrees in the xy plane. The tilting mechanism can be realized by using a wobble motor (the Q-PEM motor) and simple mechanical parts, such as one cam and one shaft fixed to the vision system.

The cam system transforms the rotational action of the motor in a linear action to the shaft. The vision system can be tilted by the shaft if two diametrically opposed points of the vision system itself are fixed to the body capsule. The entire system, including optic and electronic components, will be inserted in the capsule body.

The Q-PEM motor can be controlled with a precision of 300 steps for each complete round. A motor with overall dimensions of 4 mm of diameter and 3 mm of thickness has been designed and realized (see Fig. 9).

The main objective of the "**expert system**" subsystem is to increase the expert's ability in identifying suspicious regions and decrease the need for intervention while

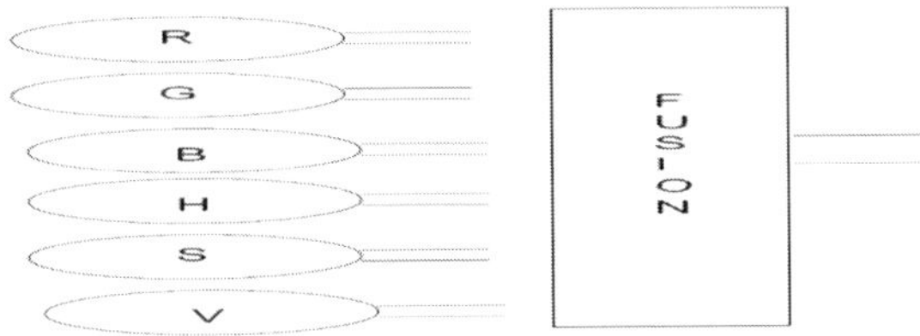

Figure 10. Proposed fusion scheme.

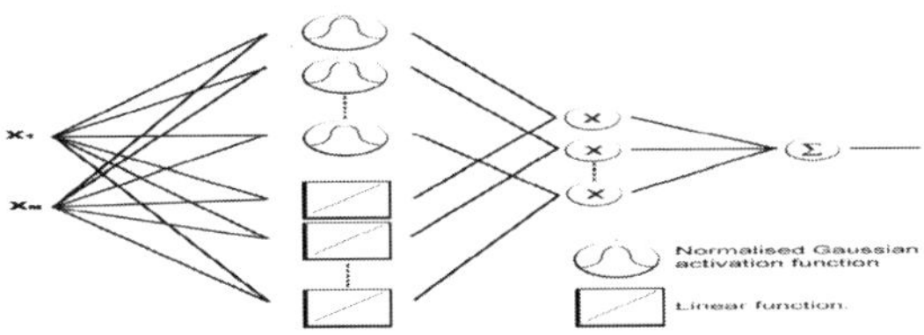

Figure 11. ENRBF scheme.

maintaining the ability for accurate diagnosis. Computer-assisted image analysis can extract the representative features of the images together with quantitative measurements and thus can ease the task of objective interpretations by a physician expert in endoscopy. The proposed methodology is considered in two phases. The first implements the extraction of image features while in the second phase an advanced neural network is implemented / employed to perform the diagnostic task. Texture analysis is one of the most important features used in image processing and pattern recognition. It can give information about the arrangement and spatial properties of fundamental image elements. The definition and extraction of quantitative parameters from endoscopic images based on texture information in the chromatic and achromatic domain is being proposed. This information is initially represented by a set of descriptive statistical features calculated on the histogram of the original image. For this reason, we focused our attention on nine statistical measures (standard deviation, variance, skew, kurtosis, entropy, energy, inverse difference moment, contrast, and covariance) [9]. All texture descriptors are estimated for all planes in both RGB {R (Red), G (Green), B (Blue)} and HSV {H (Hue), S (Saturation), V (Intensity)} spaces, creating a feature vector for each descriptor $D_i=(R_i,G_i,B_i,H_i,S_i,V_i)$. Thus, a total of 54 features (9 statistical measures x 6 image planes) are then estimated. In addition to the classic "histogram"-based approach, an alternative approach of obtaining those quantitative parameters from the texture spectra is proposed both in the chromatic and achromatic domains of the image. The definition of texture spectrum employs the determination of the texture unit (TU) and texture unit number (N_{TU}) values. Texture units characterise the local texture information for a given pixel and its neighbourhood, and the statistics of the entire texture unit over the whole image reveal the global texture aspects [10].

For the diagnostic part, the concept of multiple-classifier scheme has been adopted, where the fusion of the individual outputs was realised using fuzzy integral [11] (see Fig. 10).

3. Summary

The two videoprobes to be demonstrated in the IST-project IVP have been presented with its special features. The results show the feasibility of miniaturised video-endoscopes for many medical and technical applications. The major components of the autonomous capsule such as image sensor with the data compression for digital data transmission, the power system, a micro-mechanical tilting mechanism and the expert system have been developed.

Acknowledgement

The authors are grateful to the European Commission for the financial support of this work through the IST project IVP (IST-2001-35169).

References

[1] K.-M.Irion, "Endoscopes – Potential for Microsystem Technology" MST News, I-05 March 2005, p.26.
[2] Iddan G, Meron G, Glukhovsky A, Swain "Wireless Capsule Endoscopy" Nature 2000; 405:417, more ref. in http://www.givenimaging.com.
[3] http://www.olympus.co.jp/en/news, news release Nov 2004.
[4] http://www.rfnorika.com.
[5] Deutsches Bundespatent Nr. 42 09 536 granted 5.9.1996, United States Patent No. 5 608 204 granted 4.3.1997.
[6] U. Seger, H.-G. Graf und M.E. Landgraf, "Vision Assistance in Scenes with Extreme Contrast", IEEE Micro 13 (1) February 1993, pp. 50–56.
[7] D. Turgis, R. Puers, "Image compression in video radio transmission for capsule endoscopy", Proceedings Eurosensors XVIII, 12–15 September 2004, Rome, Italy, pp. 111–112 (4 pp. version on CD-ROM only).
[8] B. Lenaerts, R. Puers, "Inductive powering of a freely moving system", Proceedings Eurosensors XVIII, 12–15 September 2004, Rome, Italy, pp. 484–485 (4 pp. version on CD-ROM only).
[9] M. Boulougoura, E. Wadge, V.S. Kodogiannis, H.S. Chowdrey, "Intelligent systems for computer-assisted clinical endoscopic image analysis", 2nd IASTED International Conference on BIOMEDICAL ENGINEERING, February 16–18, 2004, Innsbruck, Austria, pp. 405–408, ISBN: 0889863792, ACTA Press.
[10] V. Kodogiannis, M. Boulougoura, "Neural network based approach for the classification of wireless-capsule endoscopic images", accepted to IEEE IJCNN conf, Montreal, July 2005.
[11] L.I. Kuncheva, Fuzzy Classifier Design, Physica-Verlag, 2000.
[12] V. Kodogiannis, H.S. Chowdrey, "Multi network classification scheme for computer-aided diagnosis in clinical endoscopy", MEDSIP 2004 - Advances in Medical Signal and Information Processing Int. Conference, 5–8 September 2004, Malta, pp. 262–267, ISBN: 0-86431-439-7.

Symposium on Imaging

Medical and Care Compunetics 2
L. Bos et al. (Eds.)
IOS Press, 2005

Fischer's Fused Full Field Digital Mammography and Ultrasound System (FFDMUS)

Jasjit S. SURI[a,1], Tim DANIELSON, Yujun GUO[b] and Roman JANER
[a]*Fischer Imaging Corporation, Denver, CO, USA*
[b]*Department of Computer Science, Kent State University, Kent, OH, USA*

Abstract. It has been well established that X-ray modality when combined with ultrasound modality increases sensitivity and specificity of breast lesion detections. Under the NIH grant, Fischer has developed a fused full-field digital mammography and ultrasound system (FFDMUS), which has ability to acquire 2-D X-ray mammogram and 3-D ultrasound images simultaneously. This novel technology generates co-registered breast images of X-ray and ultrasound images. The co-registration error between X-ray and ultrasound images acquired is within 2.00 mm in scan direction, and is 0.5 mm in anterior-posterior direction. We did the performance evaluation of the system, and concluded that the ultrasound image qualities from FFDMUS and Hand-held ultrasound (HHUS) are comparable, and the X-ray image qualities from FFDMUS and SenoScan® are also comparable. We also developed a preliminary CAD registration and segmentation system for FFDMUS datasets.

Keywords. Fusion, ultrasound, X-ray, breast lesion, hand-held ultrasound, full field digital mammography and ultrasound system

1. Introduction

Following lung cancer, breast cancer is the second leading cause of death from cancer among women in the United States [1]. X-ray mammography is the main tool used for the detection and diagnosis of breast malignancies (it is currently the only medical imaging modality used in breast screening). However it is technically difficult to consistently produce mammograms of high quality, and interpretation is subjective and can be variable among radiologists (the practice of mammography is the only clinical procedure to be federally regulated for quality assurance). Mammography, with about 70% sensitivity and 30% positive predictive value, is imperfect, but screening has been shown in clinical trials to reduce breast cancer mortality by 25% to 30% for women in the 50 to 70 age group (Tabar *et al.* [2,3]).

There are two ways for screening: film-based and digital-based. The film in film-screen mammography serves the three functions: image acquisition, display, and storage. By replacing the film-screen combination by a digital device, Full-Field Digital Mammography (FFDM) promises high detective quantum efficiency (DQE), high con-

---

[1] Corresponding Author: Dr. Jasjit S. Suri, Fischer Imaging Corporation, 12300 North Grant St., Denver, CO, 80241, USA, Tel: (303)254-2545, Fax: (303)254-2502, E-mail: jsuri@fischerimaging.com.

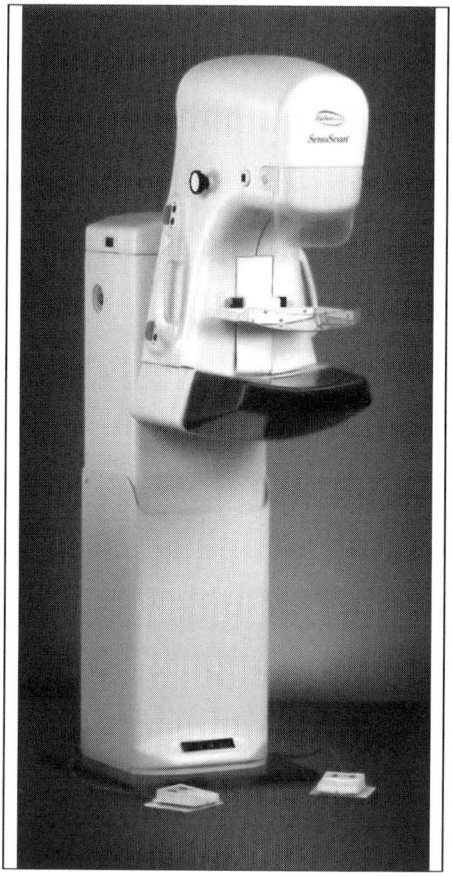

Figure 1. Fischer's SenoScan®.

trast and dynamic range, and for specific systems limiting resolution almost matching that of film (the SenoScan® images up to 16 cycles per mm, see Fig. 1). Further potential advantages include image processing versatility, direct interface to Computer Aided Detection/Diagnosis (CAD), tele-radiology, display flexibility, and long-term storage without loss of data integrity. Use of CAD, facilitated by FFDM, has shown potential for improving the accuracy of screening mammography, at least among less experienced users (Nishikawa [4], Burhenne *et al.* [5]). Use of FFDM has been demonstrated to lead to a lower rate of callbacks (Lewin *et al.* [6]).

Other technologies, including ultrasound, have demonstrated adjunctive value for diagnostic examinations, and could potentially be used in screening. Ideal detection performance may ultimately depend on multi-modality imaging, as no single imaging technology to date can accurately detect all significant lesions (Nass *et al.* [7]). The clinical significance of a fused FFDM and breast ultrasound imaging system is based on published evidence that the probability of missing a breast cancer with the combination of mammography and ultrasound is much smaller compared to mammography alone, especially in women with dense breasts. The efficacy of combining film-screen mammography with free-hand ultrasound (185 histologically confirmed invasive can-

Table 1. Clinical efficacy of mammography, ultrasound and mammography combined with ultrasound.

Diagnostic Method	Sensitivity	Specificity	Positive Predictive Value	Negative Predictive Value	Accuracy
Mammography	83.7%	68.5%	67.8%	84.1%	77.1%
Ultrasound	89.1%	79.1%	65.7%	90.1%	83.4%
Mammography + Ultrasound	94.6%	92.1%	89.7%	95.9%	93.2%

cers and 254 benign tumors) was recently investigated by Malur *et al.* [8]. Results of Malur's study are given in Table 1.

As shown in Table 1, the combination of mammography with ultrasound was shown to improve sensitivity by 13% and specificity by 34% over mammography alone. When compared to ultrasound imaging only, combined imaging resulted in a 6% improvement in sensitivity and 16% improvement in specificity. Only patients with abnormal findings as determined by palpation and/or mammographic findings and/or ultrasound findings were included in this study.

Co-registration of cross-sectional images obtained by tomosynthesis from digital mammograms and breast ultrasonography has been studied most recently by Kapur *et al.* [9]. Fusion of FFDM and ultrasound has also been studied by Elbakri *et al.* [10,11] and Suri *et al.* [12].

In this paper, we discuss Fischer's approach to development of novel fused full field digital mammography and ultrasound system (FFDMUS). Two sets of acquisitions are performed in FFDMUS: 2-D X-ray projection mammogram and 3-D ultrasound slices. The nature of the fused system puts a high pressure on image quality assessment of ultrasound and X-ray images. The image quality of X-ray image should be comparable with the mammogram from state-of-art FFDM system, such as Fischer's SenoScan®. The image quality assessment of ultrasound images is even more critical when the lesions of the breast are imaged with ultrasound transducer, where the sound waves have to travel through different material properties besides different tissue types. This leads to partial volume effect phenomenon thereby losing the edge information of the lesions in 3-D ultrasonic slices. In this paper, we not only correct the partial volume effect but also to compare with the Hand-Held ultrasound (HHUS). Beyond that, the system also provides a very preliminary computer aided diagnostic tools to help physicians.

The layout of this paper is as follows: Section 2 presents our novel FFDMUS prototype. The same section also discusses the co-registration of ultrasound and X-ray. The methods to assess the image qualities of X-ray and ultrasound images from FFDMUS are introduced and the evaluation results are presented in Section 3. CAD techniques combining the segmentation and registration techniques being developed along with the system design are presented in Section 4. Finally the paper concludes with Section 5.

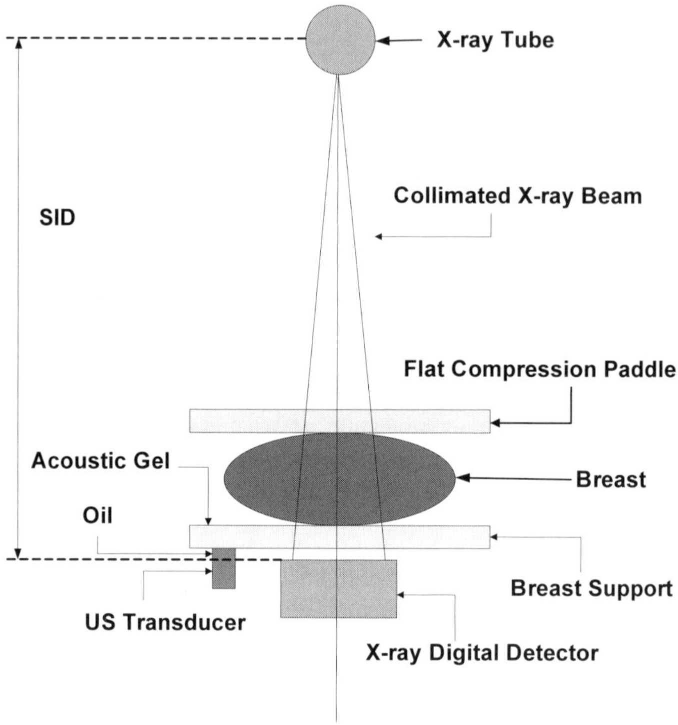

Figure 2. Sketch showing the principle of 2D X-ray and 3D Ultrasound acquisition.

2. Fusion System Design and Co-Registration

2.1. System Design

Figure 2 shows the system setup of Fischer's FFDMUS. It consists of the flat breast support on which the breast rests. The breast is then compressed via the flat compression paddle (as shown in the figure). The breast support has the thin plate tensioned around to keep it straight. Below this plate is the ultrasound transducer that scans the breast from left to right (scan direction) and in orthogonal direction (raster direction). Oil is used below the breast that helps in ultrasound image acquisition during the ultrasound scanning process, the ultrasound slices and hence the ultrasound volume is acquired. X-ray image is acquired during the X-ray scanning process. This is using full field digital mammography (FFDM) SenoScan® system.

The mechanical assembly of lower gantry of FFDMUS is shown in Fig. 3. The integrated scanning mechanism consists of a high-precision, high-rigidity linear guide with a ball screw actuator. The x-ray detector and ultrasound transducer are mounted side-by-side onto this linear actuator. A linear encoder provides closed-loop position feedback to a servomotor that drives the linear actuator. X-ray acquisition occurs during the forward stroke of the scan, at a speed of 5cm/sec with 54-micron pixel resolution. The ultrasound acquisition takes place during the back stroke, at a speed of 5mm/sec, with 1.0 mm limiting resolution. The flow chart of the whole procedure is illustrated in Fig. 4.

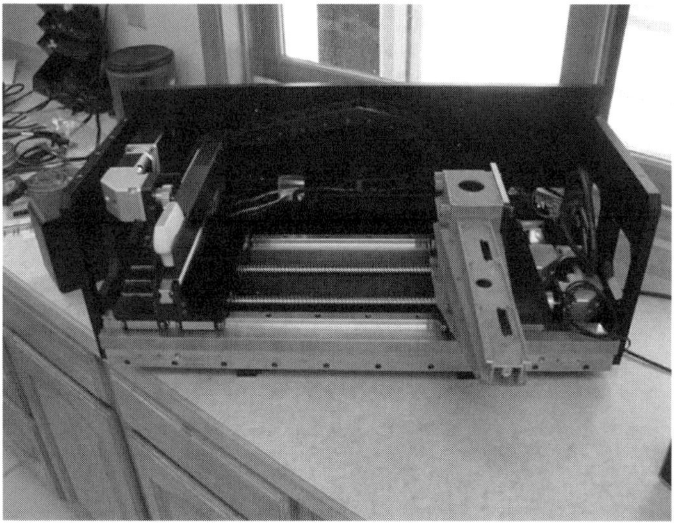

Figure 3. Assembly of lower gantry of FFDMUS showing the fusion of X-ray detector and ultrasound transducer.

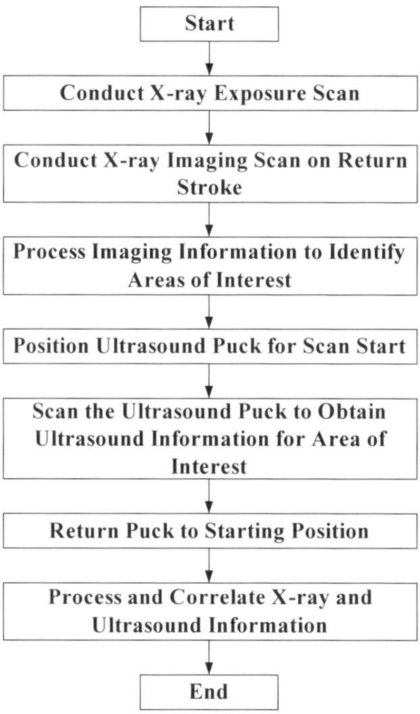

Figure 4. Flow chart of the image acquisition.

Figure 5 is the graphic interface for the image acquisition in FFDMUS. There are four scan models: AEC scan, X-ray scan, Ultrasound Full scan and Ultrasound ROI scan. At each scan model, X-ray scan and Ultrasound scan (Full and ROI) can also be

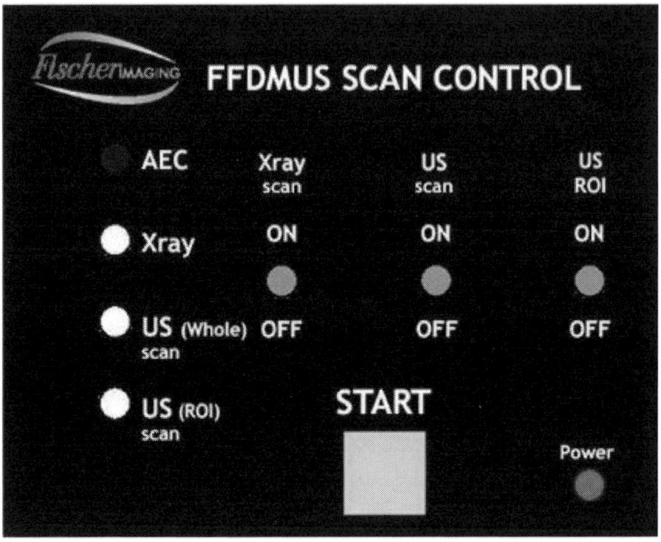

Figure 5. GUI control for digital image acquisition in FFDMUS.

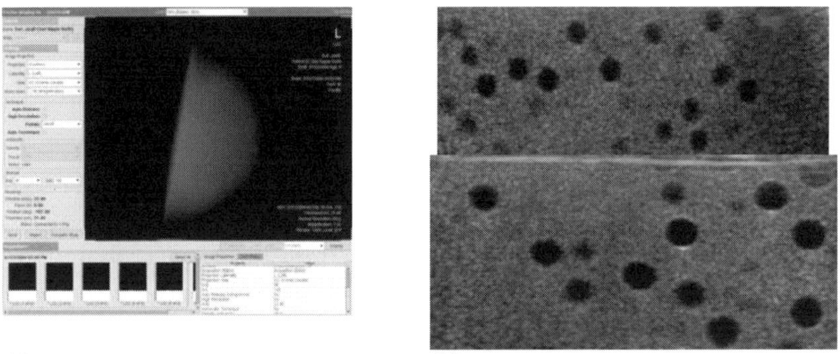

(a) (b)

Figure 6. (a) Screen shot of X-ray acquisition; (b) Sample ultrasound slices of CIRS phantom [13].

turned on or off. Button "Start" can start the scanning, and the scanning procedure can be stopped pressing the same button. By controlling the switches, X-ray and Ultrasound can be acquired at the same time. The screen shot of X-ray acquisition is shown in Fig. 6(a), while ultrasound samples from ultrasound scanning are shown in Fig. 6(b).

2.2. Co-Registration Accuracy

To determine the co-registration accuracy of the integrated system, we built a special grid phantom consisting of wire meshes at three different depths with known spacing. The wire structure was embedded in a special gel appropriate for x-ray and ultrasonic imaging. The phantom provided a large data set to examine the registration accuracy of the two modalities. Figure 7 shows the x-ray and ultrasound images of the phantom, and the wire intersections used to determine registration accuracy.

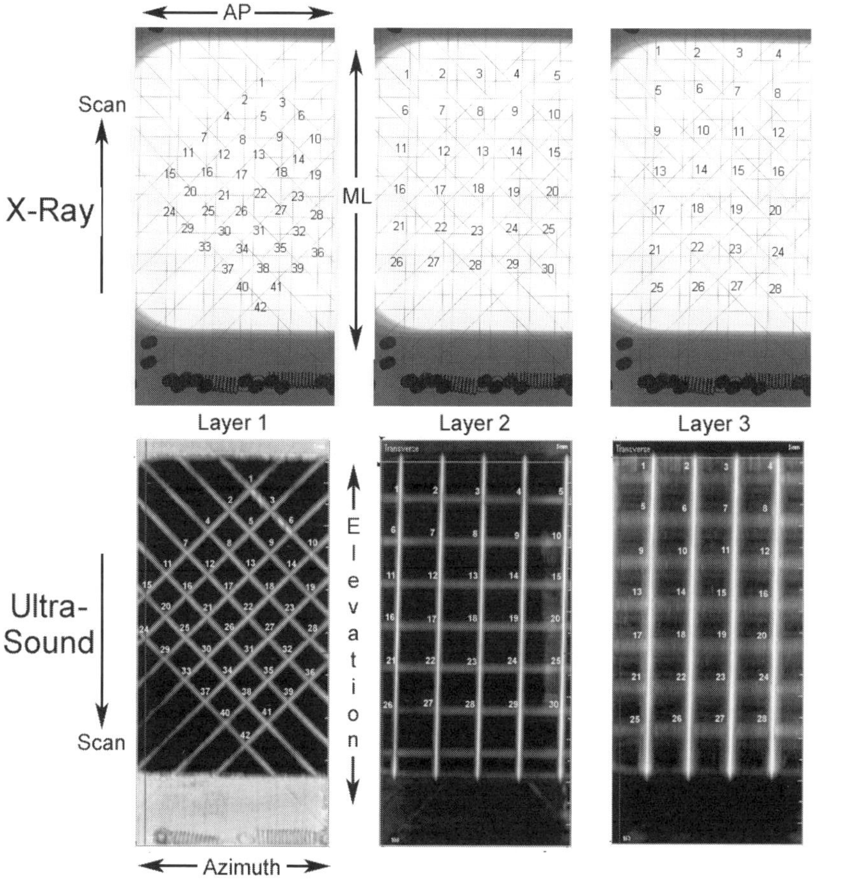

Figure 7. Wire grid phantom. The top row illustrates the x-ray projection image. The bottom row illustrates the reconstructed ultrasound transverse slices. The columns show wire intersections at different depths used to determine registration accuracy.

Knowledge of the exact dimensions of the phantom and the x-ray imaging geometry defines a geometrical transformation that maps any point of interest in the phantom to its projection in the x-ray imaging plane. For all of the wire intersections visible in the ultrasound volume (and marked in Fig. 7), we determine the projection point in the x-ray plane, and calculate the error between the computed and actual projections. Figure 8 illustrates the geometrical mapping.

The wire phantom provided 100 points (wire intersection) to determine registration accuracy. To ensure repeatability of results, we acquired several scans of the phantom. We also varied the ultrasound transducer focal depth. We obtained very similar results in all cases. We herein present the results from a representative data set.

For each point of interest in the volume reconstruction of the ultrasound data, we compute the corresponding x-ray projection. We then determine the difference error between the calculated and actual projection points in the scan and anterior-posterior (AP) directions. The wire intersections are easily identifiable in both x-ray and ultrasound. Table 2 and Fig. 9 summarize the results. In the AP direction (perpendicular to

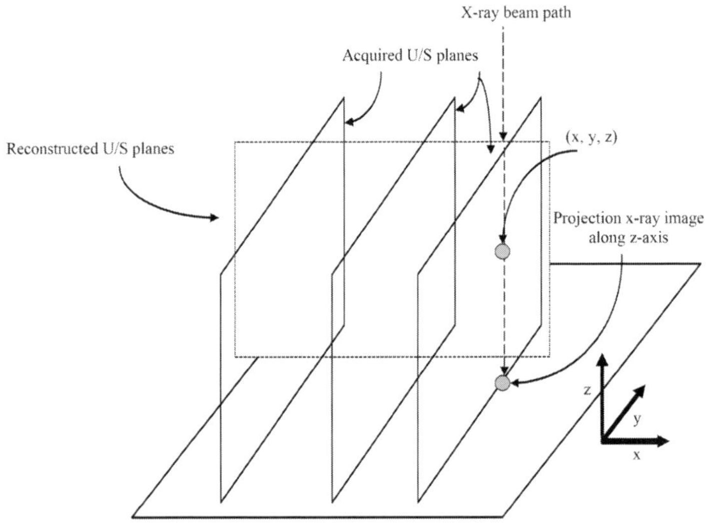

Figure 8. Ultrasound-to-X-ray geometrical mapping.

Table 2. Co-registration error.

	Scan error mean	***Scan error standard deviation***	***AP error mean***	***AP error standard deviation***
Layer 1	1.81	0.16	0.26	0.16
Layer 2	1.47	0.21	0.32	0.12
Layer 3	1.14	0.20	0.42	0.16

scan), the error is within 0.5 mm. In the scan direction, the error is within 2.0 mm. Given that the limiting resolution of the integrated system is 1.0 mm, the results thus far are very encouraging.

Figure 10 illustrates co-registered images of the CIRS phantom (Norfolk, VA). The CIRS phantom consists of cystic and solid masses, as well as microcalcifications about 250 microns in size. Imaging this phantom with the integrated US/FFDM prototype illustrates the complementary roles of x-ray and ultrasound, and the utility of acquiring co-registered images. In Fig. 10, the availability of complementary ultrasound information assists in clearly differentiated the two structures, and provides depth information.

3. Image Quality Assessment for Fused FFDMUS

Assessment of Ultrasound and X-ray images acquired using FFDMUS system is one of the most necessary protocols before the FFDMUS imaging device can be used for

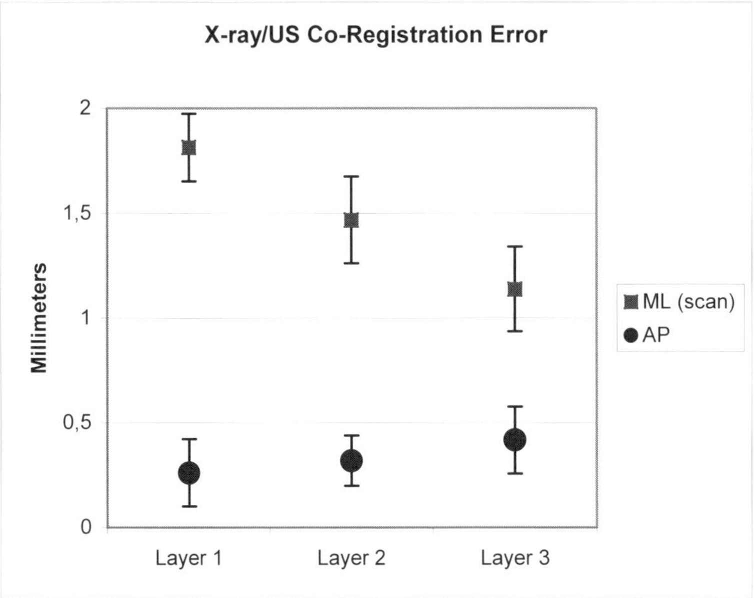

Figure 9. Co-registration error in ML and AP directions.

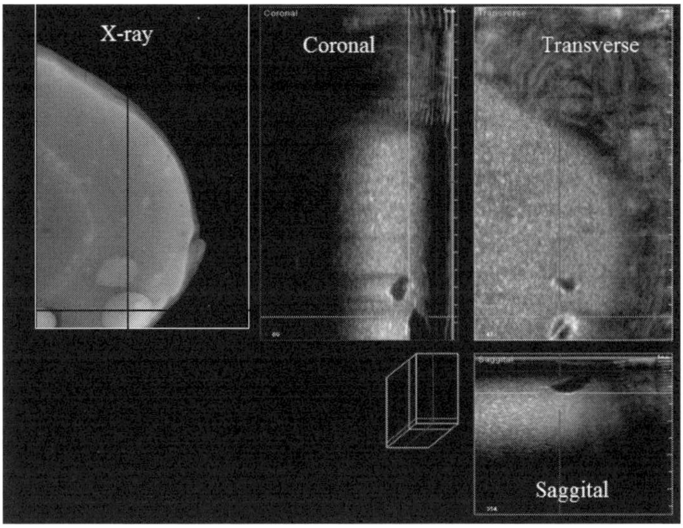

Figure 10. FFDMUS co-registered images: X-ray projection and three orthogonal ultrasound slices.

screening or diagnosis. It becomes even more important to perform IQ assessment when the two imaging modalities are tied to the same gantry while using different physical principles for image acquisition. This section presents protocols for assessment of ultrasound and X-ray image quality in the fused FFDMUS framework.

To assess the ultrasound image quality, we measured axial and lateral resolution by means of point spread function (PSF) analysis. In addition, measurements of transmission loss and near field ring-down artifact were made and compared to an equivalent

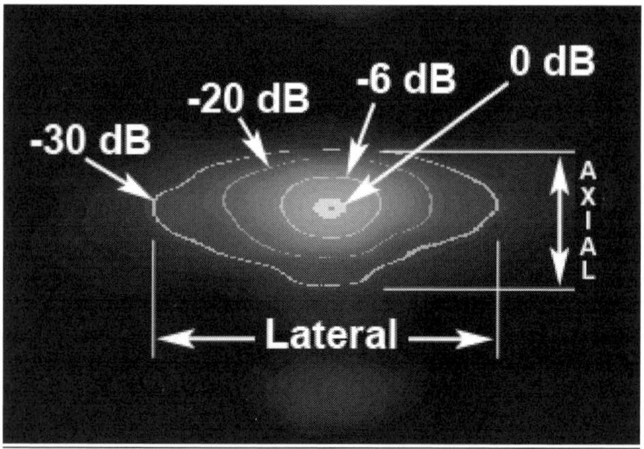

Figure 11. Ultrasound system point spread function. The dimensions labeled "Lateral" and "Axial" represent the –30 dB lateral and axial resolution.

Hand-Held ultrasound (HHUS) transducer. Finally a spherical void phantom with 3 mm and 5 mm diameter cystic lesions was used to measure the area of the observed lesion and compared that with the ideal lesion. For the X-ray image quality assessment, we measured the Modulation Transfer Function (MTF), Detective Quantum Efficiency (DQE), and Normalized Noise Power Spectrum (NNPS) of the FFDMUS and compared that to SenoScan® FFDM (Suri *et al.* [12]).

We will discuss ultrasound image quality assessment in Section 3.1 using PSF analysis, and in Section 3.2 using segmentation method. Section 3.3 presents X-ray image quality assessment.

3.1. Ultrasound Quality Assessment using PSF Analysis

This section focuses on the ultrasound image quality assessment using PSF analysis. A conventional Hand-Held L12-5 ultrasound transducer (the same type used for FFDMUS) was used as the control. The objective of the assessment was to demonstrate that the FFDMUS acoustic coupling had little or no negative effect on ultrasound (US) image quality. Parameters evaluated were (1) axial and lateral resolution; (2) transmission loss; and (3) ring-down artifact.

There are no ACR, IEC, or any other universal standards for assessing ultrasound axial or lateral resolution. Nonetheless, axial and lateral spatial resolutions are two of the most widely accepted image quality metrics [14–21]. The Philips HDI 5000 ultrasound system has internal test capability that facilitates accurate determination of the axial and lateral resolution. This is done by scanning a "string phantom" consisting of 125 mm diameter nylon monofilament strings immersed in a 10% ethylene glycol/ water mixture, which has a speed of 1540 meters per second. Since the string diameter is smaller than one ultrasound wavelength, the image of the string represents the point spread function (PSF). By tagging the image gray map with contrasting colors at known amplitudes and adjusting the gain, the resulting images display iso-amplitude contours like a topographic map, as shown in Fig. 11. The gain adjustments provide a way to measure transmission loss. The –6 dB, –20 dB, and –30 dB axial and lateral resolution are measured from the vertical and horizontal dimensions of the specified

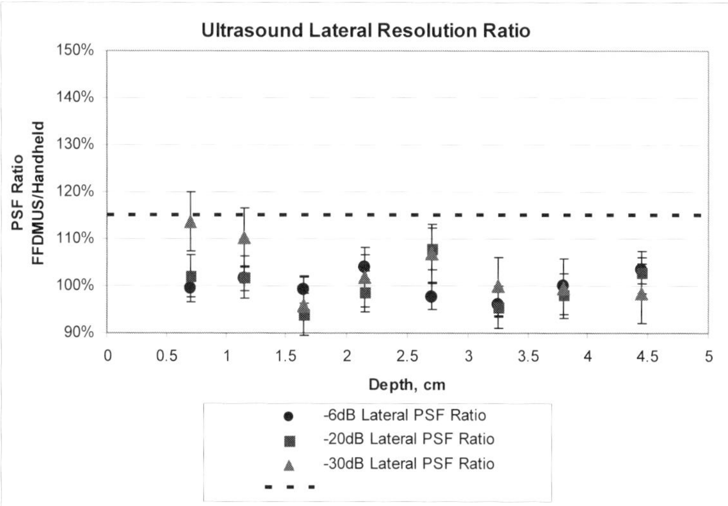

Figure 12. Lateral resolution ratio of FFDMUS relative to Hand-held US based on measurements of the system PSF.

iso-amplitude contours. These measurements were performed for both FFDMUS and the conventional L12-5 Hand-Held ultrasound transducer with seven strings at depths ranging from 0.7 cm to 4.5 cm, and repeated five times for each string. The gains were used to estimate transmission loss, and the ring-down was measured from the depth from skin line to the –30dB contour.

Because the purpose of the PSF measurements was to look for a change in resolution between FFDMUS and Hand-Held (control), the results are plotted as a ratio, as shown in Figs 12 and 13. For example, if the axial resolution ratio is 100%, it means that the results for FFDMUS and Hand-Held were the same. If the axial resolution ratio is 140%, it means that the axial PSF measurement for FFDMUS was 40% larger (worse) than for Hand-Held. The error bars represent ±1 standard deviation, which reflects an uncertainty in the measurement of about ±5%. The goal was for the ratio not to exceed the dotted line, which represents resolution loss of 15%.

Figure 12 shows that there is no systematic or significant difference in the –6 dB or –20 dB lateral resolution of the FFDMUS system, relative to Hand-Held US. The –30 dB lateral resolution of FFDMUS appears to degrade slightly relative to Hand-Held at the shallow depths of 0.7 cm and 1.15 cm. However, the degradation is less than 15%, and is therefore unlikely to be clinically noticeable.

Figure 13 illustrates the results for the axial resolution measurements. There is no systematic or significant difference for the –6 dB axial resolution of the FFDMUS system, relative to Hand-Held ultrasound.

The transmission loss in FFDMUS was measured at 4.66 dB ± 1.15 dB, relative to Hand-Held. This was within the goal of 6 dB or less, which corresponds to a penetration loss of less than 4 millimeters. The –30 dB ring-down artifact depth was measured for FFDMUS at 3.8 mm, compared with 1.7 mm for Hand-Held. This difference is mainly due to the 2mm butadiene rubber standoff, which creates an additional low attenuation reverberation path. The ring-down artifact in FFDMUS can be significantly reduced by redesign of the transducer to eliminate the standoff.

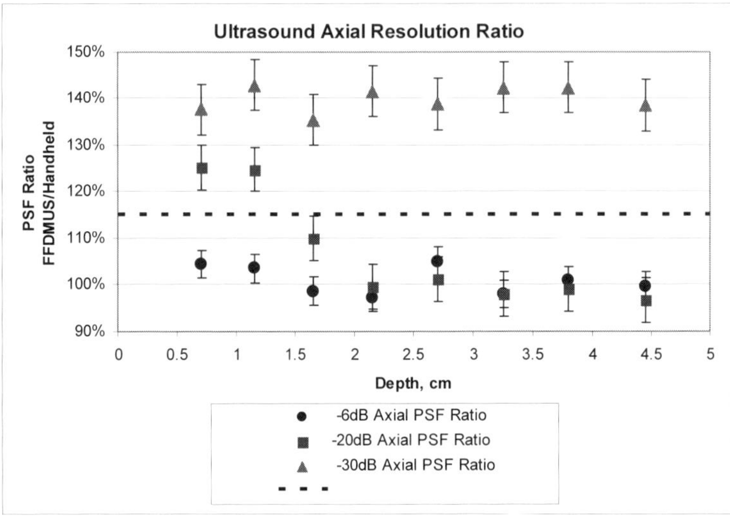

Figure 13. Axial resolution ratio of FFDMUS relative to Hand-Held US based on measurements of the system PSF.

3.2. *Ultrasound Quality Assessment using Spherical Lesion Analysis*

The purpose of this test is to evaluate the apparent size of anechoic spherical lesions of known size, embedded in a scattering medium. Although the apparent lesion size on ultrasound is expected to be smaller than the actual size (due to partial volume averaging effects), the results from FFDMUS and Handheld ultrasound should be equivalent.

CIRS Model 050 has anechoic focal lesions, 3 mm and 5 mm diameter spheres, randomly distributed inside the phantom. These "masses" are made from Zerdine® that has a different contrast and attenuation relative to the background material. We can measure the size of the lesion in the acquired ultrasound images to assess the performance of ultrasound imaging system [13]. Two sets of data were acquired: First using FFDMUS, and the second using the Hand-Held ultrasound transducer.

We adapted the following protocol for the lesion analysis: User defined region of interest (ROI) was first drawn out of the 3-D ultrasound volumetric slices acquired manually. For each group of ultrasound images acquired, FFDMUS and Hand-Held US (HHUS), one ROI of the background (without lesion) and 50 ROIs of the foreground (with lesion) were extracted respectively. Out of each 50 ROIs, half is with the lesion of diameter as 5 mm, and the other half is with the lesion of diameter as 3 mm. The method from Medson *et al.* [22] is adapted to compute the signal-to-noise (SNR) of the ROI extracted, taking the foreground as signal, and the background as noise. Then the SNR images computed are thresholded to segment the lesion area out. The threshold value was automatically calculated for each image, using Otsu's method [23]. The acquired binary image may include noise or artifacts outside the lesion area, which can be eliminated using region growing, with the seed point at the center of the image [24].

We measured the observed lesion area and compared it to the ideal lesion area to assess the ultrasound image quality. The diameter of the lesion in the phantom is already known, and we also know the pixel size in mm unit when the ultrasound image is acquired, the lesion area can be measured and compared, in pixels or mm. The percentage area error related to the ideal area is computed as following:

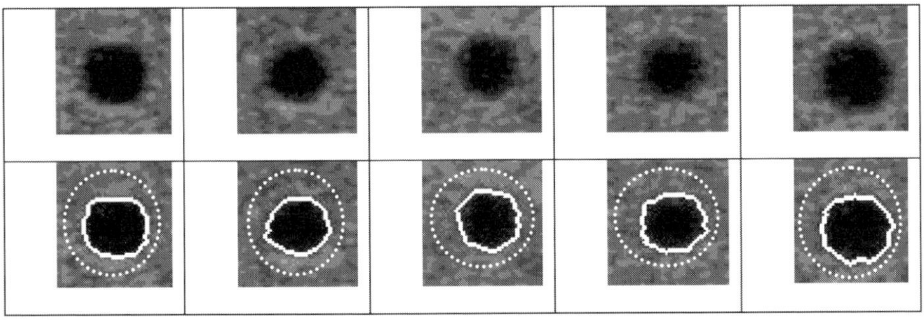

Figure 14. Samples of FFDMUS lesion with 3 mm diameter. Row #1: original images; Row #2: segmentation results with boundary Segmentation results (solid line) and true lesion size (dotted line).

Table 3. Percentage error of the segmented lesions: μ is the mean and σ is the standard deviation, both on 25 samples.

Sphere Diameter	FFDMUS	HHUS
5 mm	μ = 34.18 %	μ = 36.3 %
	σ = 3.4 %	σ = 4.5 %
3 mm	μ = 28.85 %	μ = 31.98 %
	σ = 4.42 %	σ = 4.0 %

$$Error = \frac{A_{observed} - A_{ideal}}{A_{ideal}} \tag{1}$$

where $A_{observed}$ is the area of observed lesion, and A_{ideal} is the area of ideal lesion. The area is computed using:

$$A = \sum_{i=1}^{N} \sum_{j=1}^{M} I_{i,j} \tag{2}$$

where $I_{i,j}$ is the pixel intensity from the segmented binary image of size N by M.

Figure 14 gives some examples of FFDMUS lesion with 3 mm diameter. First row is the original ultrasound region of interest (ROI). Second row shows a solid line representing the overlaid image with boundary segmentation, and a dotted line representing the true diameter of the spherical lesion.

The results of our performance evaluation are listed in Table 3. All numbers are compared with the ideal area and percentage error is computed using Eq. (1). We compare the FFDMUS with HHUS over 25 samples. For 5 mm diameter lesions: the mean percentage error and standard deviation for FFDMUS is 34.18% and 3.4%, while the mean percentage error and standard deviation for HHUS is 36.3% and 4.5% respectively. For 3 mm lesions: the mean percentage error and standard deviation for FFDMUS is 28.85% and 4.42%, while the mean percentage error and standard deviation for HHUS is 31.98% and 4.0% respectively. Taking the segmentation error into consideration, both cases show that the image qualities of the ultrasound from FFDMUS and HHUS are comparable.

3.3. X-Ray Image Quality Assessment

There are several image quality metrics that can be used to determine the impact of design changes required by the fused FFDMUS system. In this analysis, we shall consider modulation transfer function (MTF), detective quantum efficiency (DQE) and normalized noise power spectrum (NNPS).

The MTF describes the signal attenuation as a function of spatial frequency and is defined as the modulus of the Fourier transform of the line spread function. Mathematically it is defined as:

$$MTF(f) = \left|F[LSF(x)]\right| = \left|\frac{1}{\sqrt{2\pi}} \int_{-\infty}^{\infty} LSF(x)\, e^{i2\pi fx} dx\right| \tag{3}$$

where LSF(x) is the line spread function with free parameter x and f is the spatial frequency. The MTF is always scaled to unity at f=0. The LSF is the system response to a delta signal. The discrete representation of the MTF is:

$$MTF_{dis}(f) = \frac{1}{N}\left|\sum_{k=0}^{N-1} LSF(x_k)\, e^{i2\pi fx_k}\right| \tag{4}$$

where k is the sample number and N the total number of samples. The 2-D noise power spectrum (NPS) is mathematically defined as:

$$NPS(u,v) = \lim_{X,Y\to\infty} \frac{1}{XY} E\left\{\left|\iint_{XY} \sigma(x,y)\, e^{-2\pi i(ux+vy)} dxdy\right|^2\right\} \tag{5}$$

where $\sigma(x,y)$ is the standard deviation at point (x,y) and E stands for expected value. The typical technique for estimating the NPS for real images is based on averaging the power of the Fourier transform of noisy image samples taken from several images, or more routinely from a single noise image. The 1-D discrete representation of NPS is:

$$NPS_{dis}(u) = \frac{A_{pix}}{N_x N_y} \frac{1}{M} \sum_{i=0}^{M-1} \left\{\left|DFT\left(\sum_{n_y}^{N_y-1} \sigma_{n_x n_y}\right)\right|^2\right\} \tag{6}$$

The NPS in equation (6) is thus the average discrete Fourier transform of the average signal variation in the x direction scaled by the pixel size (A_{pix}) and the number of

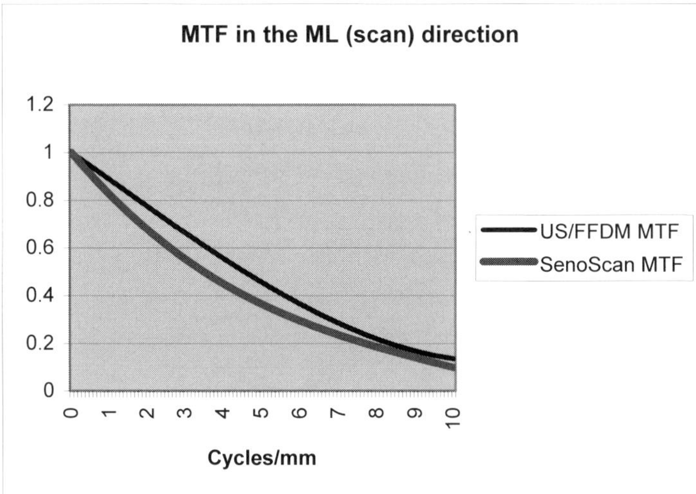

Figure 15. MTF in the medio-lateral direction.

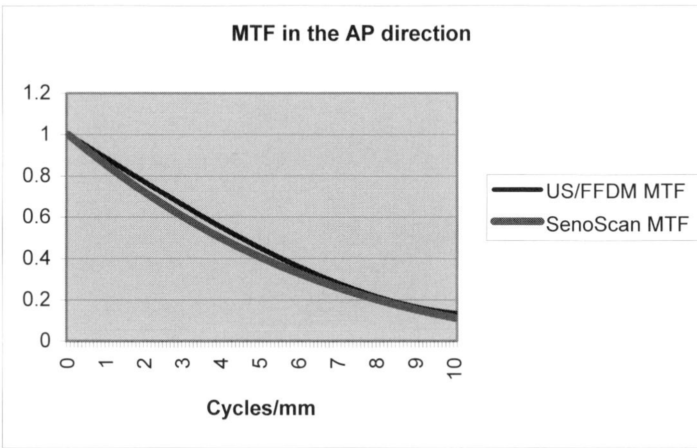

Figure 16. MTF in the anterior-posterior direction.

pixels under consideration (N_x x N_y) and M being the number of sub-images or samples under consideration.

We measured the MTF of the system in the directions parallel (medio-lateral (ML)) and perpendicular (anterior-posterior (AP)) to the X-ray scan. This is necessary to characterize any blur introduced by the scanning mechanism. We used the tilted edge method and analyzed the results according to the method of Fujita *et al*. [25]. The edge phantom consisted of 30 microns of lead embedded in acrylic for support. The edge was examined under an optical microscope to ensure it was smooth and free from defects. We compared the MTF of the FFDMUS system with those for a production qualified SenoScan®.

Figures 15 and 16 show the results of the MTF analysis for the ML and AP directions, respectively. The MTF results are actually superior to those reported for produc-

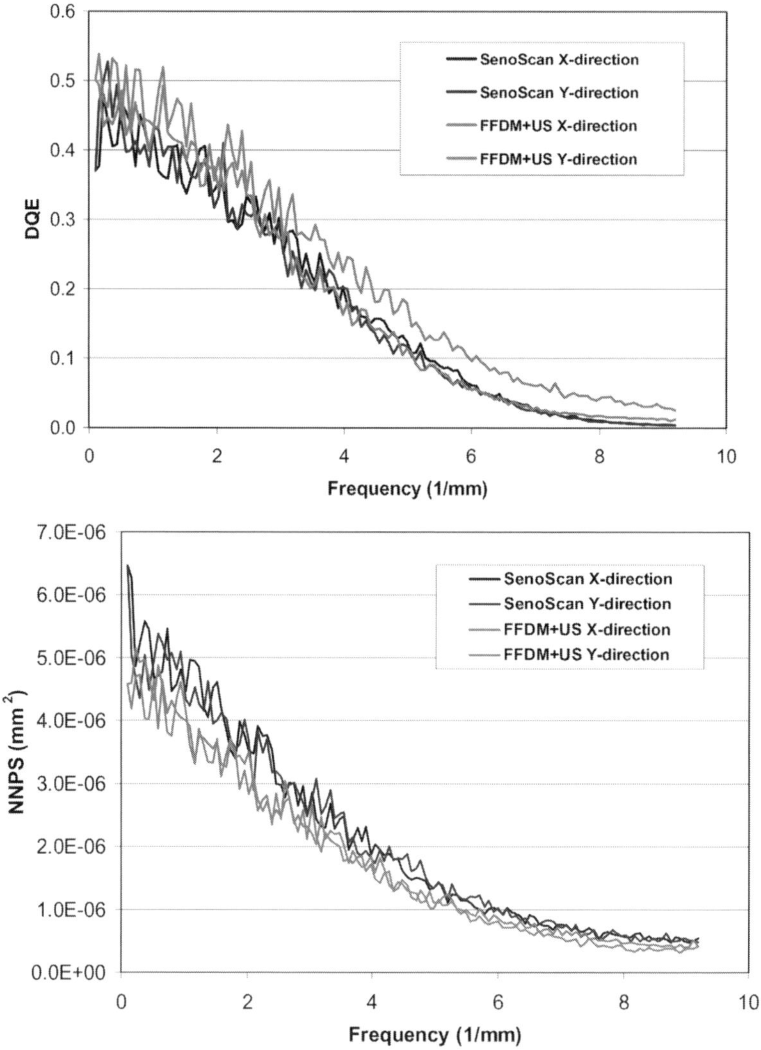

Figure 17. DQE and NNPS results. Top is DQE result, Bottom is NNPS result.

tion-qualified SenoScan® FFDM units. This improvement in MTF is due to several factors. The air gap between the scanning detector and the breast support is reduced, leading to a reduction in magnification effects in the MTF measurements. Additionally, linear scanning is used in the fused system, as opposed to a curved scan in the SenoScan®. Another factor contributing to the difference in MTF is the fact that the scan speed of the detector varies from unit to unit, and is manually optimized at installation.

Figure 17 demonstrates the experimental protocol followed for DQE and NNPS. The NNPS for the FFDMUS are lower than the SenoScan®, likely due to the slightly higher exposure used to obtain the FFDM+US measurement. (E= 6.9 mR and 6.6 mR for the FFDM+US and SenoScan® images respectively at 27 kVp and 150mA with 4.5 cm of PMMA). The DQE were similar for the two units except for the higher

FFDM+US values at the Y-direction for frequencies higher than 5 mm-1. This was likely due to the higher MTF values mentioned before.

Image quality tests on a laboratory prototype that combines X-ray and ultrasound breast scanning demonstrate that ultrasound images from FFDMUS are comparable to those from HHUS, and the X-ray images from FFDMUS are comparable those from SenoScan®.

4. Role of Advanced CAD for FFDMUS Prototype

In this section, we present CAD techniques developed under FFDMUS framework. Segmentation and registration techniques are combined into the FFDMUS to help the diagnosis.

4.1. Ultrasound Segmentation

The protocol for ultrasound image quality assessment is as follows: The system underwent the lesion segmentation from the user defined ROI samples drawn out of the 3-D ultrasound volumetric slices. The segmentation process consisted of binarization of the lesion ROI's which was implemented by computing the signal to noise ratio (SNR) of the ROI. The signal was estimated by computing the mean value of the signal in the ROI based on the method by Madsen *et al.* [22]. The noise was estimated in a background region where there was no lesion. The SNR was calculated using the following equation:

$$SNRL(j,k) = (S_L(j,k) - S_{MB}(j,k)) / (\sqrt{2}\sigma_B(j,k)) \tag{7}$$

where, S_L is calculated on the image with lesion, while S_{MB} and σ_B are computed from the image only with background material. The calculation of S_{MB} is based on a sample area pre-defined. The sample area acts as a moving window. The SNR region images were then binarized by automatic thresholding process based on Otsu's method [23]. These images underwent boundary estimation and were overlaid with gray scale ROI region image for visualization. The ultrasound segmentation procedure is illustrated in Fig. 18.

The ultrasound segmentation strategy has been used in Section 2, where the ultrasound quality from FFDMUS is compared to that from HHUS. The segmentation results are visually correct.

4.2. X-Ray Segmentation

Figure 19 shows the algorithm for X-ray lesion segmentation. Given an X-ray image, ROI with lesion was extracted first. Initial boundary was set around the lesion, and GVF-based snake was applied to converge to the final boundary [26–29]. Flood fill algorithm [30] was implemented to fill the region enclosed by the boundary points, which was the observed lesion area. Considering the noise generated in the procedure of image acquisition, PDE smoothing [31–34] was applied to the ROI first. We have shown that the PDE smoothing can improve the performance of GVF-snake based segmentation in X-ray images [35].

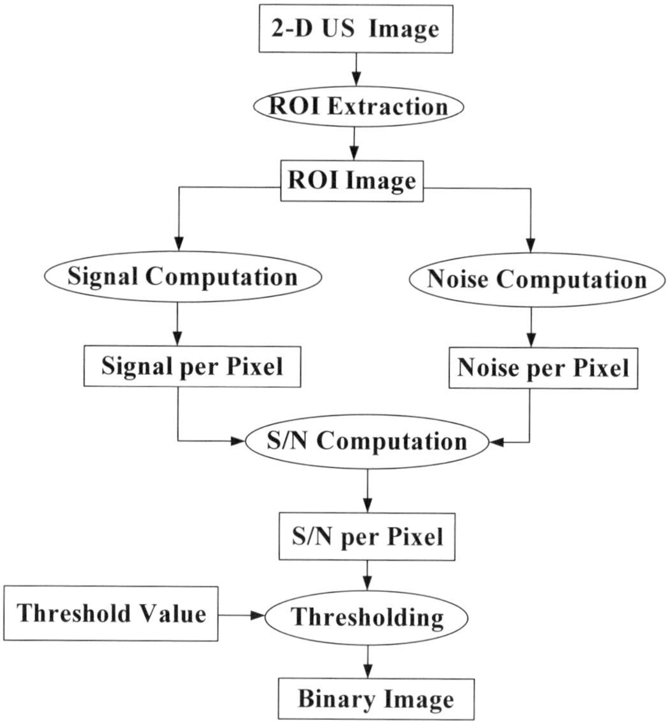

Figure 18. Ultrasound segmentation pipeline.

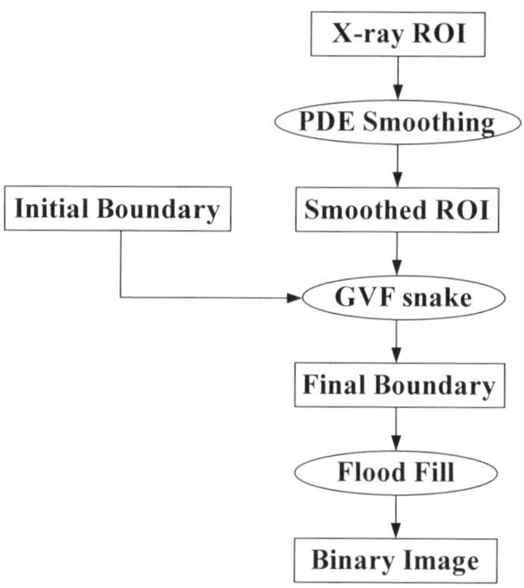

Figure 19. X-ray segmentation pipeline.

In the implementation of GVF, we used $\alpha = 0.6$ and $\beta = 0.0$ for all the snakes, $\mu = 0.2$. When the GVF is computed, the iteration is set to 60. The snakes were dynamically re-parameterized to maintain contour point separation to within 0.5–2.0 pixels. All edge maps used in GVF computations were normalized to the range [0, 1]. The

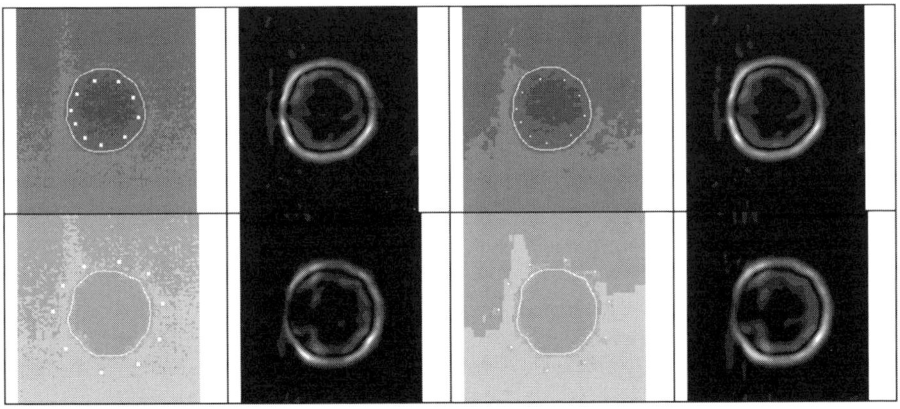

Figure 20. ROI samples with the boundary extracted before and after PDE smoother.

Gaussian blurring parameter σ is set to 3.5. The initial snake position is set manually. For each sample, two groups of points were picked around the visual boundary of the ROI with lesions, one inside and the other group outside. All the samples have two final boundaries extracted, starting from inside initial boundary or outside initial outside boundary. The parameters to be set in PDE smoother include constant K, time step t, and total number of iterations N. We used $K = 2.0$, $t = 0.1$ throughout the smoothing process. The iteration number $N = 140$, which is found to be optimal for X-ray segmentation (Suri *et al.* [35]).

Figure 20 shows the effect of PDE smoothing on GVF. The first column shows the segmentation results by running our GVF deformable model. The corresponding GVF force images are shown in column two. Note carefully that the initial boundaries in these images are complementary to each other (inside and outside). The third column shows the same noisy X-ray images but this time smoothed using PDE. The corresponding GVF forces are shown in column four. Note carefully that the GVF force images with PDE smoothed have crisper band around the central black edge. This is because PDE smoother had removed the background noise, thus the deformable model is less likely to bleed during the deformation (regaining the property of GVF). The number of iterations (n*) used for PDE smoothing was 140. The mean percentage error by GVF with PDE was 9.61%, showing an improvement of 7% over GVF without PDE.

4.3. Mutual Information Based Registration

Mutual information is derived from an information-theoretic approach to the dependence of one variable on another. It has been applied to medical image registration independently by Collignon *et al.* [36] and Wells *et al.* [37]. It is based on the shared information between the overlapping regions in the two images, which should be maximized at registration. Normalized mutual information was developed by Studholme *et al.* [38] and was proved to be a more robust similarity measure for the overlapping regions.

The definition of the mutual information I of two images A and B combines the marginal and joint entropies of the images in the following manner

$$I(A,B) = H(A) + H(B) - H(A,B) \quad (7)$$

where

$$H(A) = -\sum_a P_A(a)\log P_A(a) \quad (8)$$

$$H(B) = -\sum_b P_B(b)\log P_B(b) \quad (9)$$

$$H(A,B) = -\sum_a \sum_b P_{AB}(a,b)\log P_{AB}(a,b) \quad (10)$$

$P_A(a)$ and $P_B(b)$ denote the marginal distributions of the image intensities of A and B, respectively, and $P_{AB}(a; b)$ is their joint probability. $H(A)$ and $H(B)$ are the entropies of A and B, and $H(A;B)$ is their joint entropy, i.e., the entropy of the joint probability distribution of the image intensities.

It was shown that the mutual information measure is sensitive to the amount of overlap between the images (Studholme *et al.* [38]). NMI was introduced to overcome this problem.

$$NMI(A,B) = \frac{H(A) + H(B)}{H(A,B)}$$

where $NMI(A,B)$ is the normalized mutual information between images A and B.

Figure 21 shows the NMI-based registration framework. The transformation parameters are updated until the optimal solution that maximizes NMI is reached. Put in the terminology of Brown *et al.* [39], the feature space is the raw intensity, the search space is the rigid transformations, the similarity measure is NMI, and the search strategy is a downhill simplex method [40]. Multi-resolution approach is applied too, which may improve speed, increase the capture range and is relatively robust [41–44].

Phantom images were acquired and registered in pairs. Altogether we have registered 30 pairs of phantom images. One phantom image was taken as source image, the second phantom image as target image, and the registration was applied. The transformation parameters (rotation and translations) were determined at the end of registration procedure. Figure 22 shows the registration result of one phantom pair. The left column is the overlay images of phantom pair, and the right column is the overlay of the corresponding outlines. The first row shows the overlays before registration, and the second row shows the overlays after registration. We can see the improvement after registration.

Since there is no ground truth to compare with the computed parameters, we developed a strategy to evaluate the registration error. We used GVF snake to segment the ROIs extracted from the target image and transformed source image. The center-of-gravity of segmented lesion was computed and the distance between the corresponding CGs was calculated. The ideal distance was zero when two regions were matched perfectly. Figure 23 shows one example of ROIs and their corresponding segmentation results.

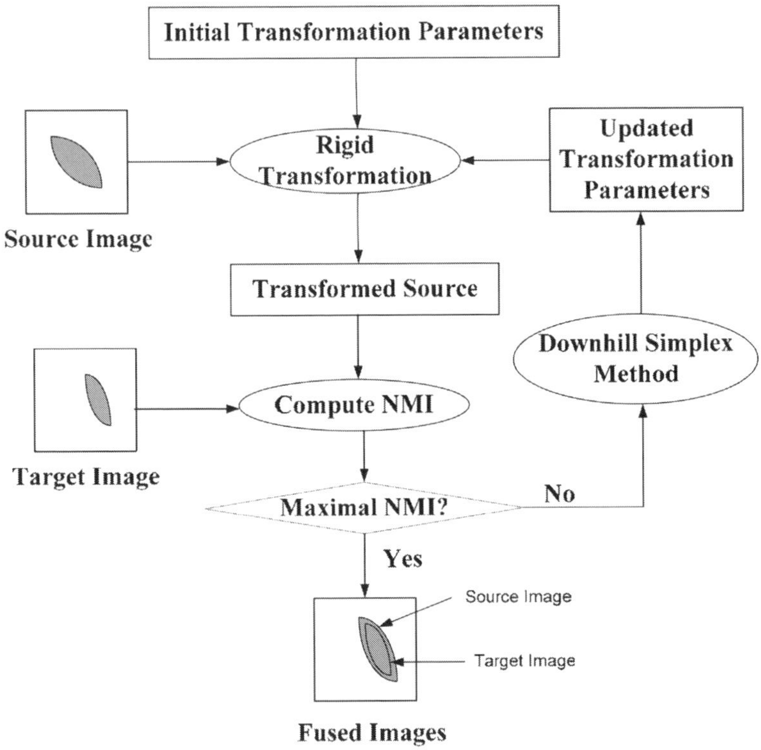

Figure 21. NMI-based Registration Framework.

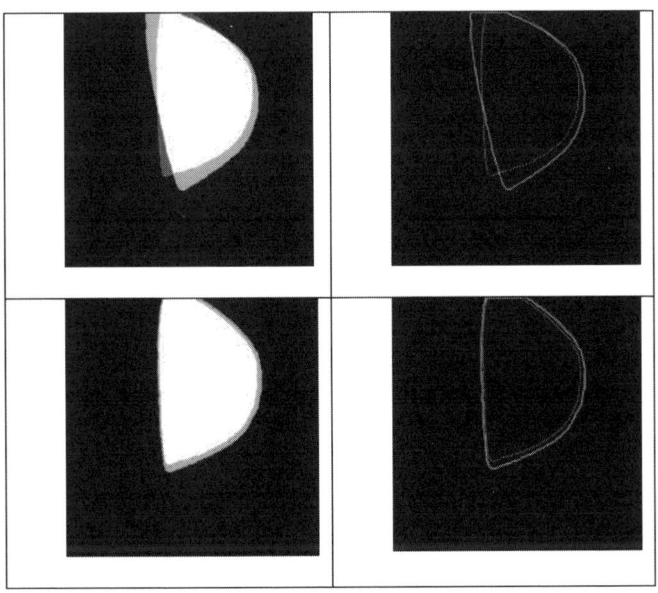

Figure 22. Overlaid images. First row: before registration; second row: after registration.

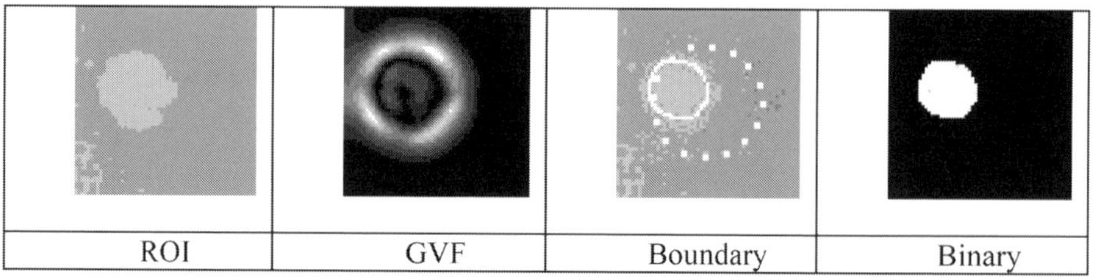

Figure 23. Segmentation of ROI extracted from phantom image. In the boundary image, dotted points were the initial boundary, and the solid line is the boundary detected. The binary image was used to compute the CG.

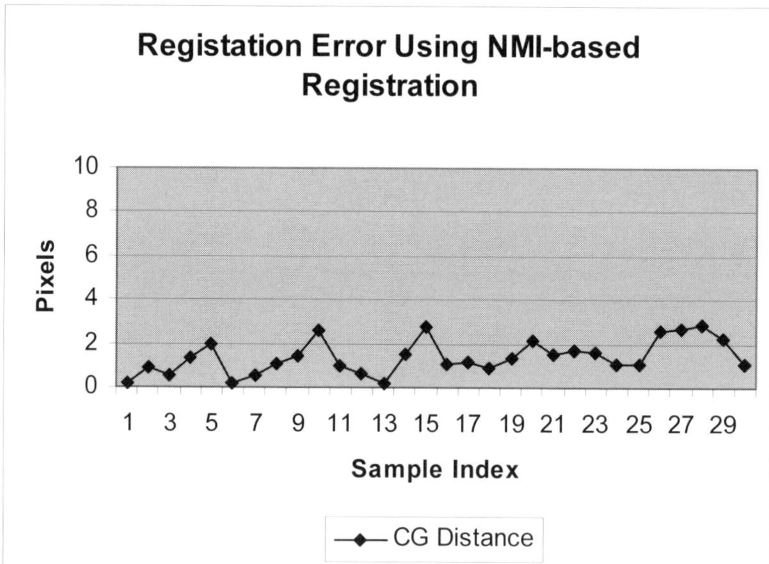

Figure 24. CG distance of ROIs after NMI-based registration (m = 1.39 pixels, s = 0.79 pixels).

The ROI extraction was applied to all the phantom images, with the same coordinates. The CG distance or the registration error curve from the phantom images registration using NMI-based method is shown in Fig. 24. Taking the segmentation error using GVF into consideration, the registration accuracy is satisfactory.

5. Conclusions

We have developed a new assembly under NIH grant to acquire 2-D X-ray mammogram and 3-D ultrasound slice simultaneously. The co-registration error is within 0.5 mm in AP direction, and 2.0 mm in the scan direction. We did an exhaustive performance evaluation and demonstrated that ultrasound image qualities from FFDMUS and Hand-held ultrasound (HHUS) are comparable, and the X-ray image qualities from FFDMUS and SenoScan® are also comparable. We also developed the CAD prototype combining segmentation and registration, and showed that the registration error is about 1.3 pixels. Our experimental results are promising.

Acknowledgments

This research is under support of NIH grant #2R44CA10059-02A1. The authors would like to thank Rob Entrekin (Philips Medical Systems) for CIRS Model 050 phantom ultrasound data acquisition.

References

[1] U.S. Department of Health and Human Service: http://www.4woman.gov/whw.

[2] Tabar, L., Vitak, B., Chen, H., Yen, M., Duffy, S. W., Smith, R. A., Beyond randomized controlled trials: organized mammographic screening substantially reduces breast carcinoma mortality. Cancer, Vol. 91, No. 9, pp. 1724–31, 2001.

[3] Tabar, L., Fagerberg, G., Chen, H., Duffy, S. W., Smart, C. R., Gad, A., Smith, R. A., Efficacy of breast cancer screening by age. New results from the Swedish Two-County Trial, Cancer, Vol. 75, No. 10, pp. 2507–17, 1995.

[4] Nishikawa, R. M., Computer-aided diagnosis complements full-field digital mammography. Diagnostic Imaging (San Franc), Vol. 21, No. 9, pp. 47–51, 1999.

[5] Warren Burhenne, L. J., Wood, S. A., D'Orsi, C. J., Feig, S. A., Kopans, D. B., O'Shaughnessy, K. F., Sickles, E. A., Tabar, L, Vyborny, C. J., Castellino, R. A., Potential contribution of computer-aided detection to the sensitivity of screening mammography. Radiology, Vol. 215, No. 2, pp. 554–62, 2000.

[6] Lewin, J. M., Hendrick, R. E., D'Orsi, C. J., Isaacs, P. K., Moss, L. J., Karellas, A., Sisney, G. A., Kuni, C. C., Cutter, G. R., Comparison of full-field digital mammography with screen-film mammography for cancer detection: results of 4,945 paired examinations. Radiology, Vol. 218, No. 3, pp. 873–80, 2001.

[7] Nass, S. J., Henderson, C., Lashof, J. C., Mammography and Beyond: Developing Technologies for the Early Detection of Breast Cancer, ed. Washington, D.C.: National Academy Press. 2001.

[8] Malur, S., Wurdinger, S., Moritz, A., Schneider, A. Comparison of written reports of mammography, sonography and magnetic resonance mammography for preoperative evaluation of breast lesions, with special emphasis on magnetic resonance mammography, Breast Cancer Res., Vol. 3, No. 1, pp. 55–60, 2001.

[9] Kapur, A., Krucker, J., Astley, O., Buckley, D., Eberhard, J., Alyassin, A., Claus, B., Thomenius, K., Myers, H., Rumsey, M., Johnson, R., Karr, S., Fusion of Digital Mammography with Breast Ultrasound – a Phantom Study, In Medical Imaging 2002: Physics of Medical Imaging. San Diego, CA: SPIE. 2002.

[10] Elbakri, I., Entrekin, R., Coad, C., Danielson, T., Janer, R., Integrated Full-Field Digital Mammography and 3-D Breast Ultrasound System, 46th AAPM Annual Meeting, July 25th – 29th, 2004.

[11] Elbakri, I., Entrekin, R., Coad, C., Danielson, T., Suri, J. S., Janer, R., Integrated X-ray and Ultrasound Breast Imaging Using Fischer Imaging's SenoScan Full Field Digital Mammography Scanner, Radiological Society of North America, 2004.

[12] Suri, J. S., Guo, Y., Coad, C., Elbakri, I., Entrekin, R., Kwan, A., Boone, J., Janer, R., Image Quality Assessment of Fused Full Field Digital Mammography and Ultrasound Imaging System (FFDMUS), Workshop on Alternatives to Mammography, September 18th – 20th, 2004, Winnipeg, Manitoba, Canada.

[13] http://www.cirsinc.com/productlist.html.

[14] Tradup, D.J., N.J. Hangiandreou, and J.P. Taubel, Comparison of ultrasound quality assurance phantom measurements from matched and mixed scanner-transducer combinations. J Appl Clin Med Phys, 2003. 4(3): p. 239–47.

[15] Dudley, N.J., *et al.*, A review of two alternative ultrasound quality assurance programmes. Eur J Ultrasound, 2001. 12(3): p. 233–45.

[16] Kanal, K.M., J.M. Kofler, and D.S. Groth, Comparison of selected ultrasound performance tests with varying overall receiver gain and dynamic range, using conventional and magnified field of view. Med Phys, 1998. 25(5): p. 642–7.

[17] Burke, E., QA in the vascular ultrasound lab. Radiol Technol, 1996. 67(3): p. 253–6.

[18] Trier, H.G., [Functional properties of diagnostic ultrasound instruments. A concept of trial building blocks for implementing quality assurance]. Ultraschall Med, 1994. 15(5): p. 223–32.

[19] Walker, J.B., G.C. Thorne, and M. Halliwell, Quality assurance of ultrasound imaging instruments by monitoring the monitor. Phys Med Biol, 1993. 38(11): p. 1601–9.

[20] Evans, J.A., *et al.*, Routine quality assurance of high frequency ultrasound breast scanners in a screening context. Br J Radiol, 1993. 66(787): p. 614–8.
[21] Metcalfe, S.C. and J.A. Evans, A study of the relationship between routine ultrasound quality assurance parameters and subjective operator image assessment. Br J Radiol, 1992. 65(775): p. 570–5.
[22] Madsen, E., Zagzebski, J., Frank, G., Rownd, J., Automated system and method for testing resolution of ultrasound scanners. Patent US 5,574,212, 1996.
[23] Otsu, N., A threshold selection method from gray level histograms. IEEE Trans. Systems, Man and Cybernetics, Vol. 9, pp. 62–66, March 1979.
[24] Haralick, R. M., Shapiro, L., Computer and Robot Vision, Addison-Wesley, 1991.
[25] H Fujita *et al.* A simple method for determining the modulation transfer function in digital radiography. IEEE Trans. Med. Imaging, 11(1):34–39, 1992.
[26] Kass, M., Witkin, A., Terzopoulos, D. Snakes: Active contour models, Int. J. Comput. Vis., Vol. 1, pp. 321–331, 1987.
[27] Ojala, T., Näppi, J., Nevalainen, O., Accurate segmentation of the breast region from digitized mammograms, Computerized Medical Imaging and Graphics, Vol. 25, pp. 47–59, 2001.
[28] Wirth, M. A., Stapinski, A., Segmentation of the Breast Region in Mammograms Using Snakes, 1st Canadian Conference on Computer and Robot Vision (CRV'04), pp. 385–392, 2004.
[29] Xu, C., Prince, J., Snakes, Shapes, and Gradient Vector Flow, IEEE Transactions on Image Processing, Vol. 7, No. 3, pp. 359–369, 1998.
[30] Foley, J. D., Van Dam, A. Feiner, S. K., Hughes, J. F., Computer Graphics in C: Principles and Practice, 2nd edition, Addision-Wesley, 1996.
[31] Perona, P., Malik, J., Scale-space and edge detection using anisotropic diffusion, IEEE Trans. In Pattern Analysis and Machine Intelligence, Vol. 12, No. 7, pp. 629–639, 1990.
[32] Suri, J. S., Laxminarayan, S., PDE & Level Sets: Algorithmic Approaches to Static & Motion Imagery, Kluwer Academic / Plenum Publishers, ISBN#: 0-306-46678-3, 2002.
[33] Suri, J. S., Liu, K., Laxminarayan, S., Zeng, X., Reden, L., Shape Recovery Algorithms Using Level Sets in 2-D/3-D Medical Imagery: A State-of-the Art Review, IEEE Trans. Info. Tech. in Biomedicine, Vol. 6, No. 1, pp. 8–28, 2002.
[34] Suri, J. S., Wu, D., Reden, L., Gao, J., Singh, S., Laxminarayan, S., Modeling Segmentation via Geometric Deformable Regularizers, PDE and Level Sets in Still and Motion Imagery: A Revisit, International Journal of Image and Graphics, Vol. 1, No. 4, pp. 681–734, 2001.
[35] Suri, J. S., Guo, Y., Danielson, T., Janer, R., Effect of PDE-based Noise Removal on GVF-based Deformation Model on Lesion Detection in Breast Phantom X-ray Images from Fischer's Fused FFDM and Ultrasound (FFDMUS) Imaging System, Accepted by SPIE 2005.
[36] Maes, F., Collignon, A., Vandermeulen, D., Marchal, G., Suetens, P., Multimodality image registration by maximization of mutual information, IEEE Transactions on Medical Imaging, Vol. 16, No. 2, pp. 187–198, 1997.
[37] Wells, W., Viola, P., Atsumi, H., Nakajima, S., Kikinis, R., Multimodal volume registration by maximization of mutual information, Medical Image Analysis, Vol. 1, No. 1, pp. 35–51, 1996.
[38] Studholme, C., Hill, D., Hawkes, D., An overlap invariant entropy measure of 3d medical image alignment, Pattern Recognition, Vol. 32, No. 1, pp. 71–86, 1999.
[39] Brown, L. G., A survey of image registration techniques, ACM Comput. Surv., Vol. 24, pp. 325–376, Dec. 1992.
[40] Press, W. H., Flannery, B. P., Teukolsky, S. A., Vetterling, W. T., Numerical Recipes in C, Cambridge University Press, 1988.
[41] Studholme, C., Hill, D., Hawkes, D., Automated 3D registration of MR and PET brain images by multiresolution optimization of voxel similarity measures, Medical Physics, Vol. 24, No. 1, pp. 25–36, 1997.
[42] Maes, F., Vandermeulen, D., Suetens, P., Comparative evaluation of multi-resolution optimization strategies for multimodality image registration by maximization of mutual information, Medical Image Analysis., Vol. 3, No. 4, pp. 373–386, 1999.
[43] Pluim, J., Maintz, J., Viergever, M., A multiscale approach to mutual information matching, Medical Imaging 1998: Image Processing, SPIE Vol. 3338, pp. 1334–1344, 1998.
[44] Lester, H., Arridge, S. R., A survey of hierarchical non-linear medical image registration, Pattern Recogn., Vol. 32, No. 1, pp. 129–149, 1999.

Symposium on Telehomecare

Medical and Care Compunetics 2
L. Bos et al. (Eds.)
IOS Press, 2005

Freeband: The Research Program for Ambient Intelligent Communication

Daan VELTHAUSZ, Program Director Freeband
Telematica Instituut, The Netherlands

Abstract. People today are surrounded by communication means. The last few decades have lead to an explosion of different means of communication. We are on the edge of a new 'paradigm change' which will move the centre of information control to the individual. He will become surrounded by "intelligent" electronic equipment that can provide almost all of their information and communication needs on demand: an ambient intelligent environment.

Keywords. Ambient intelligent communication, 4G telecommunication, technology, networking, service provisioning, generic user interaction, society, users, applications, healthcare

Freeband[1] is a national research program on mobile, personalised communication solutions, which comprises more than 30 organisations, including all-important technology providers and many representative end-user organisations. The vision for Freeband for 2010 is to consider communication and information transfer from the perspective of the user, not the provider.

Freeband addresses the entire knowledge chain of the new user-centric, ubiquitous communication paradigm. New knowledge is needed in the most important components of that chain, including:

- Enabling Technologies: No new services emerge without adequate technology; conversely, it is the technology that drives the new paradigms! We need e.g., new electronic and optical technology for broadband wireless access, house networking, optical switching, body area networks.
- Networking, Service Provisioning and Generic User Interaction: The telecommunication infrastructure viewed from the user's perspective, what are the networks and service platforms of the future?
- Society, Users and Applications: What are the new possibilities in different sectors for ubiquitous communication and ambient intelligence? What do they pre-suppose as knowledge and how can they be realised?

Freeband is especially active in the healthcare domain, researching and stimulating the use of the ambient communication paradigm to enable new applications and ways of working in healthcare practice, i.e. focusing on *Cure* (tele monitoring, tele treatment), *Care* (at home, tele care, integrated healthcare) and *Well being* (preventive, we- and family-centric). This is briefly outlined below.

---

[1] www.freeband.nl.

Teletreatment

The teletreatment initiative investigates and demonstrates the feasibility of free health treatment concepts, meaning a treatment independent of time and place utilizing a mobile service infrastructure. An important challenge in the teletreatment concept is the distribution of the intelligence in the network; i.e. to develop mechanisms within the service platform for a flexible distribution of sensing functionality, feedback and control functions and information processing algorithms. This will require a modular design of the signal processing and data interpretation chain, enabling a distributed processing which has to be optimized in relation with the bandwidth of the network and the required service level. The gained knowledge and experience will be applicable in a wide range of health care applications involving monitoring and remote treatment. The activities will be focused on Teletreatment of patients with chronic pain and will be carried out in close collaboration with rehabilitation centre Het Roessingh and homecare organization Enschede Haaksbergen.

We-Centric Services

We-centric healthcare research focuses on supporting chronically diseased patients and their professional and informal carers. Within this increasingly growing target group it is interesting to focus on elderly people who suffer from dementia. This is an interesting target group because aging presents the healthcare system with considerable challenges. Due to factors as scarcity of professionals, limited availability of homes for the elderly, and the preference of elderly to stay in their own environment as long as possible, there is a growing need for support of elderly people living in the community and their carers. We-centric service bundles may support patients in coping with their dementia, informal carers with conducting their care activities, and care professionals with supporting patients and informal carers.

Medical and Care Compunetics 2
L. Bos et al. (Eds.)
IOS Press, 2005

Use of Information and Communication Technology in Health Care

Hermie J. HERMENS[a,b], Miriam M.R. VOLLENBROEK-HUTTEN[a], Hans K.C. BLOO[a] and Rianne H.A. HUIS IN 'T VELD[a]
[a]*Roessingh Research and Development*
[b]*University of Twente*

Abstract. This report describes the possibilities of information and communication technology in healthcare. Attention is paid of how ICT can support the communication between health care professionals mutually as well as the communication between professionals and patients. Besides this some barriers that hampers implementation in everyday healthcare practice are described.

Keywords. Information availability, teleconsultation, telemonitoring, teletreatment

Introduction

There is an increasing pressure on the quality and finance of our health care system. Especially the increasing numbers of elderly and patients with chronic complex disorders who are structural dependent of care of others are responsible for this phenomenon. In the care for these patients a lot of professionals and disciplines are involved which complicates the health process. As a consequence load increases for the health care institutes whereas their capacity decreases and this leads to longer waiting lists. In order to reduce waiting lists, a considerable amount of patients will be dismissed quite earlier from the institutes with diffuse treatment advices. Other professionals get involved in treatment of these patients and care often becomes inefficient because there is a lack of tuning and cooperation between the different health care professionals and institutes.

Information and Communication Technology can bring solutions for these problems. The increasing availability of low-cost mobile devices, ad-hoc and managed wireless networks and broadband services that give access to large volumes of information offer new and unique opportunities for our health care system to increase its efficiency and effectiveness. Especially to improve the communication, in a broad sense, between professionals mutually and between the patient and the professional.

Methods

Different projects have and are performed to gain knowledge about the possibilities of ICT improve the communication, in a broad sense, between professionals and between the patient and the professional.

In more detail these projects concerns:

1. Communication between professionals mutually:

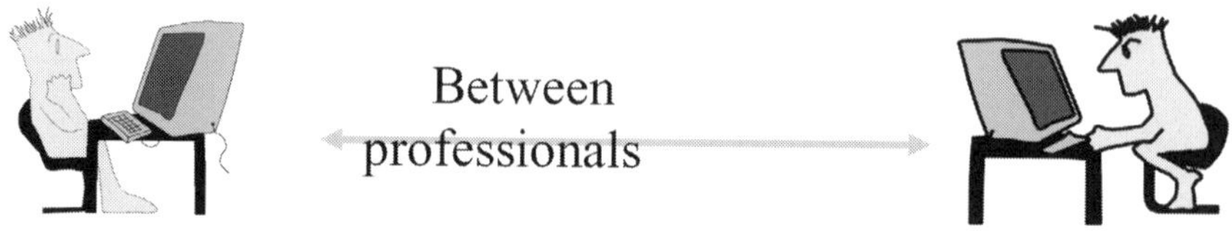

Examples are:

a) Applications that focus on the availability of patient information any place, any time (Telecare [1]).

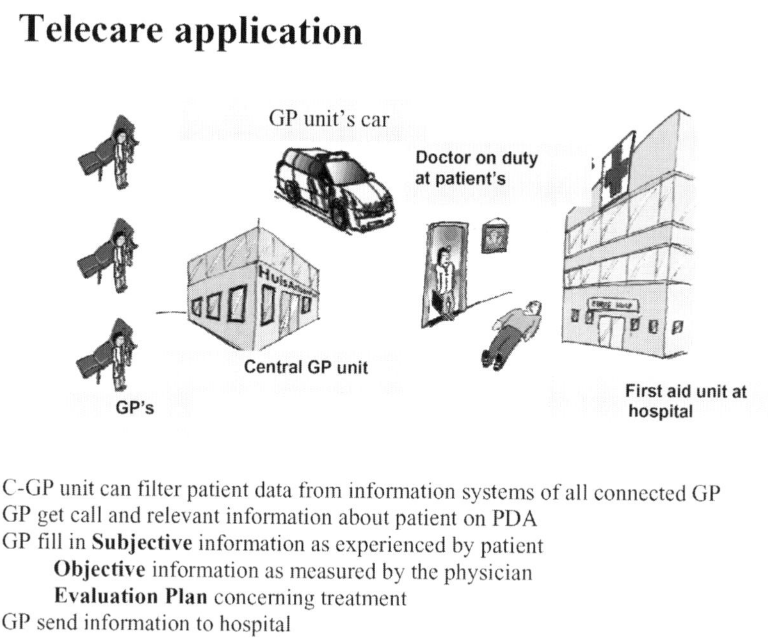

Figure 1. This figure shows the results of the Telecare project that was aimed a providing availability of patient data anywhere, anytime for general practitioners involved in the acute care around patients with a possible cerebro vascular accident (CVA).

b) Applications that focus on consultation between health care professionals (Mesh, Telefysi [2]).

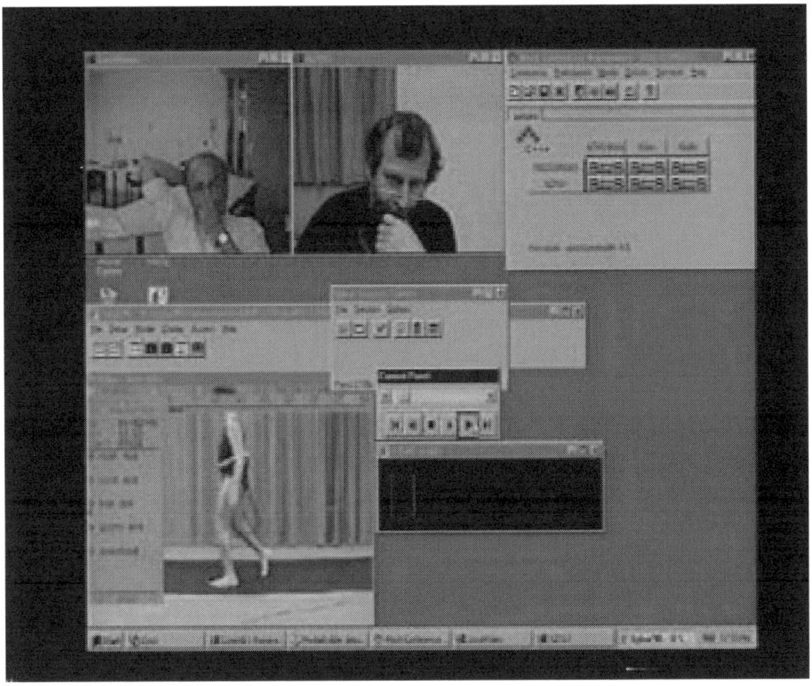

Figure 2. This picture show two rehabilitation physicians at different institutes discussion a patient by simultaneous looking at the movement patterns and other relevant kinematic parameters of this patient. This in order to come to adequate treatment operation advices.

2. Communication between professional and patient

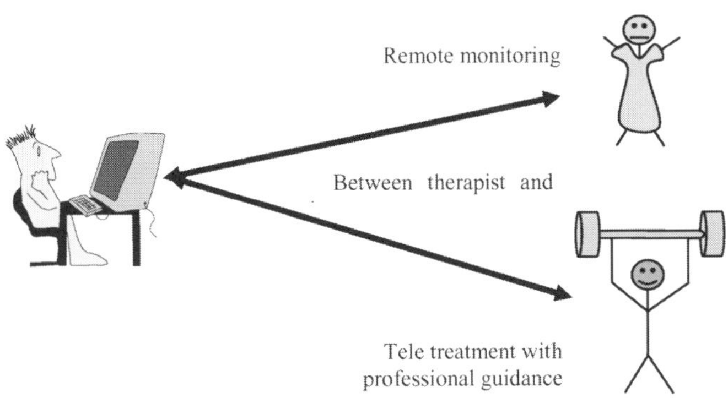

Examples are applications were patients can train their functions at their one place (home/work) at for him/her suitable times with professional guidance on distances or applications that monitor relevant body signals of the patients, guards the patient on distance and deliver care when necessary (exozorg [3], awareness).

The advantages of such teletreatment/monitoring services are 1:n relationships, more freedom for patients 'at risk', the patient is more responsible for effects of training, better translation to every day live and thus more effective treatment.

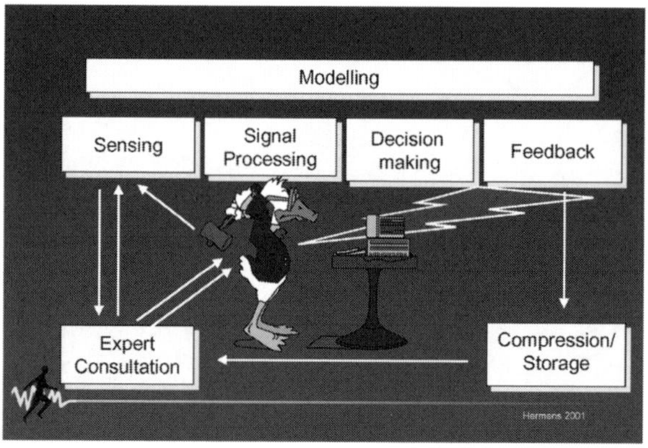

Figure 3. This figure shows a subject exercising his motor skills. His movements and other relevant characteristics are sensed and processed. Based on a comparison with training targets it is decided whether and what kind of feedback the subject gets on his performance. Simultaneously relevant data are stored and sent to a remote health care center that is able to monitor the training and to adjust the equipment anytime and anywhere. The patient will be regularly contacted to discuss the progress.

Discussion

Many initiatives have been developed showing the working mechanisms of ICT based services in clinical practice and it is the assumption that ICT can play a role in improving efficiency and effectiveness of care. Efficiency is enhanced by information exchange between professionals and by enabling 1:n relationships in telemonitoring and /or teletreatment. More effective treatment when treatment is brought at home and is likely to become more intensive. However despite these many initiatives new innovative treatments and treatment supporting concepts using ICT do hardly find their way to every day care. Reasons for this might be:

- Lack of funding for the validation part in real clinical practice.
- Health care professionals are involved only marginal; a lot of projects are 'technology driven'
- Lack of facilities to test new developments
- Lack of adequate financial arrangements from insurance companies for innovative ICT services.

Based on this it can be concluded that in new innovative treatments and treatment supporting concepts it is very important to look forward towards implementation. Health care professionals and other stakeholders need to be involved and much more adequate scientific validation studies need to be performed [4].

References

[1] Huis in 't Veld M.H.A, van Til J.A, Ijzerman M.J, Vollenbroek-Hutten M.M.R, Preferences of GPs regarding an integrated wired and wireless ICT application in acute stroke care: an illustration of an choice based conjoint analysis, Journal of Telemedicine and TeleCare Supplement, 2004 in press.

[2] L.Engbers, H. Bloo, R.Kleissen, J.Spoelstra, M.Vollenbroek-Hutten. Development of a teleconsultation system for communication between physiotherapists concerning children with complex movement and postural disorders. Journal of Telemedicine and Telecare 2003, 9: 339–343.

[3] Dijk H van, Hermens HJ. Distance training for the restoration of motor function. Journal of Telemedicine and Telecare 2004; 10: 63–71.

[4] Huis in 't Veld M.H.A, van Dijk H., Hermens, H.J., Vollenbroek-Hutten M.M.R., The methodology of telemedicine evaluation in patients with postural and movement disorders; a systematic review, Journal of Telemedicine and TeleCare, submitted.

Medical and Care Compunetics 2
L. Bos et al. (Eds.)
IOS Press, 2005

A Dynamic Interactive Social Chart in Dementia Care

Attuning Demand and Supply in the Care for Persons with Dementia and their Carers

R.M. DRÖES[a], F.J.M. MEILAND[a], C. DORUFF[b], I. VARODI[b], H. AKKERMANS[c], Z. BAIDA[c], E. FABER[d], T. HAAKER[d], F. MOELAERT[d], V. KARTSEVA[e] and Y.H. TAN[e]

[a]*Dept. of Psychiatry, VU medical centre, Valeriusplein 9, 1075 BG Amsterdam*
rm.droes@vumc.nl
[b]*Waag Society, Nieuwmarkt 4, 1012 CR Amsterdam*
[c]*Dept. of Business Informatics, Vrije Universiteit, De Boelelaan 1081a, 1081 HV Amsterdam*
[d]*Telematica Instituut, Brouwerijstraat 1, 7523 XC Enschede,*
[e]*Dept. of Economics and Business Administration, Vrije Universiteit, De Boeleaan 1105, 1081 HV Amsterdam*

Abstract. We-centric services may play an important role in the field of care and support for elderly persons with dementia and their carers. They may solve problems, such as fragmentation of care, gaps in the continuum of care and welfare services, and inefficient and uncustomized service delivery to patients and carers. In the FRUX Health Care pilot opportunities for we-centric, context-sensitive service bundles in the field of dementia care will be explored. The service on which we focus in this paper is a dynamic interactive social chart for dementia care (DEM-DISC). The feasibility of DEM-DISC will be investigated from a domain specific content perspective (needs, offerings, information and advice), an ICT perspective (ontology and application), a user perspective (persons with dementia, their carers and professionals/organizations), and an organisational perspective (necessary collaboration, governance and control, business modelling). A first demonstrator (validator) of the DEM-DISC will be designed, built and evaluated. Future possibilities to connect DEM-DISC to actual service delivery will be explored. In this paper we discuss the most important research questions from the different perspectives and the methods used to answer them.

Keywords. Dementia, (in)formal carers, we-centric services, context aware, dynamic service-bundling, user-experience, social chart

Introduction

The main objective of the project Freeband User eXperience (FRUX) is to advance the understanding of design and provision of we-centric services and service bundles. We-centric services are ICT-based services that automatically adapt to changes in the context of user groups, and push information based on group profiles. These services facilitate interaction in dynamic social networks and enable meaningful and rewarding user experiences. In the FRUX project the focus is on two issues in designing and delivering we-centric services, namely 1) context awareness, and 2) service bundling. The aim of the Health Care pilot within the FRUX project is to investigate and develop new innovative (mobile) services to support elderly people with chronic diseases who live in the community, their informal carers (family and friends that care for the patient) and formal (professional) carers. This pilot will focus on people with dementia and their (in)formal carers.

1. Opportunities for We-Centric Services in the Care for Persons with Dementia

We-centric services may play an important role in the field of care and support for elderly persons with dementia and their carers, because this field faces a number of problems now and in the near future. These problems include, in the first place, the variation, fragmentation and continuous changing of care and welfare services in a region, both public and private. Clients and referrers cannot see the wood for the trees anymore and therefore tend not to utilize the broad spectrum of available services. Possible consequences are: not receiving the specific care and support one needs, unsafe situations, social isolation of patients and frustration, overburden and illness of carers. Thus, the need for a more transparent, easily accessible and integrated offer of healthcare and welfare services is growing.

Another problem (or challenge) is the generally recognized need to create a continuum of flexible care and welfare bundles in every region in the Netherlands, that dynamically meets the care needs and wishes of individual persons with dementia and their informal carers in the different stages of the disease. Understanding of the gaps in the present offer, requires insight into the care needs and wishes of this client group and their informal carers, as well as an up-to-date overview of regional (and national) services. Recently, a first step was taken to collect this type of information: a National Dementia Programme (NDP) was developed which describes needs of the target group and examples of potential care offerings [Meerveld et al., 2004]. This NDP was produced by order of the Ministry of Public Health, Welfare and Sports in response to the latest recommendations on dementia by the Health Council of the Netherlands [Health Council, 2002]. The NDP was based on literature review and interviews with persons with dementia and (in)formal carers. This resulted in 14 problem areas (including 'feeling something is wrong'; 'being afraid, angry and confused'; 'loss experiences'; 'miscommunication with professionals'). These problem areas were clarified and care solutions found by searching successful existing care programmes and interviewing professionals. The overview of needs and care solutions in the NDP provides a good starting point for understanding the needs of persons with dementia and their informal carers in the community. However, it was based on a small sample and especially the views of the patients themselves were underrepresented (only two patients were interviewed). This is likely to have resulted in an incomplete assessment of their needs [Hancock et al., 2003].

Finally, a problem in the field of dementia care is the expected growth of the group of elderly persons with dementia, and chronically ill people in general, and as a consequence the enormous increase of informal carers in coming decades. [Health Council, 2002]. To continue to offer these groups the care and support they need, it is necessary to increase our specificity and efficiency in delivering services. This means more specific, individualized and dynamic service bundling, tailored precisely to the needs expressed by the client system (patient and carers), and the development of we-centric services for formal and informal carers.

In the FRUX Health Care pilot opportunities for we-centric, context-sensitive service bundles in the field of dementia care will be further explored.

Illustrative example

Since her mother died in 2000 from cancer, Mary, a full-time high school teacher in biology, has been looking after her 90 year old, mildly dementing, grandmother who still lives in her own home. Every weekend she drives from her hometown to the village where her grandmother lives and does the necessary shopping and cleaning. When the weather permits it, they always go to the woods, which are close to the village, for a walk. Her grandmother enjoys the countryside very much. However, the last two years Mary has noticed that her grandmother was having more difficulty walking and was becoming more and more forgetful and disorientated. For example: she no longer recognized the places in the woods where they had been together many times. Sometimes her grandmother reacted in a hostile manner when Mary arrived somewhat later than usual because of traffic, and frequently Mary found the food she had bought the week before almost untouched in the refrigerator. When one of the neighbours called Mary twice in one week to complain about her grandmother knocking on their door, late in the evening, in her pyjamas (she was afraid in her own home!), Mary decided to call her grandmother's general practitioner (GP) for consultation. She told him she was worried about the situation and felt guilty that she couldn't stay with her grandmother more often. The GP promised her he would visit her grandmother as soon as possible and would discuss the situation with her. When after two weeks Mary still had not heard from the GP, she called him again. He then explained that he had very little time, but promised her he would contact the regional ambulant mental health care institute and ask them to visit her grandmother. Two weeks passed and, again, Mary heard nothing. She decided to call the mental health care institute herself. She managed to track down the right person and made an appointment for him to visit her grandmother two weeks later.

When the social psychiatric nurse finally came to visit her grandmother, at eleven o'clock in the morning, the old lady was very bright and friendly, did not seem disorientated at all and they had a lively conversation. As promised, Mary called the nurse the next day, He told her not to worry, because her grandmother was in very good shape for her age. However, she could use some support in the household and more social contact during the week. Mary was therefore advised to organize several hours of home care a week and to organize for meals on wheels to deliver frozen meals once a week. The nurse had discussed the possibility of day care, but her grandmother had refused resolutely. As advised by the nurse, the next day, from work, between classes, Mary called the Centre for Indications in Healthcare (CIZ), for information on how to get an indication for home care. They explained she had to fill in a request form that they would send to her by post. The request form had to be returned to the CIZ where they would assess the necessity of the request after a home visit at her grandmother's house. The request form had to be signed by her grandmother. That weekend Mary discussed the situation with her grandmother, who agreed that she could use some help around the house and finally signed the form of the CIZ.

When after three weeks, on a Monday morning, Mary received the indication letter from the CIZ, she immediately called – during her lunch break – the home care organisation to make appointments. She was informed that her grandmother could have only two hours support on Tuesday afternoons and one hour early Thursday mornings. There were many persons on the waiting list and Mary was told her grandmother was very lucky that she was as old as she was, because that made her a priority. The support could already start the following week. Mary thanked the woman several times and said that she was very happy that her grandmother would receive the proposed support so soon.

Mary was indeed very happy that she finally succeeded to arrange at least 'some' support for her grandmother after almost three months of worrying, calling, telephone calls from neighbours, and making appointments with the different professionals. That evening, for the first time in weeks, she could finally relax.

The example illustrates the negative consequences of the present fragmentation of care and welfare services on a micro (client, (in)formal carers, other referrers) and meso (inter-organisational) level, and shows, among other things, the shortage of care supply in a growing elderly population (macro level). The above described scenario would have been quite different, and probably much more efficient, if there had been appropriate we-centric and context-sensitive services, that could have informed and supported Mary to find the service bundle she and her grandmother needed at that time, and that also could have facilitated the case management process for the formal carers (f.i. the GP, social psychiatric nurse).

2. A Dynamic Interactive Social Chart for Dementia Care

The service on which we focus in this paper and that could start to address the problems mentioned above, is an intelligent interactive regional social chart that is easily accessible anywhere, anytime, anyplace and that, besides providing general information on care and welfare services to persons with dementia and their (in)formal carers, is also able to respond dynamically to their individual needs with customized care and support advices and services, in short: a *Dynamic Interactive Social Chart for Dementia care (DEM-DISC)*. This is not just an ordinary social chart with an overview of (addresses of) services in a region, as they already exist in several forms in the Netherlands (e.g. on the websites of Alzheimer Nederland and 2ZW), but a service that aims to

- improve the accessibility of healthcare and welfare offerings for the target group by providing a single point of entry to information on these services: anywhere, anytime, any place, including mobile we-centric services;
- enable users (patients, informal carers, professional referrers) to find the services that meet their specific needs in different stages of the disease;
- advise patients, informal carers and professional referrers about bundles of care and welfare services depending on the specific needs, wants, and individual context (customized and context-sensitive);
- provide (in)formal carers with we-centric services to facilitate, for example, information exchange and coordination (case management) needed to realize the service offering requested by users in time, and to provide informal carers and patients with relevant information and social support;
- create a collaborative business experience between the care and welfare organizations that offer services to this target group in a region.

In other words, an integrated healthcare and welfare service that operates at a *micro level* (to support people with dementia who live in the community and their (in)formal carers by providing information and advice in a user-friendly and context-

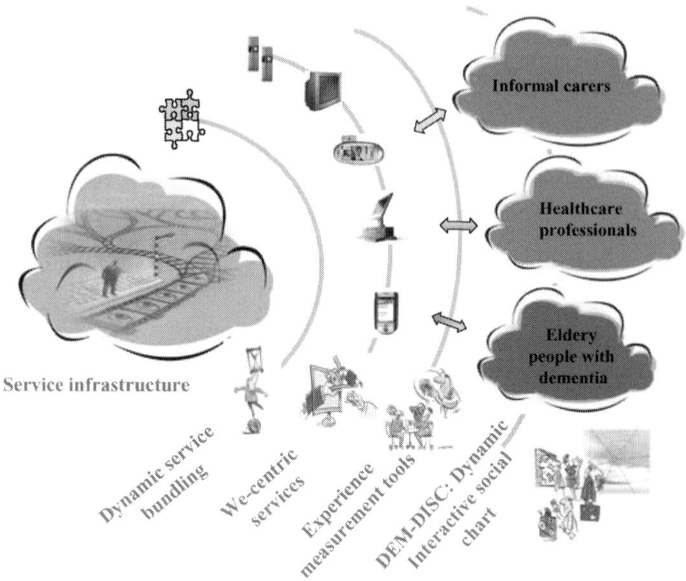

Figure 1. Dynamic Interactive Social Chart for Dementia care (DEM-DISC).

sensitive manner, as well as case management), at a *meso level* (to counteract the negative consequences of the fragmentation of services by informing and advising on possible service bundles if relevant, by stimulating the collaboration between regional care and welfare services and by detecting gaps in the continuum of services in a region), and at a *macro level* (to help people with dementia stay in their homes for a longer time, and thus contribute to a delay of nursing home admission and consequently a reduction in health care expenditure).

In the FRUX health care pilot the feasibility of such a dynamic interactive social chart for dementia care will be investigated from a domain specific content perspective (needs, offerings, information and advice), an ICT perspective (knowledge management and application), a user perspective (persons with dementia, their carers and professionals/organizations), and an organisational perspective (necessary collaboration, governance and control, business modelling). A first demonstrator (validator) of the dynamic interactive social chart will be designed, built and evaluated. Future possibilities to connect the DEM-DISC system to actual service delivery will be explored. In this paper we will discuss the most important research questions from the different perspectives and the methods used to answer them.

2.1. Domain Specific Content Perspective

DEM-DISC as described above should first of all contain a comprehensive dataset on needs of patients with dementia and informal carers formulated in the words potential users (patients, carers and professional referrers) would use, as well as a comprehensive, up-to-date dataset on care and welfare service offerings for this target group in a region. To inform/advise users on customized services and (alternative) service bundles, DEM-DISC must be able to take into account relevant personal and contextual information of its users. To find out what kind of new, mobile, we-centric services would be helpful to connect to DEM-DISC to fulfill (unmet) needs of patients and carers and/or fill gaps in the continuum of services in a region, knowledge on these unmet needs and gaps must be collected. To that end the following questions have to be answered:

1. What are the needs and demands of persons with dementia who live in the community and their carers, and which care and welfare services are offered in relation to those needs/demands?
2. Which characteristics of the patient, carer or care-giving situation are related to the needs and demands of persons with dementia and carers, and which characteristics are related to the preference for and utilization of specific care and welfare services?
3. Are persons with dementia and their carers satisfied with the care they receive or do they experience unmet needs? Where do gaps between needs/demands and care offerings seem to be located?

The (unmet) needs, as well as the characteristics possibly related to the needs and to preferences for specific services (including care recommendations of, for example, the care manager of the memory clinic), and the gaps between needs/demands and offerings, will be studied in an explorative cross-sectional design. Besides a review of the literature, persons with dementia who live in the community and their informal carers, and professionals/ experts in the field of care and welfare will be interviewed. To ensure a broad spectrum of needs in patients and carers (in different stages of the dementia process), 400 persons with dementia plus 400 informal carers will be recruited from three different settings:

- the memory clinic of the Alzheimer Centre of the VUmc in Amsterdam (50 new visitors and/or clients who visited the memory clinic in the past 3 months);
- the Centrum Indicatiestelling Zorg (CIZ) in Amsterdam (300 persons with dementia who received an indication for care 6 months ago);
- the Meeting Centres Dementia Support Programme (50 persons with dementia and their carers will be included from five meeting centres in Amsterdam (3) and Nijmegen (2)).

A sample of 45 professionals who are involved in the care of the selected persons with dementia and their carers in the above-mentioned settings will also be invited to participate in the inventory of (unmet) needs.

The inventory of the care and welfare offerings will be carried out in two regions: Amsterdam Zuid and Nijmegen. Besides studying relevant documents (of care and welfare offerings), key figures of regional care and welfare organizations that offer care and support to persons with dementia and their carers will be contacted individually for information on the services they provide.

Gaps in the regional offer will be traced by comparing the inventoried (unmet) needs with the present regional care and welfare offerings and with the needs and solutions as described in the NDP (NIZW, 2004).

2.2. ICT-Perspective

As DEM-DISC should be easily accessible anywhere, anytime and at any place by patients, carers and professionals, should provide the necessary information on the current care and welfare offer, and should provide we-centric services that fill the observed gaps between needs and offerings, a user-friendly application must be built that functions as an internet portal that is linked with the websites of all regional care and welfare services and coupled with newly proposed mobile we-centric services. To enable users to find customized and context-sensitive (bundles of) services, DEM-DISC should be able to connect (a) specific service (bundles) to the needs and demands expressed by users.

Important questions to be answered are therefore:

1. How can DEM-DISC be given form as an application (requirements, technology)?
2. How can relevant context information for DEM-DISC be gathered or measured and used within DEM-DISC?
3. What requirements for the user interface are needed to assure user friendliness?
4. How can user needs, context information and available (or to be developed) services be matched in viable dynamic service bundles?
5. What related mobile, we-centric services could fill the observed gaps in the regional care and welfare offer? What are the requirements of dementia patients and/or their (in)formal carers regarding we-centric services?
6. How can ICT help to measure user experience of we-centric services?

In answering these questions we make a distinction between Human-Computer Interaction and reasoning with domain knowledge. The requirements for the design of DEM-DISC and opportunities for other, related mobile ICT-supported we-centric services (e.g. alerts of care requests, joint scheduling of care activities, case management, contact with other patients and carers) will be studied by means of a literature review, field research, and interviews with patients, carers and key figures from regional care and welfare organizations that offer care and support to persons with dementia and their carers.

Question 4 is about reasoning with domain knowledge. To answer it, we apply structured knowledge-engineering techniques (CommonKADS, Schreiber et al., 2000) to the health domain. Specifically, we will use a semi-formal representation of domain knowledge – a so-called *ontology* – to describe customer needs and available services. This builds on earlier research on service bundling. A main advantage of ontologies is that they can be represented in a machine-interpretable form, so that software can use them to reason about a domain, in this case: about customer needs and available services. The ontology will use existing methods from the field of *Requirements Engineering* to link customer needs with available elementary services, so that the choice for a specific customer need will imply the provisioning of specific services to satisfy this need. Finally, a package (bundle) of elementary services will be designed to satisfy the customer need. We do this by using existing configuration theory, where complex components are created from smaller ones. This is achieved by describing services as components, according to configuration theory, so that service bundling is reduced to a task of component configuration. Regulatory legislation can be captured in the ontology as constraints on the bundling (configuration) process, so that no service bundles are suggested if they do not adhere to the law. This study will be used to build a validator of the DEM-DISC.

2.3. User Perspective

From a patient, carer and individual professional perspective it is very important that DEM-DISC offers, in a user-friendly and efficient manner, up-to-date, customized information on care and welfare services that can help patients face the problems they experience in daily life because of the dementia, and support carers in caring for a person with dementia. The information should include all regional services/offerings that might be useful in the different stages of the disease, as well as information on how to obtain those offerings. A potential future function of DEM-DISC that could be very helpful for carers is that it responds to service requests with direct service delivery. Mobile we-centric services will only be utilized by persons with dementia and/or his (in)formal carers if they experience them as truly supportive.

For care and welfare organizations DEM-DISC will be an important public relations medium if it contributes to reaching the target group for which they offer services, to creating a continuum of care in a region and to tracing gaps in the present care and welfare offer for persons with dementia and their carers.

Important questions to be answered from a user perspective therefore are:

1. How can DEM-DISC (including the connected mobile we-centric services) be brought into the homes of people who need it in a user-friendly manner?
2. Do users (patients, carers and professionals) find, and use, the information they searched for in DEM-DISC, and is the information experienced as useful, up-to-date and sufficiently customized? How can complaints be inventoried?
3. Does DEM-DISC help patients and carers to adapt to and cope with the consequences of dementia, and/or alleviate the caregiving task and burden of the informal carers? Does it have a preventative or therapeutic value?
4. Does DEM-DISC help organizations to keep the information on their services up-to-date? What methods could improve this?
5. What mobile we-centric services do potential users expect to be really supportive? How can user-experience be measured to evaluate those services?
6. Does DEM-DISC help organizations to reach their target group, to collaborate with other organizations by bundling services attuned to specific demands in the different stages of dementia, to create a regional continuum of care?

In order to make DEM-DISC and the connected we-centric mobile services user-friendly for the target group, the method of 'users as designers' will be used. To stimulate organizations to update their service information in DEM-DISC,organizations that neglect to update this information on a monthly basis, will be removed from the system after a warning procedure.

To study the impact of DEM-DISC on patients, carers, professionals and organizations, randomized controlled effect studies will be carried out in two regions (Amsterdam-Zuid and Nijmegen) among persons with dementia, carers and professionals/referrers who utilize, and who do not utilize the DEM-DISC. They will be recruited from the study population that participated in the needs inventory study (see Content perspective). Those who agree to participate in the effect study will be randomly assigned to the DEM-DISC group or the control group. In addition to the registration of patient and carer features, quantitative measurements will be carried out on several outcome variables in persons with dementia (behavior, mood, quality of life, nursing home admission) and their carers (feeling of competence, burden, way of coping, general health, depression). All variables will be measured with standardized instruments.

The number of nursing home admissions in the selected regions after implementation of DEM-DISC (and the connected mobile we-centric services) will be compared with the number of nursing home admissions before implementation in these regions.

To assess user experiences with DEM-DISC, persons with dementia, carers and professionals/referrers that actually used DEM-DISC will be interviewed.

2.4. Organisational Perspective

The viable exploitation of the DEM-DISC service in the future will require extensive collaboration and coordination between the participating care and welfare organizations in DEM-DISC. Apreliminary business model needs to be developed that describes how the organizations could cooperate to offer and maintain DEM-DISC. This includes governance and control, financial arrangements and legal boundaries. The proposed (alternative) service bundles suggested by DEM-DISC should not be in conflict with current rules and legislation.

Important questions to be answered are therefore:

1. What are the impacts of health-specific legislation and current (legal) organizational and financial arrangements on the options for service bundles and associated business models?
2. Is it possible to connect DEM-DISC with actual service delivery in the future? What are the present possibilities and obstacles, for example, with respect to legislation and financing?
3. What viable business models exist for DEM-DISC?

To answer question 1, domain-specific knowledge on legislation and current organizational and financial arrangements will be collected by interviewing relevant professionals in this field, studying the existing literature on the subject and utilizing the currently applied software. As mentioned, this knowledge will be incorporated in the ontology as constraints.

Additionally, to analyze the impact of current legal, organizational and financial arrangements in the health-care sector on the social chart, several business scenarios of the social chart will be analyzed. The first business scenario will represent the current business model of the health-care sector, including such parties as different healthcare and welfare service organizations, healthcare offices (in Dutch: *"zorgkantoor"*), and other parties, whose activities impact the potential users of the social chart. Furthermore, starting with the current situation, several future business scenarios for social chart will be examined, including the analysis and design of necessary governance mechanisms. For this we will apply the business modeling methodology *e^3-value* [Gordijn, 2002; Gordijn and Akkermans 2003] to describe and analyze business scenarios and the extended version of *e^3-value* [Kartseva, Tan and Gordijn, 2005] to design inter-organizational control mechanisms.

With respect to question 2 relevant key-figures in the field of care and welfare legislation will be interviewed to inventory possibilities for and obstacles to connecting DEM-DISC to actual service delivery in the future.

To study relevant business models existing methods for designing business models (FBBM [Haaker et al 2003]; [Haaker et al 2004] and e^3-value [Gordijn, 2002; Gordijn and Akkermans 2003]) will be used.

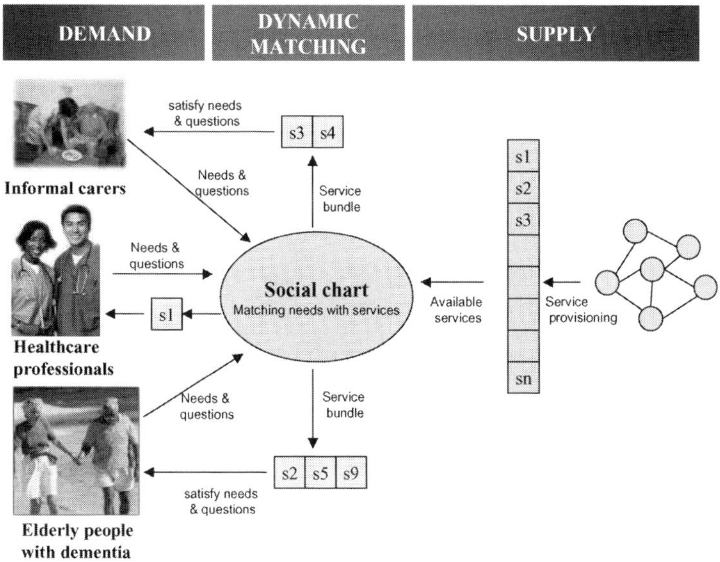

Figure 2. Creating a care continuum – bundling healthcare and welfare services.

3. Results and Conclusion

The results of the study will be published in reports and articles in scientific and professional journals, and presented at (inter)national symposia and congresses.

The main results will be: the design and implementation of the dynamic interactive social chart in dementia care coupled with mobile we-centric services, DEM-DISC; the validation of experience measurement tools, a service bundle configuration method in healthcare; business models, and outcome of the effect studies into the introduction of DEM-DISC and the developed we-centric services for patients and (in)formal carers.

This Health Care pilot of the FRUX project [FRUX flyer, 2004] started in February 2005 and will end in March 2008. The results will be published on the project website http://frux.freeband.nl.

Acknowledgement

This work is part of the Freeband FRUX project (http://frux.freeband.nl). Freeband is sponsored by the Dutch government under contract BSIK 03025.

References

[1] Meerveld, J., Schumacher, J., Krijger, E., Bal, R., Nies, H. (2004). *Werkboek Landelijk dementie Programma.* NIZW, Utrecht, The Netherlands.
[2] Health Council (2002), *Dementia.* Health Council, The Hague, The Netherlands.
[3] Hancock, G.A., Reynolds, T., Woods, B., Thornicroft, G., Orrell, M. (2003). The needs of older people with mental health problems according to the user, the carer, and the staff. *Int J Geriatr Psychiatry.* Sep;18(9):803–11.

[4] Schreiber, A. T., Akkermans, J. M., Anjewierden, A. A., Hoog, R. de, Shadbolt, N., Velde, W. van der, & Wielinga, B. J. (2000). *Knowledge engineering and management*. Cambridge, MA: The MIT Press.

[5] Haaker, T., Bouwman, H., Faber, E. (2004). *Customer and network value of mobile services: balancing requirements and strategic interests*. Paper presented at the International Conference on Information Systems (ICIS 2004), December 12–15 2004, Washington, DC, USA.

[6] Haaker, T., et al. (2003). *Freeband Business Blauwdruk Methode©: handleiding voor succesvol samenwerken bij het ontwikkelen en exploiteren van innovatieve (mobiele) ICT diensten.* Telematica Instituut, Enschede.

[7] Gordijn, J., Akkermans, J.M. (2003). Value based requirements engineering: Exploring innovative e-commerce idea. *Requirements Engineering Journal* (web version available), Springer Verlag, Vol 8, 2:114–134, 2003.

[8] Gordijn, J. *e3value in a Nutshell*. International workshop on e-business modeling, HEC Business School, Lausanne, 2002 (on invitation), PDF document.

[9] Kartseva, V., Gordijn, J., and Tan, Y. Towards a Modelling Tool for Designing Control Mechanisms in Network Organisations, *International Journal of Electronic commerce*, to be published, 2005.

[10] FRUX flyer 2004: http://frux.freeband.nl.

Medical and Care Compunetics 2
L. Bos et al. (Eds.)
IOS Press, 2005

Personal Networks Enabling Remote Assistance for Medical Emergency Teams

F.T.H. DEN HARTOG[1], J.R. SCHMIDT and A. DE VRIES
TNO Information and Communication Technology, The Netherlands

Abstract. Personal Networks provide the technology that is needed to interconnect the various private networks of a single user (home network, car network, office network, Personal Area Network, and others) seamlessly, at any time and at any place. This can be useful in many business sectors. In case of medical emergencies, it can provide a means to enlist remote assistance from peers wherever they are in the world at that particular moment. To illustrate this, we have analyzed the use case of a medical emergency surgery and have built a demonstrator.

Keywords. Personal network, medical emergency team, personal area network, mobility provider, personal network gateway

Introduction

Operating theatres are called like that because, in early times, students and other specialists could attend medical operations live, in an operating room with stands around the table (see Fig. 1). Because of modern demands on hygiene, today's surgeries are heavily protected environments with few facilities for physical communication with the outside world. Especially in cases of medical emergency, when there is little time to prepare the operation, this limits the amount of assistance the medical team can call upon.

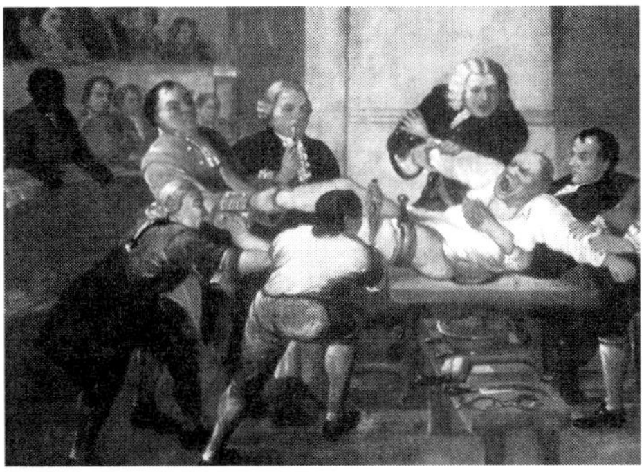

Figure 1. Surgery performed in the operating theatre of old St. Thomas Hospital, London, about 1775. Students and peers are physically present in the room to ask questions or to give helpful advice.

[1] Corresponding Author: TNO Information and Communication Technology, Brassersplein 2, P.O. Box 5050, 2600 GB Delft, The Netherlands; E-mail: F.T.H.denHartog@telecom.tno.nl.

Personal Networking technology can provide a means to enlist remote assistance from peers wherever they are in the world at that particular moment. Depending on the available networks and equipment, the peers can have voice, data and video communication with the operating room, and also remotely control the cameras that record the treatment.

This paper first discusses the general concept of Personal Networks, its various application domains, the current state of the technology and the research challenges ahead. In the second section we treat the use case of the medical emergency team in more detail and describe a demonstrator that we have built. In the final section we summarize the main conclusions and provide an overview of the user studies we are currently performing.

1. Personal Networks

1.1. The Concept of Personal Networks

Personal Networks (PNs) is a concept that has been introduced only recently [1,2]. It is based on the following trends:

- People possess more and more electronic devices, such as mobile phones, laptops, Personal Digital Assistants (PDAs), digital cameras, MP3 players, gaming consoles, digital video recorders, set-top-boxes, broadband modems, media centers, TV screens, desktop PCs, tablet PCs, PC accessories, navigation systems, DVD players, and white goods.
- More and more electronic devices have networking functionality that enables the device to share content, data, applications, and resources with other devices, and to communicate with the rest of the world.
- In the various private domains of the user (home, car, office, workplace, etc.) clusters of networked devices ("private networks") appear that indeed share content, data, applications, and resources with each other, and communicate with the rest of the world by means of a common gateway, for instance the broadband modem [3].
- With increasing wealth, people are becoming more mobile and carry an increasing number of (portable) electronic devices with them. Often these devices can relatively easily be connected to the public mobile network, but local interaction between them is still rather limited. In the near future, however, it is expected that these devices will form a Personal Area Network (PAN) with the help of recently developed Wireless Personal Area Networking (WPAN) technologies such as Bluetooth [4].

A PAN can therefore be defined as a network of devices in the personal operating space of the user. A schematic representation of a PAN is given in Fig. 2. The user is carrying a laptop, a PDA, a mobile phone, a wireless headset and a digital camera. The devices are networked with each other by means of high-data-rate WPAN technology (>200 kbps) [4], here depicted as "802.15". The mobile phone, the laptop and the PDA can also communicate to the rest of the world by means of Universal Mobile Telecommunications System (UMTS) technology or Wireless Local Area Network (WLAN) technology. This configuration enables e.g. pictures taken by the digital cam-

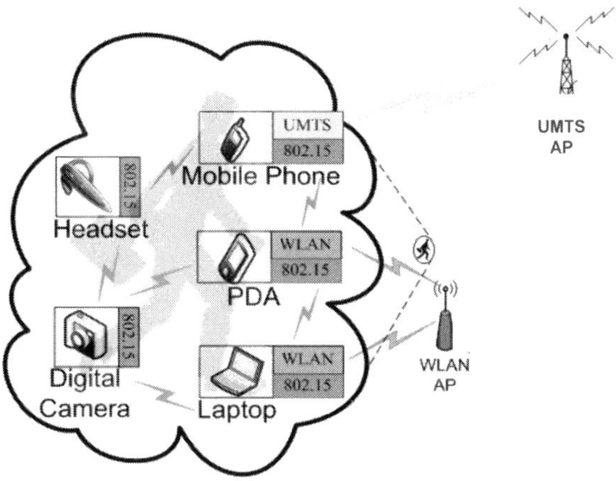

Figure 2. Example of a Personal Area Network.

era to be emailed by means of the email client on the PDA and the UMTS connection of the mobile phone.

A Personal Network (not to be confused with a Personal Area Network, or PAN), is envisaged as the next step in achieving unlimited communication between peoples electronic devices. A PN provides the technology needed to interconnect the various private networks of a single user seamlessly, at any time and at any place. Such private networks are, as mentioned before, home networks, car networks, company networks, PANs, and others. Often, a user wants to remotely access content, applications, or resources that are located in one of his private domains. For example, a business man who is at a conference wants to take pictures of the various demonstrators without having to worry where the pictures should be stored: on the memory card of the camera, the hard disc of the laptop, the content server in the office, or the desktop computer at home. A PN should solve the current limitations that inhibit (user-friendly) access to the personal devices that are not physically close to the user at the moment of need.

A schematic view of a PN is given in Fig. 3. In the figure, the clouds represent the various private and public infrastructures involved in creating a PN. The PN itself is drawn as an overlay over the multiple domains that should hide the underlying network and business complexity from the user. At the heart of the PN is the core-PAN, which is physically associated with the owner of the PN. The core-PAN consists of networked personal devices carried by the user. Depending on the location of the user, the core-PAN can interact with devices in its direct environment or with remote devices in the user's other private networks to create a PN. A key element of the core-PAN is therefore the PN Gateway (PNG). The PNG is the device that contains the functionality needed to create a PN from the core-PAN and the other private networks. This functionality might include, amongst others, local storage, local intelligence, and multiple wireless (mobile) access network interfaces. The PNG can be a single dedicated device, or added functionality of other devices in the core-PAN. In the example of Fig. 2, the PNG functionality is distributed over the laptop, PDA, and mobile phone.

Another important factor for enabling a fully functional PN will be the Mobility Provider (MP) [5]. The MP is not a device or a specific application, but a new business

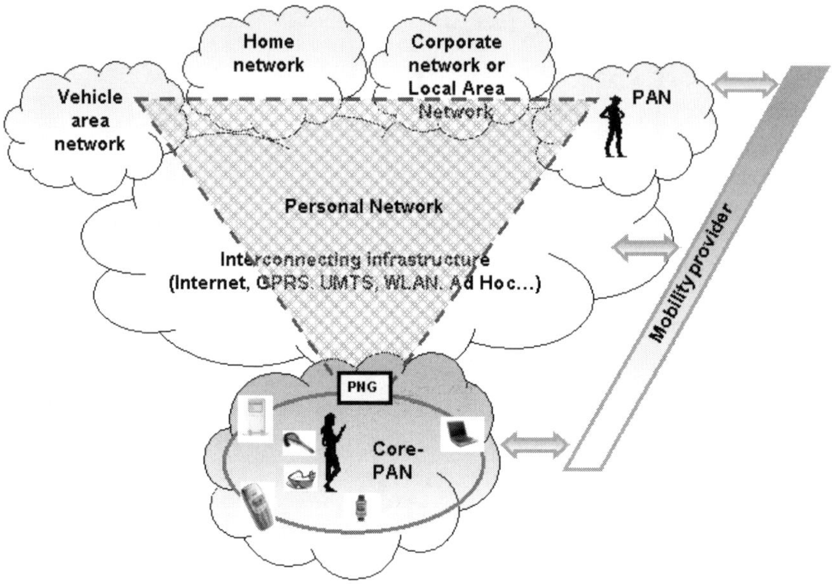

Figure 3. A Personal Network (PN) is a personalized overlay over multiple network domains. The Mobility Provider offers the PN service. The PNG connects the core-PAN to the other private networks, thus creating a PN.

role. It is basically the service provider offering the PN service and providing an operational environment to manage user, service, content and network related issues. For that purpose the MP might use a service platform like that described in ref. [6], which communicates with the PNG and offers service control functions that enable end users to easily gain and maintain access to services, while roaming between different interconnecting public infrastructures. For other service providers, the MP can act as a one-stop shop for providing their services to the PN. The MP could also take care of the billing, depending on the subscriptions with the various network and service providers, and on the authentication of the devices and content belonging to the PN.

1.2. State of the Art, Research Challenges, and Application Domains

The goal of the Freeband Personal Network Pilot 2008 project (PNP2008) [7] is to develop the concept of Personal Networking. The generic research question is how to create a PN to support, in a meaningful way, users in their private and professional activities. This involves investigating the desired user experience and finding solutions to a range of technical problems, but also business problems. These research and development challenges basically arise from the fact that current networks often support user mobility within a single network domain (a single cloud in Fig. 3), but not between the different network domains. Users can therefore not switch between the different networks whilst automatically retaining their session and information. Furthermore, in PNs we no longer have single terminals wanting to establish co-operation with the other infrastructures (like in current cellular systems or WLANs), but very dynamic and heterogeneous mobile PAN networks. Finally, there are no suitable business models in place for PNs, because current business parties are usually dedicated to a single network or application domain.

A PN should result in a distributed personal environment, consisting of clusters of geographically dispersed devices, that dynamically changes according to the context and needs of the user. It offers users access to their personal applications, devices and content depending on the role of the user (employee, private person, member of a community, etc.). Therefore, a PN should not only be non-specific to the underlying network domains, but also to the application domains. In ref. [8] we have studied the value that PNs can add to various business market sectors, based on the sectors' need for integration of dispersed resources, the level of complexity a PN can hide for their employees, the number of different contexts in which the employees are acting and that the PN can adapt to, and the size of the market. We found that PNs should be especially attractive to the construction sector, the transportation sector, the manufacturing sector, the health care sector and the emergency services sector. In the first year of the PNP2008 project we have decided to develop the concept of PNs in more detail for the latter two sectors. This resulted in a demonstrator that will be described in the following section.

2. Use Case and Demonstrator

2.1. Use Case

Healthcare professionals indicate that information and communication is crucial to their functioning. The information should be complete, covering all subjects, and if possible be available in the doctor's office whenever needed. Doctors especially need a wide range of data from different perspectives and supplied by several parties. Some examples are the patient's history, transfer data by nurses and other doctors/specialists, and information on medication. Currently, however, this information is often not available when and where it is needed. It can be concluded that in the healthcare sector ICT is not yet supporting the complex internal and intramural work processes sufficiently and does not yet ensure adequate information and communication. Personal Networks might be a very helpful tool in this situation. This can be illustrated by the following use case.

In medical emergency operations, the medical staff involved has only limited time to make a diagnose and to collect all the information needed. Quite often, therefore, the operating surgeon has to consult a colleague by physically leaving and re-entering the operating theatre, which is fairly time consuming because of the tight hygiene regulations. A PN consisting of the PANs of the surgeon and the peer, extended with the appropriate cameras and screens in the vicinity of the people involved, might improve the communication significantly. This use case is the basis of the first PNP2008 demonstrator, as described in the following section.

Other stages in medical emergency cases desire communication of voice, data, and video that can also be improved by the use of PNs. A medical emergency often consists of the following stages:

1. The emergency call center is contacted by a bystander
2. Medical emergency team is notified
3. The ambulance is on the way

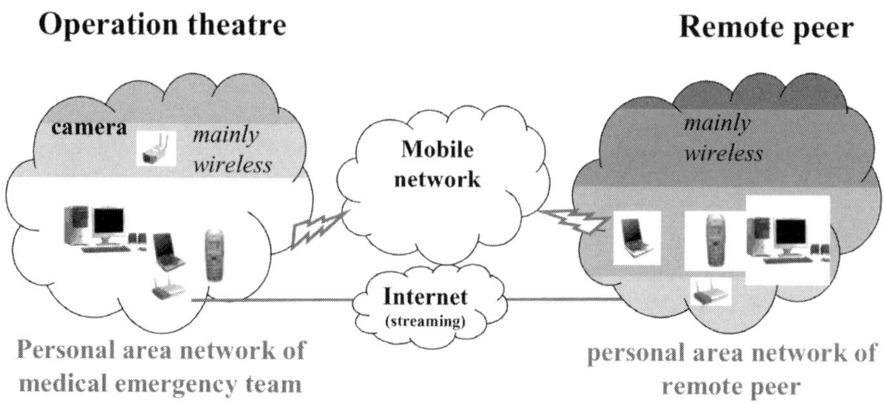

Figure 4. Schematic overview of the demonstrator set-up.

4. The ambulance is on the spot
5. The ambulance doctor contacts the intensive care doctor for an expert opinion
6. The ambulance is on the way back to the hospital
7. The patient is transferred to the emergency room
8. More diagnostic measurements are done
9. The patient is operated

PN technology can also be useful in stages 3–6. The PN then consists of the PANs of the ambulance personnel, the ambulance network, the PAN of the intensive care doctor, and the hospital network. When the ambulance is on its way, updated status reports and the medical background of the patient can be automatically and continuously exchanged between the ambulance and the hospital and the personnel involved. At the spot, the first diagnosis can be discussed with the intensive care doctor, who also has a video connection to the scene via the cameras of the ambulance. Any data measured by medical equipment on the spot is directly communicated to the doctor and the hospital, where the data can be processed by various intelligent systems, and immediate medication be suggested to the ambulance personnel. It can then also be decided, for example, to transport the patient directly to an academic hospital instead. On the way back to the hospital, the patient is continuously monitored, and the information is shared with the hospital and the surgeon.

2.2. Demonstrator

The use case to which the demonstrator refers is based on step 9 of the medical emergency case of Section 2.1. In this case, the PN consists of the PANs of the surgeon and his remote peers (containing various mobile devices), the local area network of the emergency room (containing controllable high quality cameras), and the local network of the peers (containing any type of screen). This setup is drawn in Fig. 4.

We assume a medical emergency team working in the operation theatre. A number of controllable digital video cameras are recording the scene. The cameras and the streaming server become part of the surgeon's PAN as soon he enters the operating theatre. The surgeon controls the streaming server with his mobile phone or another device in his PAN that, for instance, enables him to operate the cameras by means of voice recognition. The surgeon is then in control of the recording, i.e. he decides what is recorded and when. On demand the surgeon is also able to deliver the live streaming content to the outside world. In this particular case the surgeon wants to consult a few peers around the world about a patient he is operating on. A previously constructed list of peers is then used (based on their phone numbers) to make an invitation phone call. The invited peers receive an SMS message with the invitation to join the group. The surgeon receives the confirmations indicated by, for instance, highlighted list items. From that moment on the medical emergency team and the remote group members are able to talk to each other.

After briefly describing the problem at hand, the operating team sends a message to the peers containing a web address and login details. The group members can then access the live streaming video by temporarily absorbing any local device with a screen into their PAN (e.g. their home TV screen) and using the web address. Based on this web address, the video (with audio stream) could in principal be received on any screen devices connected to the Internet. The invited group is now able to discuss the problem with the surgeon watching live video images. Moreover, the surgeon can delegate the control (pan, tilt, zoom) of one or more cameras to one of the invited peers to have an optimal interaction.

The architecture of the demonstrator can be briefly described as follows. The emergency room has a wireless local area network, based on the IEEE 802.11a standard, that is connected to the Internet by means of a router/gateway. The wireless network consists of a high quality networked camera with a stream server and a control interface. It also contains a PC that can play the camera image and that registers the camera so that it can be automatically discovered by other devices that enter the theatre. This PC can also be used to collect other health data of the patient. The PAN of the surgeon consists of a GPRS and Bluetooth enabled mobile phone and a Bluetooth and IEEE 802.11a enabled laptop or PDA. The laptop/PDA is used to discover the camera (by using the Zeroconfig autodiscovery and – configuration protocol standardized by the Internet Engineering Task Force (IETF) [9]). The phone is used for inviting group members and setting up a group conversation by using a Push-to-Talk service [10]. There exists an open standard for Push-to-Talk over cellular networks, but this is not implemented yet by most operators. We therefore use proprietary software, licensed by SPING B.V. [11], that enables Push-to-Talk over GPRS. For Push-to-Talk an extra server is needed that is deployed and maintained by e.g. the Mobility Provider. Via the Bluetooth connection between phone and laptop, the camera can be controlled and the camera details (web address, login details) can be retrieved and sent to the message server. This message server is based on the Simple Object Access Protocol and Remote Procedure Call (SOAP-RPC [12]), and is also to be deployed and maintained by the Mobility Provider.

The architecture of the peer's networks is very simple. The peer has a PAN containing a similar mobile phone and laptop/PDA. The mobile phone is used for the Push-to-Talk session, and the IEEE 802.11a enabled laptop/PDA is used for discovering a screen with a video player nearby and for receiving the camera instructions from the mobile phone. The screen might be connected to the Internet by its own broadband connection (the home network or the hospital network). In that case the camera images can be routed to the screen via the broadband fixed network. If the screen is stand-alone, the images might be streamed via the much slower GPRS and Bluetooth connection. In that case, some content adaptation should be performed by, e.g. the Mobility Provider. In both PANs involved, the PNG functionality is distributed over the mobile phone and the laptop or PDA.

3. Conclusions and Future Work

People want to access more and more electronic devices that reside in their personal domains. At this moment, these devices form networked clusters that can be relatively easily connected to the public network. However, context aware interaction between these clusters and with remote personal content and applications is not possible yet. A Personal Network should provide the technology needed to interconnect the various private networks of a single user seamlessly, at any time and at any place.

A PN is not really an end-user application, but merely a sector non-specific service enabler. We found that PNs should be especially useful for stimulating voice, data, and video communication in the construction sector, the transportation sector, the manufacturing sector, the health care sector and the emergency services sector. We have shown some of this added value with a demonstrator that is based on the use case of a medical emergency team that can communicate with remote peers by using a PN. Further evidence will be acquired by conducting a number of user studies, in which we will interview a number of medical specialists and have the demonstrator tested by them on usefulness and usability.

Ultimately, PN technology should enable a truly user-centric ambient communication environment in a highly heterogeneous world of devices, operators and network technologies. This is a challenging research task, but it has a strong industrial potential, since it would enable a whole new class of applications.

Acknowledgement

The work presented in this paper is supported by the Freeband Communication technology program of the Dutch Ministry of Economic Affairs.

References

[1] G. Niemegeers and S.M. Heemstra de Groot, Research issues in ad-hoc distributed Personal Networking, *Journal on Wireless and Personal Communication* **26** (2003), 149–167.

[2] I.G. Niemegeers and S.M. Heemstra de Groot, From Personal Area Networks to Personal Networks: A user oriented approach, *Journal on Wireless and Personal Communications* **22** (2002), 175–186.

[3] F.T.H. den Hartog, M. Balm, C.M. de Jong, and J.J.B. Kwaaitaal, Convergence of Residential Gateway technology, *IEEE Commun. Mag* 42 (2004), 138–143.

[4] T. Cooklev, *Wireless communication standards*, Standards Information Network IEEE Press, New York, 2004.

[5] N.H.G. Baken, E.F.M. van Boven, F.T.H. den Hartog, and R. Hekmat, A four-tiered hierarchy in a converged fixed-mobile architecture enabling Personal Networks, *Proc. FITCE 2004*, Ghent, 2004, also in *The Journal of The Communications Network* **3** (2004) part 3.

[6] D.-J. Plas, M. Bargh, J. Laarhuis, J. van Vugt, J. Brok, and H. van Kranenburg, The 4GPLUS project; overview and main results, *Proc. of ECUMN 2004*, Porto, 2004.

[7] Pnp2008.freeband.nl.

[8] A. de Vries, J. Kort, M.S. de Jonge, and L.L.M.L. Kuiper-Hoyng, Professional target groups for a Personal Network, *Deliverable 4.1 of the PNP2008 project*, 2004.
[9] www.ietf.org/rfc/rfc3927.txt.
[10] Push-to-Talk on a mobile phone, GSA opinion paper, www.gsacom.com/downloads/pdf/gsa_opinion_paper_015.php4.
[11] www.imfree.nl.
[12] www.ietf.org/rfc/rfc3288.txt.

Medical and Care Compunetics 2
L. Bos et al. (Eds.)
IOS Press, 2005

Context Aware Tele-Monitoring and Tele-Treatment Services

Miriam M.R. VOLLENBROEK HUTTEN[a], Hermie J. HERMENS[a,b] and Rianne M.H.A. HUIS IN 'T VELD[a]
[a]*Roessingh Research and Development*
[b]*University of Twente*

Abstracts. This report describes the Awareness project which attempts to make a step forward new kind of e-health services by realizing remote monitoring of health functions and by demonstrating the feasibility of free health treatment concepts; meaning monitoring and treatment independent of time and place utilizing a mobile service infrastructure.

Keywords. Tele treatment, tele monitoring, context aware services

Introduction

There is a considerable pressure on both the quality and quantity of our health care system. The increasing availability of low-cost mobile devices, ad-hoc and managed wireless networks and broadband services providing access to large volumes of information offer new and unique opportunities for our health care system to increase its efficiency and effectiveness. Probably more important is the pressure, related to the increasing number of subjects who need health care services for a longer period of time such as elderly, patients with rather complex chronic disorders and subjects with work related disorders. As a consequence there is an increasing load for the health care institutes whereas their capacity decreases resulting in longer waiting lists. In order to reduce waiting lists, a considerable amount of patients will be dismissed quite earlier from the institutes with diffuse treatment advices. This indicates that care needs to be delivered more and more at the patient's own environment.

The Awareness project [1] attempts to make a step forward into enabling this new kind of health services by realizing remote monitoring of health functions and by demonstrating the feasibility of free health treatment concepts; meaning a treatment independent of time and place utilizing a mobile service infrastructure. Such treatment is supported by an M-health service platform, which enables a continuous bi-directional data stream between the patient and a healthcare professional. The M-health service platform conveys the health signals collected by a Body Area Network (BAN) worn by the patient to a healthcare professional. Based on his performance, the patient will receive feedback to optimize the treatment goals.

The generalized concept of personal telemonitoring and teletreatment is shown in Fig. 1.

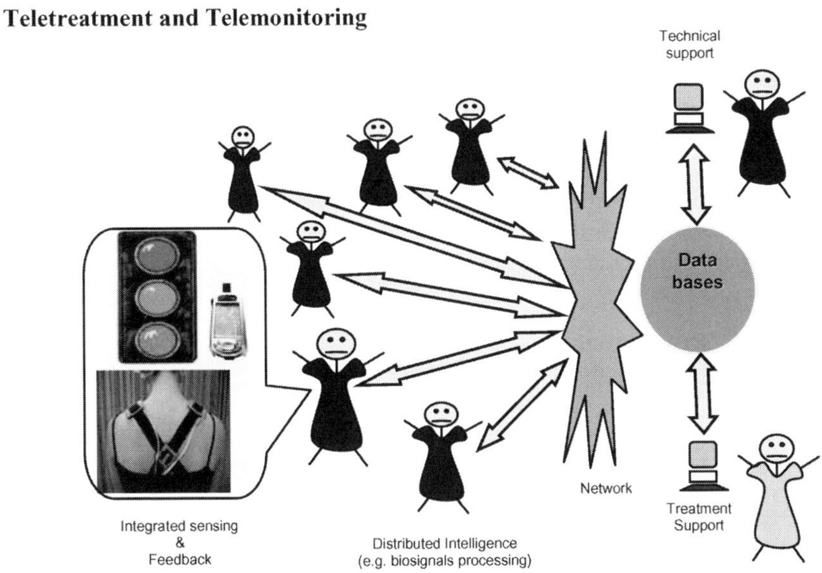

Figure 1. Illustration of teletreatment and telemonitoring concept.

This figure shows that many subjects are monitored/treated outside the traditional intramural care institutions. All subjects are equipped with a personalised interface consisting of a sensor system, which continuously measures relevant health functions and simultaneously provides the subject with feedback on his functioning. Biosignals originating from the sensors are conditioned, processed, compared with criteria and interpreted. In the different steps of these processes, the required bandwidth decreases but the required intelligence increases. Intelligence is required to detect failures in the sensing and to derive medical alarm conditions from the biosignals in their context.

Research is focused on people in the need of continuous monitoring of their health status (tele-monitoring) and continuous treatment of their health (tele-treatment). Telemonitoring will focus on affected neuromuscular functions because of sudden and only partly predictive exacerbations. Applications for telemonitoring concern epileptic seizures and the uncontrolled movements in spasticity. Tele-treatment focuses on treatment of patient with chronic pain.

The Awareness activities will result in an advanced ubiquitous attentive service and network infrastructure. Awareness integrates ubiquitous computing, information processing and exchange of context parameters with a framework that supports proactive responsiveness of applications. For the monitoring services the datastream is largely unidirectional, whereas the personal teletreatment services require full bidirectional transfer of data to be able to monitor the patient status, to control and adjust the treatment and to provide the patient adequate feedback about his health condition. In addition, concepts of distributed intelligence are required to create a stable and reliable system in varying conditions and context. Depending on the context for example, intelligence should be located more close to the subject (limited intelligence and bandwidth) or more to the central server system (higher intelligence, including modelling but requiring higher bandwidth).

Methods

To develop knowledge about such monitoring and treatment services, research is needed into which contextual information is relevant to combine in a meaningful way and how this information can be sensed in a reliable way. Proper sensing, inferring, reasoning, decision making and communicating the patient's spatiotemporal condition and symptoms must be followed by quick communication of the treatment-needed information to either the medical helpers or e.g. implanted medicine-delivering-devices. In other words, the systems should be ubiquitously aware of all relevant contextual information and attentive to address the relevant actions. Tele-treatment requires very reliable and secure ways to communicate with actuators. Main topics of research concern:

1. Which contextual information is essential and how can this be sensed, modeled, measured and represented in a reliable way?
2. What are the requirements for and how is the design of the data management process (intelligence) to address aspects as automatic adaptation, flexibility, security, privacy, reliability?
3. What are the system requirement specifications and how to design the application UA components that realize the above-mentioned applications?
4. How to distribute the processing of health signals? Especially in the case of tele-treatment where at the start if a treatment the processing and configuration of the tele-treatment will be done by a health professional, but later in the treatment this processing will be more done locally with the patient.

Results

Sofar, scenarios have been developed for both the tele-treatment and telemonitoring. Based on this specifications for the applications will be derived. Scenarios are described in Fig. 2.

A Tele-Treatment Scenario – Treatment of Chronic Pain

Jitske is a 28 years old girl with serious chronic complaints in her neck and shoulder. Due to her intelligence and her personality she became the management assistant of the director of a big company and she really enjoyed her work. Up to last year. Then the complaints in her neck and shoulder started and rapidly increased. After six months she was really not able to do her work anymore properly due to the terrible pain which built up during the day and did hardly vanish during the night. The frustration about this pain often made her try to ignore it and work very hard to show that she could handle it. But always, she had to pay for such behaviour the next days with an increase of pain disabling her completely.

She went to a rehabilitation centre specialised in chronic pain where she was treated for the pain and also was teached how to handle when pain occurs during work. She felt really relieved after this period and started full confidence again with her work.

But, sadly, the pain returned very quick. It became clear that she was not able to use what she had learned in the rehabilitation centre in her daily activities. She felt back to her old habits.

After consulting her specialist, she volunteered to participate in a new tele-treatment program. At a visit to the rehabilitation centre she received the portable equipment and was taught how to use it. It consists of a garment with integrated sensors which can be invisibly worn under her clothes. A portable computer is connected to these sensors and is able to collect the biosig-

nals, to process them and to send them to the rehabilitation centre. In addition Jitske gets continuously feedback about her health status and how she should behave. It provides her with crucial information how to behave in terms of the tight balance between underactivity and overactivity which are both harmful and increase the pain. At the rehabilitation centre, the specialists are able to monitor her health status and to adapt her treatment according to her particular abilities and progress she is making. Especially at the start of the treatment a broadband connection is used to obtain all raw signals to feed these signals into a complex model to obtain a first setting of the treatment parameters. In the first week(s) this is often repeated in order to obtain the best treatment settings for Jitske.

Jitske is quickly used to the equipment which hardly limits her in her daily activities. She learns to react on the feedback she is continuously being provided. In addition she has regular sessions during which she remotely communicates with her specialist by voice while at the same time relevant courses of her health data are provided on her pda. After a few weeks she is starting to notice the changes. She is well capable to maintain a good balance in her daily activities, her pain is decreasing and she feels a growing self-confidence that she will be better.

A Tele-Monitoring Scenario – Monitoring Epileptic Seizures

Sandra is a 24 years old girl with epilepsy. She has this disease already for many years. From time to time she has serious epileptic seizures, which manifest themselves as a complete unconsciousness combined with strong muscle contractions and shaking. Sandra cannot foresee these seizures nor can she remember what has happened looking back. This accounts especially for the periods in which her medication has to be adapted as a consequence of the increasing occurrence of seizures. In such period, she hardly dares to go on the street alone, too afraid of a seizure to occur in a strange environment and with unknown circumstances.

As Sandra wants to life an independent life as much as possible she volunteers to participate in a pilot tele-monitoring service. She gets a garment which she can wear under her clothes, with embedded sensors which are able to monitor her heart, her muscles and also her activity level, so whether she sits, walks or runs. This garment is connected to a small computer at her belt which is able to record these signals and send them to the institute where she is being treated for her disease. There, her health signals are continuously monitored and an alarm goes off when she is having a seizure. The doctor on duty is then able to directly have a look at her signals and to obtain relevant information on her condition as well as on her environment. He is able to observe where she is but also in what kind of environment (car, in house, street). Based on all this information, he is able to decide whether to send assistance, what kind of assistance and from which closest place.

Sandra is very quickly used to the equipment and she does not even feel she wears it. When she is aware of it, it makes her feel very confident that someone is keeping an eye on her and in this way provides her an opportunity to have a more independent life, like the girls of her age.

Figure 2. Scenarios.

Using these scenarios, the different application framework components are defined (see Fig. 3) [2] and a start is made to come to the technical and functional specifications of each of these components.

The Health BAN is one of the application components. For this part, literature reviews were performed to get insight in biosignals which are able to detect epileptic seizures. Heart frequency together with activity monitoring are probably important [3]. The next step is to identify the most reliable way of sensing and development of the algorithms which can be used for the clinical decision making process. This will be done based on experiments.

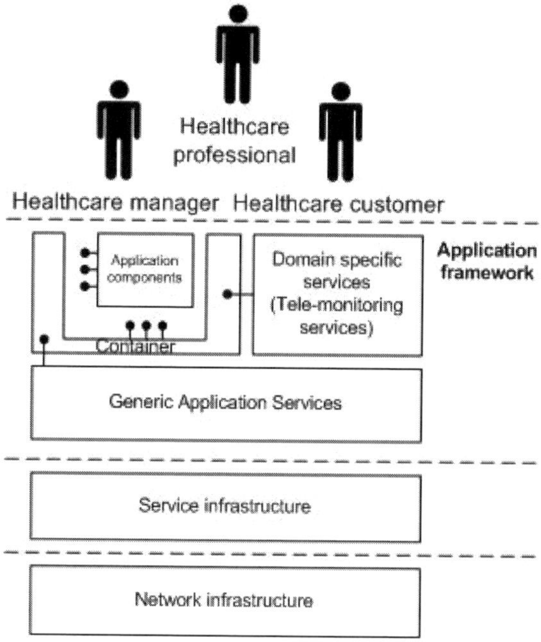

Figure 3. Application components [4].

Acknowledgement

This work is part of the Freeband AWARENESS project (http://awareness.freeband.nl). Freeband is sponsored by the Dutch government under contract BSIK 03025.

References

[1] Awareness flyer http://awareness.freeband.nl.
[2] Deliverable 4.2: Context aware application components: Http://awareness.freeband.nl.
[3] Deliverable 4.1: Tools and methods for reliable measurement of of sensory input information: http://awareness.freeband.nl.
[4] Broens, T., Halteren, A. van, Sinderen, M. van, Wac, K., Towards an application framework for context-aware m-health applications, Proceedings of EUNICE 2005, Madrid, Spain, 2005.

Medical and Care Compunetics 2
L. Bos et al. (Eds.)
IOS Press, 2005

Tele-Cardiology for Patients with Chronic Heart Failure: The 'SHL' Experience in Israel and Germany

Arie ROTH[a], Ronen GADOT[b] and Eric KALTER[c]
[a] *Tel Aviv Sourasky Medical Center, Dept. of Cardiology*
[b] *SHL-Telemedicine International LTD*
[c] *Dutch Healthcare Insurance Board*

Abstract. Chronic heart failure (CHF) is an example of a disease that can benefit to a great extent from a combination of disease management, telemedicine and outreaching care by professionals. This article summarizes how experience has been built up since 15 years and how cost-effectiveness could be demonstrated in several studies. Tele-cardiology for CHF has proven it's value and is currently being applied successfully in Israel and Germany by SHL-telemedicine International LTD. The Dutch Ministry of Health has recently issued a positive recommendation to Health Insurance Companies to promote the use of telemedicine where feasible in these types of chronic ailments.

Disease Management

Disease Management is a system of coordinated healthcare interventions and communications for populations with conditions in which patient self-care efforts are significant [1]. Disease management supports the physician or practitioner/patient relationship, emphasizes prevention of exacerbations and complications utilizing evidence-based practice guidelines and patient empowerment strategies, and evaluates clinical, humanistic, and economic outcomes on an ongoing basis with the goal of improving overall health.

Typically, Disease Management programs aim at monitoring and treatment for Cardiovascular Diseases, Asthma and COPD, Diabetes Mellitus and Psychiatric Disorders.

It is the goal to offer the patient totally integrated, protocol-driven, pro-active care, aimed at reaching pre-defined targets as a result of long-term treatments in large populations with chronic ailments.

Telemedicine

The advent of telemedicine has added even more dimensions to disease management programs: It increases quality of care at lower costs and enhances patient education and compliance. Moreover on the basis of frequent monitoring in the home situation, decreases in the condition of the patient can be detected early thus enabling timely interventions by dedicated medical personnel. It not only provides the patient with a higher level of safety and quality of life, but also decreases the workload of the medical support systems. Finally, telemedicine truly enables the patient to make the transition to demand-driven care. This will be illustrated below with chronic heart failure as an example.

Experience in Chronic Heart Failure

Chronic heart failure (CHF) is a typical example of a chronic disease that qualifies for a disease management program with telemedicine support and self-monitoring at the home situation. It is estimated to affect about 2% of the population.

Already in 1995 interesting observations have been published from a telemedicine service program ('Shahal') with patients who were trained to use a device for trans-telephonic transmission of an EKG [2]. In the majority of calls an emergency pick up by an ambulance could be avoided and thus a fair number of emergency room visits too. In contrast, time elapsed between onset of cardiac symptoms and the decision to call for medical help was markedly shortened. Therefore the 'Shahal experience' proved to be a double edged sword, reassuring most (85%) of the patients calling in and helping those truly in need faster (15%) whilst avoiding unnecessary involvement of medical attention at emergency rooms.

Shortly thereafter, in 1997, it was reported that intensive contact by telephone, on the basis of consensus guidelines was able to increase patient compliance to therapy and to reduce emergency room visits for heart failure by 67% and hospitalization rates by 87% [3].

Thereafter several studies demonstrated fewer hospitalizations and fewer total days of hospitalization by implementing homecare strategies [4–8].

In 2001, a pilot study was published in which 10 patients with CHF were monitored with fully automated data transmission of blood pressure, heart rate and weight, to a central server, proving that this concept could work in daily practice [9].

Recently, Roth et al published a larger series of 118 patients with CHF, who's blood pressure, heart rate and weight were transmitted automatically to a medical service centre, to be monitored with the aid of a software algorithm, in conjunction with a 24 hour emergency call service on demand, in case of medical complaints, and an elective biweekly call from nursing staff to promote adherence to therapy [10]. When comparing the observed data with those obtained retrospectively from the same group of patients during the preceding year, a 66% reduction in hospitalization days were observed, together with an improvement in reported quality of life.

Meanwhile, this program has taken off in Germany too, where a telemonitoring service centre has been established by SHL TeleMedicine Ltd at Düsseldorf[1]. The local Healthcare Insurance Company 'Taunus Betriebskrankenkasse', has calculated that it will save at least € 2.8 million in 5 years on hospitalization costs with the use of such services for their region [11].

The Dutch Ministry of Health has recognized the importance of telemedicine services for chronic patient care and urges the health care insurance companies to positively support these initiatives in The Netherlands [12].

---

[1] http://www.shl-telemedicine.com/content.asp?id=3.

Also from an economic point of view the use of telemedicine has recently been recommended as one of the possible options to increase labour-productivity in health-care in The Netherlands [13].

Conclusion

In conclusion it can be stated that telemedicine in general and more specifically tele-cardiology for chronic heart failure, has made great progress with the advent of telemonitoring equipment and the possibility of automated central monitoring. It has been shown that it can be effectively applied in the home situation and that it improves quality of life at a more efficient use of medical resources simultaneously.

References

[1] Definition from: Disease Management Association of America (DMAA).
[2] Roth A, Herling M, Vishlitzki V, Aitkin I. The Impact of 'SHAHAL' (a new Cardiac emergency service) on subscribers' requests for Medical Assistance: Characteristics and Distribution of Calls. *Eur Heart J* 1995;16:129–133.
[3] West JA, Miller NH, Parker KM, e.a. A Comprehensive Management System for Heart Failure improves Clinical Outcomes and reduces Medical Resource Utilization. *Am J Cardiol* 1997;79:58–63.
[4] Hanumanthu S, Butler J, Chomsky D, e.a. Effect of a Heart Failure Program on Hospitalization Frequency and Exercise Tolerance. *Circulation* 1997;96:2843–8.
[5] Stewart S, Pearson S, Horowitz J. Effects of a Home Based Intervention among Patients with Congestive Heart Failure discharged from Acute Hospital Care. *Arch Intern Med* 1998;158:1067–72.
[6] Stewart S, Pearson S, Horowitz J. Effects of a home based intervention among patients with congestive heart failure discharged from acute hospital care. Arch Intern Med 1998;158:1067–72.
[7] Stewart S, Marley JE, Horowitz JD. Effects of a Multidisciplinary Home-Based Inter-vention on Planned Readmissions and Survival among Patients with Chronic Congestive Heart Failure: a Randomized Controlled Clinical Trial. *Lancet* 1999;354:1077–83.
[8] Cordisco ME, Beniaminovitz A, Hammond K, Mancini D. Use of Telemonitoring to decrease the Rate of Hospitalization in Patients with Severe Congestive Heart Failure. *Am J Cardiol* 1999;84:860–2.
[9] De Lusignan S, Wells S, Johnson P e.a. Compliance and Effectiveness of 1 year's Home Telemonitoring. The Report of a Pilot Study of Patients with Chronic Heart Failure. *Eur J Heart Fail* 2001;3: 723–30.
[10] Roth A, Kajiloti I, Elkyam I e.a.: Telecardiology for Patients with Chronic Heart Failure: the 'SHL' Experience in Israel. *Int J Cardiol* 2004;97:49–55.
[11] Neuer Vertrag deckt Telemedizin für chronisch Herzkranke ab. *Ärzte Zeitung* 2005; March 23.
[12] Letter IBE/I 2564494, 2005;March 4th.
[13] Schoone M, van Boxsel JAM. Kansen voor technologische innovatie. In: Dossier Arbeidsproductiviteit in de Zorg. *ESB* 2005 February 10; dossier #4452:D28–29. (http://www.economie.nl/index_go.html?ESBdossiers.htm).

Medical and Care Compunetics 2
L. Bos et al. (Eds.)
IOS Press, 2005

Hybrid and Customized Approach in Telemedicine Systems: An Unavoidable Destination

Manuel PRADO[a,1], Laura M. ROA[a] and Javier REINA-TOSINA[b]
[a] *Biomedical Engineering Group, University of Seville, Seville, Spain*
[b] *Signal Theory and Communications Group, University of Seville, Seville, Spain*

Abstract. Several important problems in the majority of industrialized countries have challenged the centralized and overburdened current model of healthcare. Telehealthcare systems are presented as a new paradigm, offering high expectations to provide effective solutions to this picture. With this paper we present a new methodological approach for telehealthcare systems that pursues the generation of clinical and physiological knowledge of the patient in a real time and personalized manner. This approach is based on a computational component, identified as patient physiological image (PPI), which is responsible for generating an image of the state of the patient and therapy devices. Three key issues of the proposed methodological approach are evaluated. With the objective to validate the capability of the PPI to determine the internal state of a patient, a digital simulation experiment over the mathematical model of a PPI is done. Numerical results are compared to those obtained by a validated mathematical model. Secondly, a laboratory prototype of a novel human physical activity monitor that follows the designed methodological approach will be tested, in order to evaluate the trade-off between processing capacity, portability, and cost-efficiency and power consumption, which are necessary to assure its compliance with the methodology. As a third key issue, the capability of our methodology to integrate physiological information belonging to different scales is analyzed. This is done by means of a case study related to the integration of the regulation of water function of AQP2 channels (genomic, proteomic and cellular levels) into a kidney collecting duct epithelium mathematical model of a PPI. The analysis and preliminary evaluation of the proposed telehealthcare methodological approach, featured by an advanced personalization of health assistance, have been satisfactory.

Keywords. Telehealthcare, hybrid signal processing, personalized healthcare, patient physiological image, modelling and simulation

Introduction

Several important problems in the majority of industrialized countries have challenged the centralized and overburdened current model of healthcare. The aging of population together with the growth of chronic pathologies such as diabetes mellitus, end stage renal disease, or cardiovascular disease [1–4], may be considered two of the reasons for

[1] Corresponding Author: Grupo de Ingeniería Biomédica, Universidad de Sevilla, Sevilla, Spain; E-mail: mpradovelasco@ieee.org.

this situation. Moreover the increase of quality of life and the change of social models and the structure of the families incorporate more social and healthcare requirements.

Telehealthcare systems are presented as a new paradigm, offering high expectations to provide effective solutions [5] to this picture. These systems pursue the decentralization of healthcare, allowing the geographical separation between patient and physician by means of modern multimedia services and communications networks. Telehealthcare systems may improve the supervision of the patient without a reduction in the quality of life associated to the hospital stays, reduce the waiting times, and facilitate the post-hospital follow-up, what can help to reduce the length of the hospital stays.

There is a trend towards the convergence and overlap of functions among the different types of telemedicine systems, what although complicates the classification process, is maximizing the possibilities that these systems offer to the healthcare model. A complete review of telemedical information systems from a technological perspective can be read in Horsch and Balbach [6]. A more clinical review about their capabilities and limitations was published recently by Wootton [7]. According to the cited evolution, modern telehealthcare systems are adding functions related to the management of patient's clinical information [8], pushing the concept of knowledge-based telehealthcare.

Nevertheless, current telehealthcare systems still have many limitations, and many of them only offer an effective system of multimedia services based on wide-band communications [9]. Among the main areas of research in telehealthcare, the systems for the assistance to patients with diabetes mellitus can be cited. The UTOPIA (Utilities for Optimizing Insulin Adjustment) project is a representative example in this area [10]. This project was initially designed as a computer aided system for the insulin administration to the diabetic patient, although was subsequently extended to account for the telehealthcare concept [11]. UTOPIA generates therapeutic advices for the insulin dose from the solution of a linear equation system. This linear model is in turn obtained from the relationships between the insulin intakes and the glucose trend temporal patterns calculated from blood glucose measurements.

Regarding the application of telehealthcare to the elderly, between a 20 % and a 40 % of this population group report some inability to be alone and one third of them say that their quality of life is low or very low [12]. In addition, morbidity is also very high, as the mean of three diseases and ten different complaints reported by the study group of the aforementioned study [12], of which pain and impaired mobility were the most frequent. The fear of falling and the effect of these ones in morbidity and mortality is also an important issue in the elderly [4,13,14]. These problems are growing in industrialized countries due to the aging of the population, what is propelling the research and development in telehealthcare systems focused in elderly and people with mobility impairment [15], and in portable systems for falling detection. The latter have evolved towards portable monitors that enable movement analysis [16–19], facilitating the necessary research about the causes and conditions that produce instability and falling [20].

The number of telehealthcare systems devoted to the care of the chronic renal disease patients is still low, being a remarkable reference the HOMER-D (Home Rehabilitation Treatment – Dialysis) project, which started under the fourth framework program of the European union (EU), and which has surpassed different technical and clinical evaluations [21,22]. The primary objective of HOMER-D is to provide an alarm management system based on a modern communication link that overcomes the lack of supervision in home hemodialysis (HD). Current research lines in telehealthcare for home HD assistance are mainly oriented to alarm telemonitoring [23,24]. Stroetmann and colleagues published a similar system for telehealthcare of patients submitted to continuous automated peritoneal dialysis (CAPD) [25]. The latter allows videoconference facilities by means of an Integrated Services Digital Network (ISDN) channel (128 Kb/s). The outcomes of all these systems was positive, both in the response of the patient and in their integration into the clinical environment.

There is a explosion of new solutions and advances of non-invasive and portable biosensors for the measurement of different clinical variables, including hemodynamical variables as blood oxygen level, blood pressure, heart rate, or blood glucose level [26–28]. Continuous monitoring is a concept acquired by many of these new biosensors, allowing real time knowledge generation in a growing set of biosignals.

Discovery and extraction of knowledge from biosignals and clinical data is also a very important area [29], however it is mainly directed to the off-line processing of the data with the aim to detect and classify patterns. These tools use to be based on expert systems [30]. As a consequence, there is a lack of methodologies and technologies that allow the extraction of useful medical information in a real time mode from on-line biosignals, despite these knowledge could increase notably the capacity of supervision of telehealthcare systems, adding new values for this healthcare model that are not available in the classical centralized healthcare model.

The cost-effectiveness of telemedicine systems has been addressed in many studies and application areas such as elderly, diabetes mellitus and renal chronic disease, obtaining good outcomes, although many of these studies do not include a sensibility study into the economical analysis and perhaps some methodological aspects of them must be improved, according to Whitten and colleagues [31]. Moreover, many studies indicate an improvement on clinical outcomes and patient satisfaction, although a larger analysis including both client and provider perspectives will be required to properly explore this issue [32].

In spite of all these advances, diffusion of telemedicine is still very scarce. The barriers to its diffusion have a technical, economical, organizational, and behavioural nature [33]. One of the factors that contribute to limit the diffusion of telehealthcare is the perception that this new model only offers a decentralization of the patient healthcare.

With the goal to change this perspective we have developed a new methodological approach for a telehealthcare system that pursues the generation of clinical and physiological knowledge of a patient in a real time manner. This methodology allows a very efficient customization of the supervision of a patient, using a distributed and hybrid computational architecture to process the information. This approach has been applied to the development of a prototype of a telehealthcare system for renal support, whose technological aspects and previous clinical review have been published recently [34,35].

This paper presents an evaluation of three key issues of our proposed methodological approach. The first of them refers to the knowledge generation method. This is based on a computational component named PPI (Patient Physiological Image). The essential aspects of PPI will be summarized in the following Section. Its ability to compute personalized knowledge will be subsequently evaluated by a simulation experiment over a PPI's prototype.

The processing of biosignals to generate a customized knowledge of the patient comprises also the sensor layer. According to this approach, and as a second issue, a

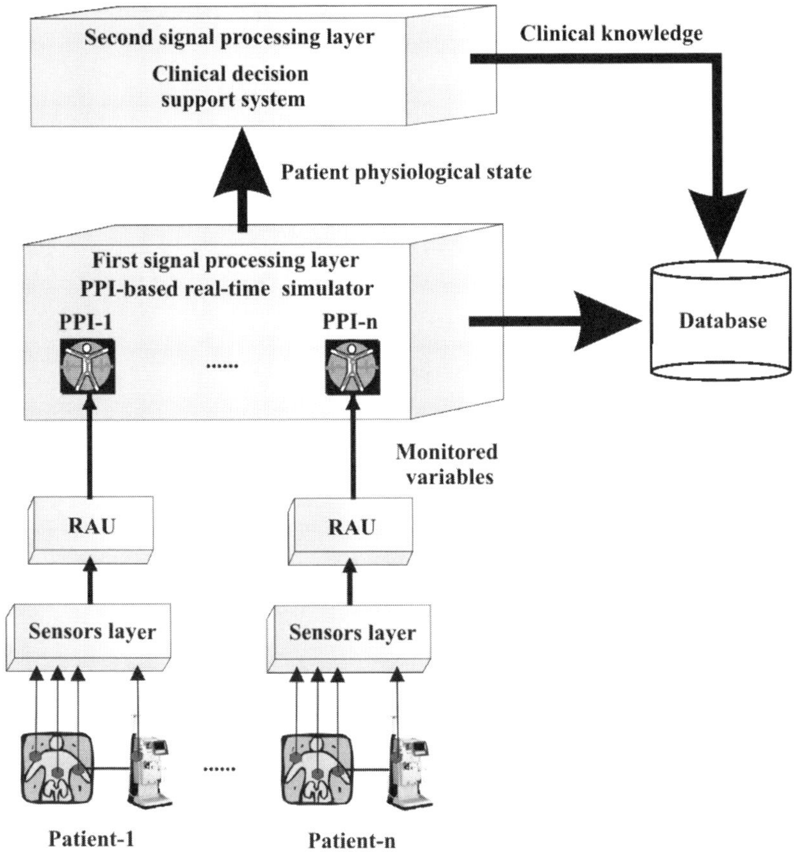

Figure 1. Signal processing according to the telehealthcare methodology presented. The first layer is a real-time simulator based on PPIs, which is able to build an integrated image of patients and their connected therapy devices. This knowledge is utilized in a second layer to generate warnings and alarms, and to feed the clinical decision support system.

novel human physical activity monitor that follows this concept will be presented and a laboratory prototype will be subsequently validated. This customizable monitor has important applications both in patients with chronic pathologies such as chronic renal disease and diabetes mellitus, and in persons with mobility impairment and falling risk, as the elderly.

The capability of the PPI to built knowledge from the dynamics mathematical models that represent the internal state of the patient is an essential property that can be exploited to allow the integration of physiological information pertaining to different scales, from genomic and proteomic level to organ and systemic level. This feature will be analyzed by means of a case study.

1. Methodological Approach

Figure 1 shows a simplified block diagram with the processing stages followed by the monitored variables and the knowledge generated according to the developed method-

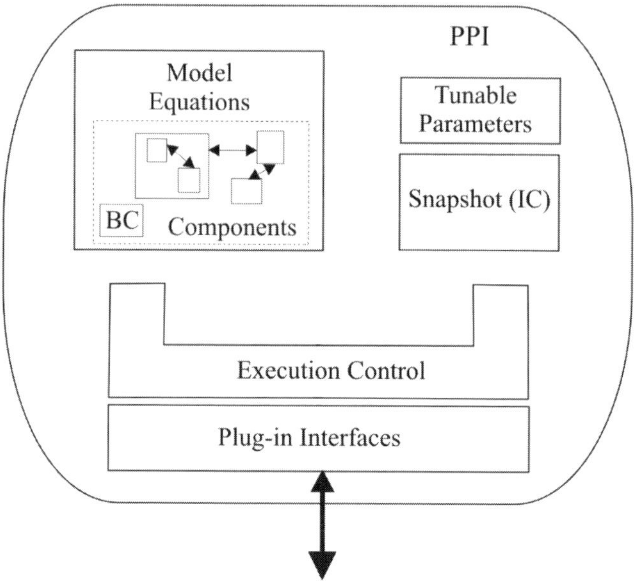

Figure 2. Simplified block diagram of a PPI.

ology. A sensors layer gets relevant information from the patient and associated therapy devices and forwards the data through a remote access unit (RAU) to a service provider center, where all signals are processed. The upper layer performs a clinical decision support which can be implemented by an expert system, following a reasoning method based either on rules (RBR), cases (CBR), models (MBR) or multimodal strategies [30]. It also includes an algorithm-based mathematical module for the analysis of the state. This layer is not unusual in modern telemedicine, as for example the UTOPIA project aforementioned. However, unlike current state-of-the-art systems, in which this layer directly applies to patient's recorded data and monitored variables, an additional processing layer has been included in this methodology. This layer is based on PPIs, which are responsible for generating an image of the state of the patient, and therapy devices. As shown in the same figure, each PPI is an autonomous simulator with real time execution capability, associated with only one patient.

Figure 2 outlines a block diagram of a PPI. As indicated this computational component is composed of a mathematical model together with two additional elements. The mathematical model is represented in that figure by a set of equations, related to a certain representation of the physical or physiological structure of the system. It is organized in a set of virtual components [36], a set of parameters customized to each patient and the values of the variables which define the state of the system in a particular instant (*snapshot*). The interfaces block (plug-in) provides the connection of the PPI to the outer world, i.e. databases and other computational objects, relying on different application protocols. Finally the execution control block is responsible for the simulation control of the PPI, based on the aforementioned model, and attends external commands.

A PPI can be executed either in observation mode or in predictive mode. In addition, multiple instances of a PPI can be linked to a single patient in a particular instant. In this case at least one of them is always operating in the observation mode, obtaining in real time the evolution of the internal state of the patient and that of the associated therapy machines. This technique allows a very efficient knowledge generation from the monitored signals, providing at the same time an exhaustive supervision of the health state of the patient. The concept of mathematical observer is an essential part within the adaptive and optimum control theory [37], and has been widely applied to the control of industrial processes. During the last decade it has also been used in research applied to automatic diagnostic techniques and to the on-line evaluation of efficiency in energy plants, with successful results [38]. In predictive mode, instead of being synchronized with the real-time clock, the PPI allows the calculation of the short-time future evolution of the patient. For instance this technique can be applied to obtain the state of the physiological variables of a patient at the end of an HD session using the information available 15 minutes after the beginning of the HD. An experiment of digital simulation of this functionality has been reported by Prado and colleagues [34]. This operation mode can be started by explicit request of the physician or automatically every certain time period, allowing anticipation to the events together with the on-line trials of different therapeutic actuations over the computational image of the patient.

Knowledge representation in PPI is based on dynamic systemic mathematical models. This approach describes the structure of causal relationships of the physiological system under representation and therefore its methodology is completely different from that of data-driven approaches like linear regressive models, neural networks or rule-based systems. The last models are also known as functional models and they are frequently used within the clinical decision support module, providing a high precision in the therapeutic recommendations whenever the input variables take values that have been considered in the parameterization of the model or during its training phase. This kind of model is utilized in the UTOPIA system aforementioned. On the other hand, the kind of mathematical model selected for the PPI provides a higher predictive capability besides offering a more complete image of the dynamics of the represented physiological system.

PPIs offer other advantages associated with the applied technology, which are key issues to guarantee the feasibility of this methodology. These are described in detail in a recent paper of Prado and colleagues [34]. Among them we emphasize the modular architecture and the reusability of the mathematical models. The latter refers to the capability of reusing a mathematical model, or even a part of this one, in the representation of other system sharing some similarities. It also eases the incorporation of new knowledge to existing models.

In order to accomplish this capability we have applied modelling techniques based on virtual prototyping [36,39], which guarantee the most perfect possible isomorphism between the virtual prototype (mathematical submodel) and the component or physical subsystem, removing the restrictions associated with the way how the variables are calculated. The last property defines the so-called non-causal modelling languages, where the causality concept refers to the flux of determination of the mathematical variables. We have taken advantage of this methodology together with the capability of the object-oriented hierarchical representation that these languages provide, to define a methodology of partition of the system to be modeled (space discretization) which distinguishes the physical processes in one or several lower layers, from the physical components where they are included, placed in the upper layers. This approach is a simple way to the integration of new physiological knowledge at different scales in the existing models.

The measurement of the physical activity and particularly certain kinetic parameters like walking speed, are related to the loss of independence in the elderly population, their admission to residences or even their mortality. On the other hand, the monitoring of postural and kinetic parameters together with measurements of vibration allows the detection of falls, which represent a valuable risk and challenging trauma for elderly people [4,13,14]. The risk of falls is emphasized when suffering from different chronic pathologies like end stage renal disease, due to secondary effects on the deterioration of mobility as a consequence of muscular loss and lack of D vitamin, as well as a higher incidence of arthropathy by $\beta 2$-microglobulin [2]. In this sense a recent study [40] has proven the relationship of walking speed with Kt/V and the level of albumin in blood, which are two key parameters in End Stage Renal Disease (ESRD) patients subjected to periodic HD. In the case of individuals with diabetes mellitus, energy expenditure related to physical activity is also a relevant variable. Different researchers have demonstrated the possibility of measuring energy expenditure by physical activity, falling detection and obtain the postural and kinetic state of the individual by means of the monitoring of the corporal acceleration near the gravity center [16,18,41]. In agreement with our methodology for personalized knowledge generation, we have developed an intelligent monitor of the physical activity in humans, which overcomes some of the existing limitations in previous designs [42]. Its architecture is conceived as a wireless personal area network (WPAN) integrating a server device (PSE), and an intelligent sensor unit for the acquisition of corporal accelerations (IAU). The PSE is responsible for the access to the personal network, being in charge of the real-time processing of the signals measured by the IAUs, with which it communicates using a master-slave protocol over a low power wireless link. It also manages the communication with the RAU. In order to make available the permanent functioning and connection between the movement monitor and the service provider center of the telemedicine system, the architecture includes an additional client element, designated as router, which can be connected to a mobile phone by a serial port. This approach allows the separation of the accelerometric sensor from the elements that configure the interface with the patient, which are supported by the PSE. Indeed the IAU has been conceived to be attached to the body using an adhesive patch. The architecture is outlined in Fig. 3.

2. Materials and Methods

2.1. Assessment of a Customized Supervision

We have accomplished an experiment by digital simulation over the mathematical model of a PPI, based on the aforementioned methodology. The objective of this experiment is the validation of the capability of the PPI to determine the internal state of an end stage renal disease patient during an HD session. To that aim we developed a pharmacokinetic library using the non-causal EcosimPro language (EL) [43]. The components of this library were applied to the definition of a three-pool urea kinetic model, with variable volumes, representing the vascular, interstitial and cellular compartments of the patient. Moreover this model can be connected to a dialyzer model, also developed with the components of the library, through the vascular compartment. Figure 4 shows an iconic diagram of the described model.

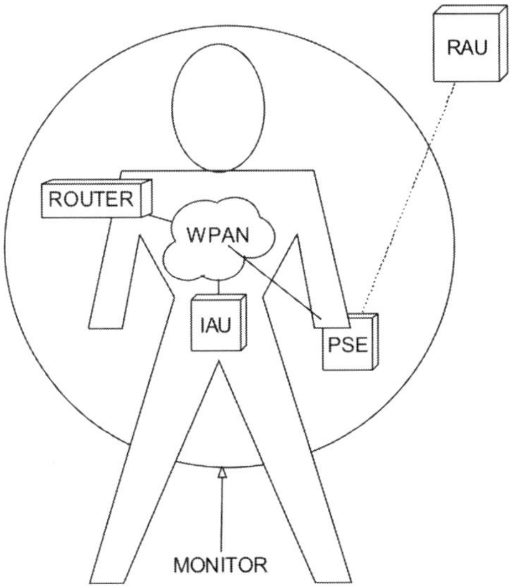

Figure 3. Diagram with the major components of the physical activity monitor.

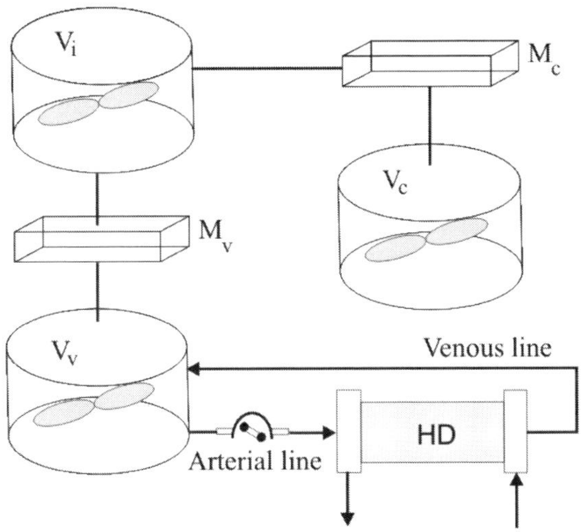

Figure 4. Iconic diagram of the tree-pool variable-volume urea kinetic model, representing vascular, interstitial and cellular human compartments, connected trough a vascular access to the hemodialyzer.

Variables V_v, V_i and V_c represent the volume of the vascular, interstitial and cellular compartments, respectively, while M_v and M_c are the vascular and cellular membranes. The importance of urea kinetic in the quantization and adequacy of hemodialysis has been demonstrated in multiple studies [44], and therefore the election of this particular type of simplified physiological model as a base of PPI prototype in ESRD patients is justified in this experiment.

The experiment was performed off-line using data monitored from a patient submitted to periodic HD, randomly selected from a group of 30 patients with similar clinical conditions and number of sessions per week. The selected patient was a 50 years non-diabetic man, weight 95 kg and height 179 cm, reporting anuria. Access recirculation measured with the two-needle urea-based method [45] was below 10 %. We selected the Wednesday session for this study. Measurement data included blood urea concentration, BUC, plasma protein concentration, Cp_p, and hematocrit, HTO, corresponding to blood samples extracted before the HD (point 1), at the end of the session (point 2), and thirty minutes before the end (point 3). Standard analyzers were utilized for all measurements. The postdialysis sample was taken approximately one minute after completion of the HD, keeping the flow in the arterial line at 50 ml/min. The values of BUC_1 BUC_2 and BUC_3 were 169, 59 and 67 mg/dl, being Cp_{p1}, Cp_{p2} and Cp_{p3} equal to 6.8, 8.6, 7.1 g/dl, and HTO_1, HTO_2 and HTO_3 values of 29.8, 35.8 y 33.5 %, respectively. The operating conditions remained constant during the whole session. The dialyzer flow rate was established at 500 ml/min and blood flow rate fixed at 300 ml/min.

A PPI was adjusted to the patient's kinetic and subsequently executed to evaluate the evolution of urea concentrations in the corresponding compartments. Urea concentrations and related dKt/V were compared with those estimated by a classical two-pool kinetic model. Index dKt/V refers to the product of the dialyzer effective urea clearance by the total HD session time over the urea distribution volume. The accuracy of the urea concentration obtained by the reference model in the accessible compartment has been demonstrated in the study of Canaud and colleagues [46]. The methodology of adjustment of the parameters of the two-pool model applied in this experiment is similar to the methodology used in a previous study [47].

2.2. Wearable and Customizable Technology for Physical Activity Monitoring

An important characteristic of the proposed activity monitor is its personalization capability for the user. This customization is a trade-off among processing capacity, portability, low cost and power consumption, which are necessary to assure its feasibility. In order to evaluate these key issues, together with precision, we have developed a prototype of monitor, which has been tested using the setup shown in Fig. 5.

The developed IAU provides four-measurement axis, three of which form an orthogonal system, and can be fixed at the back of the individual, at the height of the sacrum, by means of a waterproof adhesive patch. This location is very near from the gravity center, and is recommended in several recent studies [16,41]. This device consists of a low-cost, low-power microcontroller with embedded code (ROM) and RAM memory (PIC16LC66 from Microchip), two capacitive biaxial accelerometers (ADXL202E from Analog Devices), prepared to measure static and dynamic accelerations, a non volatile external memory (EEPROM), an integrated wireless transceiver, and other additional elements [42]. Sampling frequency for each of the four channels was adjusted at 40 S/s to optimize the capability to detect impacts [42]. The microcontroller provides the necessary processing capacity to the IAU for attending requests from the PSE, and for customizing a small signal analysis that is executed before signals will be sent to the PSE.

The set-up shown (Fig. 5) has been applied to evaluate different strategies to read the accelerations, evaluating both precision and power consumption with each method. The latter has been optimized keeping the microcontroller in the sleep mode and the sensors switched off for the largest possible time between successive sampling instants, but without affecting the evaluated measurement procedure. The images shown at the

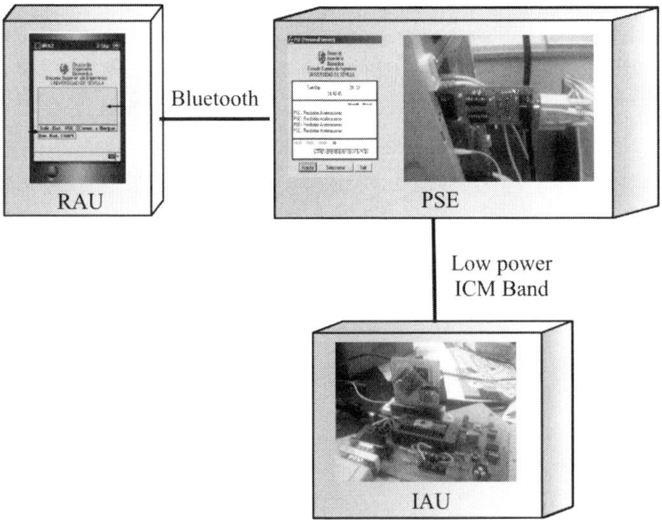

Figure 5. Set-up for the evaluation of the physical activity monitor.

top of the blocks in the aforementioned figure refer to photographies of the devices or to captured screens of the software applications. This way, the picture representing the RAU refers to the main window of the RAU's application implemented in a Compaq iPAQ Pocket PC H3970 PDA, equiped with 64 MB of RAM and a PXA250 400 MHz processor. The PSE block shows a screen of the PSE simulated in a personal computer, and one of the electronic devices used to communicate the IAU with the simulated PSE. A detail of a laboratory prototype of the IAU is shown over the IAU's block.

2.3. Integrating Different Physiological Scales by Virtual Prototyping

The hydraulic permeability, L_p, of the microvascular walls is not governed only by diffusion through channels (mainly intercellular) shared with low molecular weight compounds (urea, sodium, etc), but also there are specific channels for water, which are not shared with other low molecular weight solutes. These are responsible for an average percentage lower than 10 % of the overall value of L_p [48]. In certain tissues, like the renal one, these channels play a very important role and they can increase the value of L_p by a factor of four or even more, depending on the systemic and homeostatic conditions. Moreover recent studies have shown that vascular permeability is increased in renal and diabetic patients [49,50].

Water specific channels are associated with proteins of the MIP class, with function of water channel, which are known as aquaporins (AQP). These proteins were discovered a decade ago and among them two groups may be distinguished, being represented by AQP2 and AQP3 respectively [51]. An important advance has been accomplished in the characterization of the structure, functions and mechanisms of regulation of the channels that these proteins form, specially of the AQP2, which plays a key role in the regulation of water absorption by the renal tubules under antidiuretic conditions (concentrated urea).

Diabetes mellitus is the first cause of ESRD in industrialized countries [52], and therefore mechanisms of regulation of AQP2 channels in the kidney collecting duct

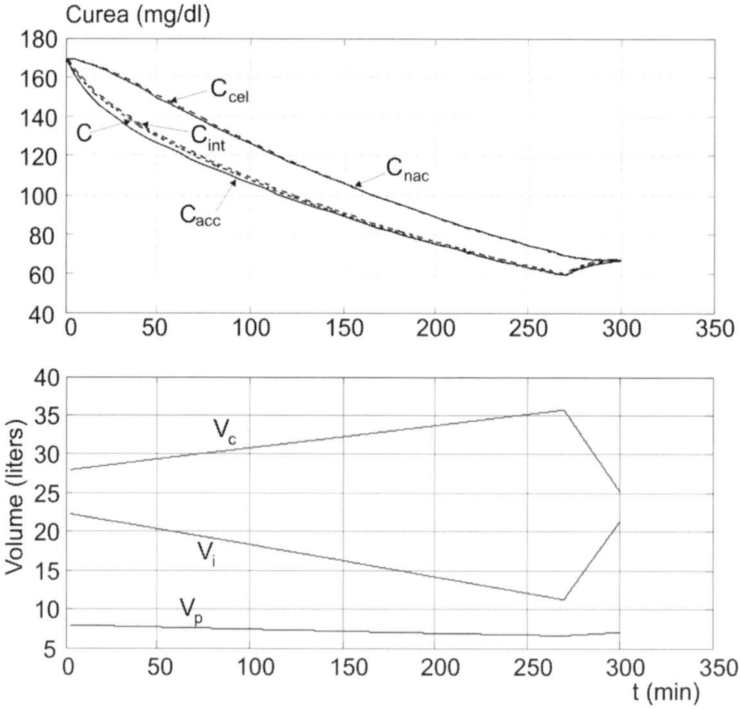

Figure 6. Evolution of the urea concentrations calculated by the two-pool model (solid lines in the upper graph) and with a PPI based on a three-pool model (dashed lines in the upper graph), during the HD session and the period of subsequent rebound for the selected patient. The lower graph depicts the evolution of the compartmental volumes.

cells could be considered in PPIs linked to diabetic patients with functional kidneys, with the aim to study their clinical evolution. The methodology of integration of the genomic, proteomic and cellular mechanisms of regulation of AQP2 channels on the hydraulic permeability of the kidney collecting duct epithelium, will be analyzed using a diagram that shows a simplified hierarchical structure of this membrane, together with the associated EL source code. The component of the hydraulic permeability associated with AQP2 channels in the kidney collecting duct epithelium will be referenced as L_p*.

We do not pretend to present a complete mathematical model that describes the water flow through the kidney collecting duct epithelium, because this objective exceeds the scope of the present work, and moreover there are other proteins that regulate the hydraulic permeability of kidney collecting duct epithelium, as AQP3 and AQP4 in the basolateral membrane of the kidney collecting duct cells.

3. Results

The upper graph of Fig. 6 shows the evolutions of the urea concentrations c, c_{int} and c_{cel} corresponding to the patient's vascular, interstitial and cellular compartments, respectively, calculated by the PPI. In the same graph we have also included the concentrations obtained with the two-pool model, c_{acc} y c_{nac}, corresponding to the accessible and non-accessible compartments, respectively. A value of 1.28 for dKt/V was calculated by the PPI, while the two-pool reference model yields 1.30. This small difference is due to the fact that the extracellular urea concentration depletion during HD calculated by PPI is slightly lower than that calculated by the reference model. In any case, urea dynamics computed by the three-pool model-based PPI accurately agrees with that of the reference model.

The lower graph of Fig. 6 represents the variation of the volumes calculated by the PPI. It can be observed that the interstice behaves as a buffer, moderating the loss of vascular volume and therefore reducing the risk of hypotension events [53], especially under the conditions of the session, during which the cellular compartment did not contribute at all supplying ultrafiltrated liquid (4600 ml). This moderate reduction of V_v is in agreement with measurements reported in recent studies [54].

With regard to the evaluation of the physical activity monitor, when samples were acquired in parallel for the four channels, in order to reduce the power consumption at the minimum level, the dispersion of the measurements was much higher than the 5 % target value specified during the design. The high value of this error is associated with the delay in the process of management of interruptions in the microcontroller and the high requirements that the concurrent reading of all the channels impose. However, dispersion dropped below 4 % once the channels were attended sequentially following a polling scheme. This solution is still compatible with low power consumption. The IAU presents autonomy above 2 months using a non-rechargeable Lithium button battery (CR2450, 500 mAh, 6 grams), without considering the integrated transceiver. This autonomy can be doubled if particular energy-saving strategies are accounted for, like switching the IAU off during the night, with a command from the PSE. Power consumption in the integrated transceiver depends on the transmission level and is currently under optimization in order to keep high values of autonomy in the monitor.

Figure 7 shows the value of gravitational acceleration in static conditions, expressed in units of g, as a function of the angle θ formed between one of the IAU measurement axis and the horizontal reference. The dispersion referred above has been removed averaging the samples at the point of measurement, every 15 degrees, in order to validate the precision of both the calibration and the measurement algorithm in static conditions. Deviations between each point (measurement) and the theoretical value (circle with unit radius) are practically negligible.

Finally, and in agreement with the method previously stated, Fig. 8 shows the hierarchical structure associated to a virtual component representing kidney collecting duct epithelium. This diagram is focused on the hydraulic permeability of the membrane. A virtual component is a mathematical submodel that can be linked to other submodels by means of its connection ports. Components and ports are the main elements of a non-causal modelling language-based library, as EcosimPro. As described in that figure, the kidney collecting duct epithelium can connect both of its faces with two compartments through the ports represented as rectangles with solid border lines. This membrane is asymmetric, in such a way that AQP2 channels are in epithelium cell apical membrane (duct side), while epithelium cell basolateral membrane, at interstice side has AQP3 and AQP4 channels. This asymmetry can be associated to mi and mo ports. The inside of the component includes the two major physical processes related to the hydraulic permeability of the component: L_p, which refers to the hydraulic permeability associated with the normal diffusive channels, usually paracellular paths, not controlled by AQP, and L_p*, which is the component of the hydraulic permeability associated with AQP channels. According to this methodology, physical processes are also represented

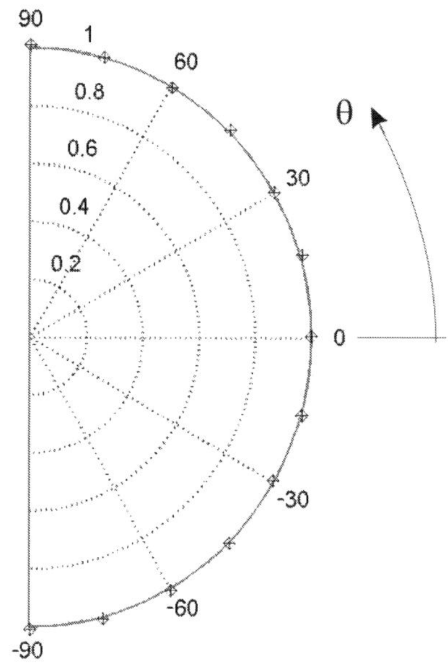

Figure 7. Gravitational acceleration measured in one axis of the IAU as a function of the angle with the horizontal reference.

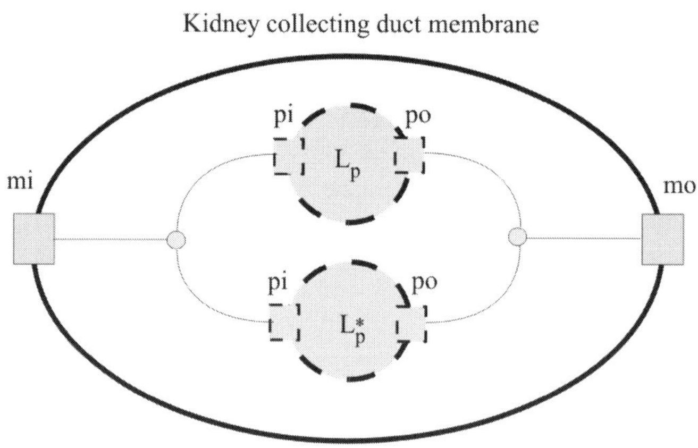

Figure 8. Hierarchical structure of a kidney collecting duct membrane component.

by non-causal components and ports. This is another advantage since it is possible to increase the complexity or modify the behaviour of a virtual component adding or changing the physical processes of the lower layers. As can be seen in the aforementioned hierarchical diagram (Fig. 8), the physical processes are connected in parallel through their ports.

The EL source code of L_p process (Box 1) is formed basically by the declaration of two port variables corresponding to pi and po ports (PORT block), together with the equations that describe the physics. The latter are represented here by the law of mass conservation and the law of transfer mass (CONTINUOUS block). The last law has been simplified in this example to consider only static pressure difference, given by pi.ptotal-po.ptotal. The other blocks are mainly related to variables and parameters definitions.

Box 1: EL code of a virtual component that represents the physics process Lp.

```
COMPONENT LpProcess
PORTS
    IN physics pi                  "Input port"
    OUT physics po                 "output port"
DATA
    REAL Lp   "Hydraulic permeability (m3/s/Pa)"
DECLS
    REAL atrans    "Transfer area (m2)"
TOPOLOGY
    PATH pi TO po
CONTINUOUS
    -- Law of conservation of mass
    pi.wbulk=po.wbulk
    -- Law of mass transfer
    pi.wbulk=Lp*(pi.ptotal-po.ptotal) — water flow
END COMPONENT
```

The virtual component associated to the kidney collecting duct membrane is denoted as KidneyCollectorMembrane, and can be formed by simply aggregating simulation components representing physical processes, as is shown in the following EL code (Box 2). This task can be done declaring and connecting components. The resulting virtual component will pertain to an upper hierarchically layer, as indicated in Fig. 8.

Box 2: EL code (simplified) of a virtual component that represents the kidney collecting duct membrane

```
COMPONENT KidneyCollectorMembrane
PORTS
    IN physics mi  "Input side"
    OUT physics mo  "output side"
TOPOLOGY
    LpProcess LpPromedio (atransfer=200)
    LpStarProcess LpAQP
    CONNECT LpPromedio.pi TO LpAQP.pi
    CONNECT LpPromedio.po TO LpAQP.po
    ...
END COMPONENT
```

Virtual component representing the physical process L_p* has been denoted as LpStarProcess, and it has been instanced once under the name LpAQP. Two fundamental strategies are defined to incorporate the behaviour of the AQP channels into the component LpStarProcess. The first one, called functional strategy, defines this physical process using phenomenological equations that describe the variation of L_p* without considering the feedback relationships related to regulation mechanisms. This is a simple approach to include new knowledge in the model. The second procedure, called structural strategy, accounts for the feedback relationships that define the regulation mechanisms affecting the value of L_p* at different scales.

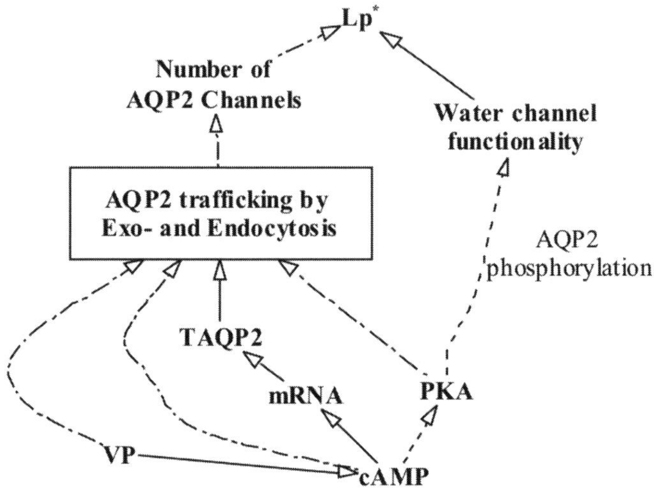

Figure 9. Diagram showing in a simple way the major regulation mechanisms of L_p* related at genomic level (solid arrows), proteomic (dotted arrows) and cellular level (dashed-dot arrows).

Figure 9 describes in a simple way the main regulation mechanisms known for L_p*. The type of line used in the arrows is used to distinguish the level of regulation. According to this diagram, the mechanism at the genomic level shows that an increase of vasopressin (VP) stimulates the formation of intracellular cyclic adenosine monophosphate (cAMP) through membrane receptors, which stimulates the transcription of the AQP2 gene, increasing thus the concentration of its associated mRNA, and therefore the total of AQP2 (TAPQ2), which in turn has been demonstrated that increases the value of L_p*, possibly increasing the number of AQP2 channels. At the proteomic level, it has been proven that VP stimulates phosphorylation of AQP2, through the kinase cAMP-dependent protein (PKA). Phosphorylated AQP2 protein increases the permeability of the channel to water. Finally, at the cellular level, it has been demonstrated the existence of a traffic of AQP2 in vesicles, which formation and fusion by endocytosis and exocytosis with apical membrane, increase or decrease the number of available AQP2 channels. The mechanisms are not completely known and therefore they have been included as a box in the referred figure.

These mechanisms are implemented into LpStarProcess component, using a structural modelling technique, as bond graph [55,56]. This structural component can be used instead of the functional component by means of a simple aggregation. This technique can be extended to account for more anatomical details in physiological models.

4. Discussion

The simulation experiment presented was designed to show the capability of PPI as mathematical observer and predictor of the internal dynamics state of the patient. The selection of a compartmental urea kinetic model is justified by the proved ability of these models to improve clinical outcomes of renal replacement therapies [44,57]. Moreover we selected an ESRD patient submitted to periodic HD, given the increasing importance of this disease and the new advances of telemedicine in nephrology, propelled by daily and nocturnal HD therapies [58–60], among other reasons.

According to our outcomes, extracellular and intracellular urea dynamics calculated by PPI agrees accurately with the reference two-pool model. Urea concentration shows an abrupt depletion in the extracellular compartment, during HD, followed by a rebound during the subsequent 30 minutes after the HD end. This is due to the non-uniform distribution of urea between the different compartments and also to the low blood perfusion in some tissues. The last mechanism can be observed from the three-pool model that forms the PPI (Fig. 4), formulating vascular and cellular membranes by means of their characteristic geometries, and solving an equivalent average cellular diameter. The comparison between computed cellular diameter and the human average cellular diameter gives a measure of the influence of blood regional mechanism. A preliminary advance of this model has been presented in Prado and colleagues [61].

In addition, the evolution of compartmental volumes shows the importance of interstice to moderate the blood volume reduction due to ultrafiltration during HD, reducing this way the risk of a hypovolemia event. The hypotension complication appears in 30 % of all HD treatments, and although the genesis of this problem is multifactorial, hypovolemia is the major responsible mechanism [53]. Several studies indicate that blood pressure can be controlled by a proper management of the extracellular volume (ECV) [62,63]. This fact suggests that the ability of a PPI to predict excessive plasma volume depletion can be used to avoid the occurrence of hypotension events.

Blood volume can be monitored by means of the HTO value [64], which in turn can be measured by optic reflection, allowing a non-invasive and on-line monitoring of blood volume [65]. However, HTO measurements could be better utilized as input variables by a customized PPI, providing an integral and correlated image of the three compartmental volumes and even other state variables of the patient. This greater knowledge can help to know the causes that originate a more abrupt depletion in plasma volume for some patients, and provides a better control of ultrafiltration velocity, avoiding for example, the occurrence of backfiltration due to low transmembrane pressure [66].

Several research works support the ability of dynamics mathematical models to predict hypotension events in patients submitted to intermittent dialysis therapy, being a remarkable reference the study from Cavalcanti and Marco [67]. Regarding other important chronic pathologies in telemedicine, as diabetes mellitus, glucose and insulin kinetic models have been successfully applied in support systems for therapy of insulin [68]. Mathematical dynamics models are also utilized to analyze the falling risk in subjects with motor control impairment by means of the study of the relationships between postural and kinematic states [69].

Signal monitoring is a key issue in any telehealthcare system. We have presented a laboratory evaluation of a novel physical activity monitor for humans. This device is mainly featured by its ability to customization and distributed process based on intelligent sensors, performing a monitoring non limited to local environments, neither to the corporal position of the sensors nor to particular clothing. This way it overcomes several limitations of other monitors [16–19]. The design has been based on modern microelectromechanical-system (MEMS) technologies and wireless communication. Vibratory artefacts related to bouncing and jolting are removed because of its permanent contact with the subject skin.

The first results of the laboratory prototype were satisfactory. The accuracy of dynamic measurements was greater than 4% of g for the algorithm selected to read and calibrate the sensors. The remaining processing capacity of the IAU's microcontroller is available for customizing it to the client, satisfying this way the requirements of the telehealthcare methodological approach. We have evaluated the different noise sources proving the possibility to improve the previous accuracy using the CCP (Capture/Compare/PWM) module in the microcontroller. The communication links indicated in Fig. 5 were also validated. Power consumption of IAU, without the integrated transceiver, and according to the selected algorithm for measurement, provides more than two months of autonomy for IAU for a Lithium non-rechargeable battery type CR2450. We are optimizing the power consumption of the transceiver taking profit of the very low range necessary for the WPAN, by hardware and software techniques. These outcomes suggest that the physical activity monitor will accomplish the whole economical and functional specifications needed to be applied under the novel telehealthcare methodology presented.

The capability to measure energy expenditure and extract postural and kinematic information from accelerations measured at waist and chest has been demonstrated in several studies [41,70,71]. The relationship between the corporal position of the accelerometric sensor axis and suitable postural and activity classifications has also been analyzed by Foerster and Fahrenberg [72] with successful conclusions. Finally, the monitor has been designed with the aim to process acceleration signals captured by the IAU in a real time manner. This objective is achieved by a modern digital signal processor (DSP TMS 320 C6713 from Texas Instrument) that joins high power process together with low cost and low power consumption. Moreover we have distributed the signal processing between the IAU and the PSE [42]. This device is currently under international patent process.

This telehealthcare methodology provides an opportunity to give new technological and scientific solutions to human physiology simulation environments, as the one represented by the Physiome project [73]. These simulation environments are emerging as a trend that is also known as System Biology [74,75]. Modelling and simulation tools are essential in this new area, because they assist us forward integrating and connecting information from several domains and scales [75,76].

Multiscale integration in virtual prototyping is a very powerful capability that has been analyzed in the framework of our telehealthcare methodology. Some preliminary aspects of the modelling and simulation methodology developed to the PPI were presented in Prado and colleagues [77]. In this work we have briefly studied the compatibility of the PPI methodology with multiscale knowledge integration approaches by means of a virtual component that describes the hydraulic permeability of the kidney collecting duct epithelial membrane. We have presented two types of strategies to integrate the hydraulic permeability associated to AQP2 channels. The concepts have been clarified by means of the simplified EL source code of the kidney collecting duct epithelial membrane virtual component. The EL codification of the connection ports is not shown here because it exceeds the scope of the paper.

5. Conclusions

We have presented a new methodological approach in telehealthcare systems based on the on-line, customized, and dynamics generation of knowledge about the physiological and internal state of patients or clients of the system and the associated therapy devices. This approach modifies the current focus in telemedicine and telehealthcare systems, which is directed to optimize remote monitoring, process biosignals to generate alarms and warnings, and speed up the clinical information management, by means of advances on information and communication technologies.

The study has been based on three key aspects of the methodology that have been previously and briefly described. Firstly, we have evaluated the capability of the PPI for building an image of the internal state of its associated patient. With that aim we have performed a simulation experiment over a urea kinetic model-based PPI associated to a patient during an HD session. The outcomes were in agreement with those obtained by a validated reference mathematical model.

The processing of biosignals to generate customized knowledge of the patient comprises also the sensor layer. A novel physical activity monitor that follows this concept has been presented and a laboratory prototype has been validated.

Finally, we have analyzed the manner to integrate multiscale knowledge into the mathematical models that form the PPI, using a simplistic virtual component of the kidney collecting duct membrane, together with the genomic, proteomic and cell regulation mechanisms of AQP2 channels.

As a major conclusion the study presents a new telehealthcare model in which the goal is not the decentralization but the personalization of the health assistance by means of modern technologies both in communications and in mathematical modelling and simulation.

Acknowledgments

This work was partly supported by the Spanish National Board of Biomedical Research (Instituto de Salud Carlos III, Fondo de Investigación Sanitaria), under Grants 01/0072-01 and PI040687.

References

[1] Harvey JN. Diabetic nephropathy. BMJ 2002;325(7355):59–60.
[2] Sims RJA, Cassidy MJD, Masud T. The increasing number of older patients with renal disease. BMJ 2003;327(7413):463–464.
[3] Parmar MS. Chronic renal disease. BMJ 2002;325(7355):85–90.
[4] Swift CG. Care of older people: Falls in late life and their consequences-implementing effective services. BMJ 2001;322(7290):855–7.
[5] Wootton R. Telemedicine: a cautious welcome. BMJ 1996;313(7069):1375–7.
[6] Horsch A, Balbach T. Telemedical Information Systems. IEEE Transactions on Information Technology in Biomedicine 1999;3(3):166–75.
[7] Wootton R. Recent advances: Telemedicine. BMJ 2001;323(7312):557–60.
[8] Raghupathi W, Tan J. Strategic IT applications in health care. Communications of the ACM 2002;45(12):56–61.
[9] Bronzino JD. The biomedical engineering handbook. 2nd ed. Florida: CRC Press; 2000.
[10] Deutsch T, Roudsari A, Leicester H, Theodorou T, Carson E, Sonksen P. UTOPIA: a consultation system for visit-by-visit diabetes management. Med. Inform. (Lond) 1996;21(4):345–58.
[11] Carson ER, Cramp DG, Morgan A, Roudsari AV. Clinical decision support, systems methodology, and telemedicine: their role in the management of chronic disease. IEEE Transactions on Information Technology in Biomedicine 1998;2(2):80–8.
[12] Hellström Y, Hallberg IR. Perspectives of elderly people receiving home help on health, care and quality of life. Health & Social Care in the Community 2001;9(2):61–71.
[13] Slobounov SM, Moss SA, Slobounova ES, Newell KM. Aging and time to instability in posture. Journals of Gerontology. Series a, Biological Sciences and Medical Sciences 1998;53(1):B71–8.

[14] Howland J, Lachman ME, Peterson EW, Cote J, Kasten L, Jette A. Covariates of fear of falling and associated activity curtailment. Gerontologist 1998;38(5):549–55.
[15] Rialle V, Duchene F, Noury N, Bajolle L, Demongeot J. Health "Smart" home: information technology for patients at home. Telemed J E Health 2002;8(4):395–409.
[16] Mathie MJ, Basilakis J, Celler BG. A System for Monitoring Posture and Physical Activity Using Accelerometers. In: 23rd Annual International Conference of the IEEE Engineering in Medicine and Biology Society; 2001 Oct. 25–28; Istanbul, Turkey; 2001.
[17] Naemura K, Hosaka H, Iseki H, Itao K. Development of a new wearable multi-channel sensing unit. In: 23rd Annual International Conference of the IEEE Engineering in Medicine and Biology Society; 2001 Oct. 25–28; Istanbul, Turkey; 2001.
[18] Sekine M, Tamura T, Fujimoto T, Fukui Y. Classification of walking pattern using acceleration waveform in elderly people. In: Engineering in Medicine and Biology Society, editor. Proceedings of the 22nd Annual International Conference of the IEEE; 2000 23–28, Jul; Chicago, Illinois, USA; 2000. p. 1356–1359.
[19] Nakahara AK, Sabelman EE, Jaffe DL. Development of a second generation wearable accelerometric motion analysis system. In: Engineering in Medicine and Biology Society, editor. Proceedings of the 21nd Annual International Conference of the IEEE; 1999 23–28, Jul; Atlanta, GA, USA; 1999.
[20] Woolf AD, Akesson K. Preventing fractures in elderly people. BMJ 2003;327(7406):89–95.
[21] Agroyannis B, Fourtounas C, Romagnoli G, Skiadas M, Tsavdaris C, Chassomeris C, et al. Telemedicine technology and applications for home hemodialysis. The International Journal of Artificial Organs 1999;22(10):679–83.
[22] Skiadas M, Agroyiannis B, Carson E, Cramp D, Fourtounas C, Darnige A, et al. Design, implementation and preliminary evaluation of a telemedicine system for home haemodialysis. Journal of Telemedicine and Telecare 2002;8(3):157–64.
[23] Stokvis S, Verhallen A, Meijer P, de Graaff M, Kooistra M. Online Monitoring of Nocturnal Home Hemodialysis. Hemodialysis International 2003;7(1):73–104.
[24] Kooistra MP. Frequent prolonged home haemodialysis: three old concepts, one modern solution. Nephrol. Dial. Transplant. 2003;18(1):16–18.
[25] Stroetmann KA, Gruetzmacher P, Stroetmann VN. Improving quality of life for dialysis patients through telecare. J Telemed Telecare 2000;6(Suppl 1):S80–3.
[26] Zhang Y, Yang B-H, Asada HH. Cuff-less ambulatory monitoring of beat-to-beat blood pressure based on a hemodynamic model. In: Engineering in Medicine and Biology Society, editor. Proceedings of the 19th Annual International Conference of the IEEE; 1999 Oct 13–16; Atlanta, GA, USA; 1999.
[27] Hayes MJ, Smith PR. A New Method for Pulse Oximetry Possessing Inherent Insensitivity to Artifact. IEEE Trans. Biomed. Eng. 2001;48(4):452–461.
[28] Koschinsky T, Heinemann L. Sensors for glucose monitoring: technical and clinical aspects. Diabetes Metab Res Rev 2001;17(2):113–23.
[29] Kovalerchuck B, Vityaev E, Ruiz JF. Consistent Knowledge Discovery in Medical Diagnosis. IEEE Engineering in Medicine and Biology 2000;19(4):26–37.
[30] Torasso P. Multiple representations and multi-modal reasoning in medical diagnostic systems. Artificial Intelligence in Medicine 2001;23(1):49–69.
[31] Whitten PS, Mair FS, Haycox A, May CR, Williams TL, Hellmich S. Systematic review of cost effectiveness studies of telemedicine interventions. BMJ 2002;324(7351):1434–7.
[32] Mair F, Whitten P. Systematic review of studies of patient satisfaction with telemedicine. BMJ 2000;320(7248):1517–20.
[33] Tanriverdi H, Iacono CS. Diffusion of telemedicine: a knowledge barrier perspective. Telemedicine Journal and e-Health 1999;5(3):223–44.
[34] Prado M, Roa L, Reina-Tosina J, Palma A, Milán JA. Virtual Center for Renal Support: Technological Approach to *Patient Physiological Image*. IEEE Transactions on Biomedical Engineering 2002;49(12):1420–1430.
[35] Prado M, Roa L, Reina-Tosina J, Palma A, Milán JA. Renal telehealthcare system based on a patient physiological image: a novel hybrid approach in telemedicine. Telemedicine Journal and e-Health 2003;9(2):149–165.
[36] Tiller M. Introduction to Physical Modelling with Modelica. Boston: Kluwer Academic Publishers; 2001.
[37] Stengel RF. Optimal control and estimation: New York Dover; 1994.
[38] Rapún JL, López N. Application of a PMAX System on a Biomass Plant. In: 2000 Performance Software Users Group Meeting Proceedings; 2000; Idaho Falls, Idaho, USA; 2000.
[39] Vara RP, Herrero PC, Parrilla AG. Ecosim: a State-of-the-art Continuous Simulation Tool for TCS and ECLSS. In: International Conference On Environmental Systems; 1999 July; Denver, CO, USA: Society of Automotive Engineers; 1999.

[40] Johansen KL, Chertow GM, Da Silva M, Carey S, Painter P. Determinants of physical performance in ambulatory patients on hemodialysis. Kidney International 2001;60(4):1586–91.
[41] Bouten CVC, Koekkoek KTM, Verduin M, Kodde R, Janssen JD. A Triaxial Accelerometer and Portable Data Processing Unit for the Assessment of Daily Physical Activity. IEEE Transactions on Biomedical Engineering 1997;44(3):136–47.
[42] Prado M, Reina-Tosina J, Roa L. Distributed intelligent architecture for falling detection and physical activity analysis in the elderly. In: 24th Annual International Conference of the IEEE-EMBS and Annual Fall Meeting of the BMES; 2002 Oct 23–26; Houston, TX, USA; 2002. p. 1910–1911.
[43] Empresarios-Agrupados. EL Modelling Language (EcosimPro) version 3.2: EA International, http://www.ecosimpro.com/; 2002.
[44] Gotch FA, Sargent JA, Keen ML. Whither goest Kt/V? Kidney International 2000;58(Suppl 76): S3–S18.
[45] Hester RL, Curry E, Bower J. The determination of hemodialysis blood recirculation using blood urea nitrogen measurements. Am J Kidney Dis 1992;20:598–602.
[46] Canaud B, Bosc JY, Cabrol L, Leray Moragues H, Navino C, Verzetti G, et al. Urea as a marker of adequacy in hemodialysis: lesson from in vivo urea dynamics monitoring. Kidney International 2000;58 Suppl 76:S28–40.
[47] Prado M, Roa L, Palma A, Milán JA: A novel mathematical method based on urea kinetic modelling for computing the dialysis dose. Computer Methods and Programs in Biomedicine 74:109–128, 2004.
[48] Michel CC, Curry FE. Microvascular Permeability. Physiol. Rev. 1999;79(3):703–761.
[49] Fauchald P, Norseth J, Jervell J. Transcapillary colloid osmotic gradient, plasma volume and interstitial fluid volume in long-term type 1 (insulin-dependent) diabetes. Diabetologia 1985;28(5):269–73.
[50] Harper S, Tomson C, Bates D. Human uremic plasma increases microvascular permeability to water and proteins in vivo. Kidney Int 2002;61(4):1416–22.
[51] Sasaki S, Ishibashi K, Marumo F. Aquaporin-2 and -3: representatives of two subgroups of the aquaporin family colocalized in the kidney collecting duct. Annu Rev Physiol 1998;60:199–220.
[52] USRDS. U.S. Renal Data System: Annual Data Report. Bethesda, MD: National Institute of Health, National Institute of Diabetes and Digestive and Kidney Diseases; 2000 June 2000.
[53] Johner C, Chamney PW, Schneditz D, Kramer M. Evaluation of an ultrasonic blood volume monitor. Nephrology, Dialysis, Transplantation 1998;13(8):2098–103.
[54] Fenech M, Maasrani M, Jaffrin MY. Fluid volumes determination by impedance spectroscopy and hematocrit monitoring: application to pediatric hemodialysis. Artificial Organs 2001;25(2):89–98.
[55] Broenink JF. Object–oriented modelling with bond graphs and Modelica. In: ICBGM '99, International Conference on Bond Graph Modelling and Simulation, part of the WMC '99, the Western MultiConference; 1999 January 17–20; San Francisco, CA; 1999.
[56] Margolis DL. An Introduction to Bond Graph Techniques for Biomedical System Modelling. Simulation 1975;25(1):22–26.
[57] Gotch FA. Evolution of the single-pool urea kinetic model. Seminars in Dialysis 2001;14(4):252–6.
[58] Chan C. Nocturnal hemodialysis: an attempt to correct the "unphysiology" of conventional intermittent renal replacement therapy. Clin Invest Med 2002;25(6):233–5.
[59] Pierratos A. Daily hemodialysis: an update. Curr Opin Nephrol Hypertens 2002;11(2):165–71.
[60] Agroyannis B, Tzanatos H, Fourtounas C, Kopelias I. Telematics application for home hemodialysis. Kidney International 1999;55(1):338.
[61] Prado M, Roa L, Palma A, Milan JA. (Clinical Validation of the Normalized Single Pool Urea Kinetic Model). In: XVIII Congreso Anual de la Soc. Esp. de Ingeniería Biomédica (CASEIB); 2000 27–29 Sep; Cartagena, Murcia, Spain; 2000. p. 283–286.
[62] Katzarski KS, Charra B, Luik AJ, Nisell J, Divino Filho JC, Leypoldt JK, et al. Fluid state and blood pressure control in patients treated with long and short haemodialysis. Nephrology, Dialysis, Transplantation 1999;14(2):369–75.
[63] Katzarski KS, Filho JCD, Bergström J. Extracellular Volume Changes and Blood Pressure Levels in Hemodialysis Patients. Hemodialysis International 2003;7(2):135–142.
[64] Steuer RR, Leypoldt JK, Cheung AK, Harris DH, Conis JM. Hematocrit as an indicator of blood volume and a predictor of intradialytic morbid events. Asaio Journal 1994;40(3):M691–6.
[65] de Vries JP, Kouw PM, van der Meer NJ, Olthof CG, Oe LP, Donker AJ, et al. Non-invasive monitoring of blood volume during hemodialysis: its relation with post-dialytic dry weight. Kidney International 1993;44(4):851–4.
[66] Ofsthun NJ, Leypoldt JK. Ultrafiltration and backfiltration during hemodialysis. Artificial Organs 1995;19(11):1143–61.
[67] Cavalcanti S, Marco LYD. Numerical Simulation of the hemodynamic response to hemodialysis-induced hypovolemia. Artif. Organs 1999;23:1063–1073.

[68] Nucci G, Cobelli C. Models of subcutaneous insulin kinetics. A critical review. Comp. Meth. Progr. Biomed. 2000;62:249–257.

[69] Ramos C. How models help us to understand the interactions between posture and voluntary movements. IEEE Engineering in Medicine and Biology Magazine 1992;11(4):91–92.

[70] Najafi BA, K.; Paraschiv-Ionescu, A.; Loew, F.; Bula, C.J.; Robert, P. Ambulatory system for human motion analysis using a kinematic sensor: monitoring of daily physical activity in the elderly. Biomedical Engineering, IEEE Transactions on 2003;50(6):711–723.

[71] Foerster F, Smeja M, Fahrenberg J. Detection of posture and motion by accelerometry: a validation study in ambulatory monitoring. Computers-in-Human-Behavior 1999;15(5):571–583.

[72] Foerster F, Fahrenberg J. Motion pattern and posture: correctly assessed by calibrated accelerometers. Behav Res Methods Instrum Comput 2000;32(3):450–7.

[73] Bassingthwaighte JB. Strategies for the Physiome Project. Ann Biomed Eng 2000;28:1043–1058.

[74] Kitano H. Systems Biology: A Brief Overview. Science 2002;295:1662–1664.

[75] Noble D. Modeling the Heart–from Genes to Cells to the Whole Organ. Science 2002;295:1678–1682.

[76] Csete ME, Doyle JC. Reverse Engineering of Biological Complexity. Science 2002;295:1664–1669.

[77] Prado M, Roa L, Palma A, Milan JA. Space Discretization in Multipool Kinetic Models Used for Telehealthcare. In: 4th International workshop in Biosignals Interpretation; 2002 June 24–26; Villa Olmo, Como, Italy; 2002. p. 363–366.

Medical and Care Compunetics 2
L. Bos et al. (Eds.)
IOS Press, 2005

Standardization of Demographic Service for a Federated Healthcare Environment

I. ROMÁN[a], L.M. ROA[b], L.J. REINA[b] and G. MADINABEITIA[a]
[a] *Group of Telematic Engineering, University of Seville, Spain*
[b] *Biomedical Engineering Group, University of Seville, Spain*
isabel@trajano.us.es

Abstract. The main objective of this paper is to contribute into the process of the standardization of a demographic service in a federated healthcare environment. Our approach is based on semantic web techniques and aimed at the reconciliation of several previous standardization works.

Keywords. Demographic service, EHR, standardization, semantic WEB

Introduction

Throughout everybody's lifetime any person may have episodes of care provided by many health-care professionals. This is mainly due to the increasingly specialization of medicine practice and to the growth of population mobility, among other factors. On the other hand, new information and communication technologies (ICT) are being used in the healthcare tasks making these easier and more efficient. The aid of ICT is having a clear impact in the transition to the digital hospital being the management of multimedia clinical information systems an essential issue.

In this new scenario patient's clinical information is distributed among several information systems, geographically dispersed. These are usually autonomous and heterogeneous systems developed with different objectives, and consequently with diverse data models, platforms, standards and semantics. The interest is that they work in a collaborative environment as a federated environment.

In order to collect the patient's healthcare information distributed in all the federation (the Electronic Healthcare Record, EHR) a resolution of incompatibilities between the systems of the federation must be accomplished. These conflicts can be classified into three levels: semantic, functional and instance [1–7].

1. The Demographic Service

In order to collect the patient's healthcare information within an autonomous system from the federation, the patient must be uniquely identified first. Usually a system will allow the user to submit a search for a patient's record using some combination of identity parameters for the person and when the identification is finished this is translated into an unique identifier (ID) used in the whole system to reference this patient.

Most of these systems assign and maintain patient IDs autonomously. This management style suit the purposes of recording and retrieval of patient's records for the local organization. However for efficient collection or correlation of health records in a federated context a more sophisticated management of patient IDs must be performed.

After the identification of the person, the demographic data about the patient has to be requested over the federation in order to have an unique view of his/her demographic knowledge. Only after these first tasks, which are carried out by a Demographic Server, the whole EHR would be visualized. This shows the importance of this server, which objective is to manage the identification of a person and query his demographic data. Notice that the service is not centered in the patient but in the identification of every person involved in a global healthcare system.

In this paper, both identification and demographic data query are addressed. Our objective is to get an open and optimal specification for a demographic server in a federated environment. By an open specification we mean that the changes performed in a system of the federation should not involve changes in the management of the unique identification of the patient and the introduction of a new system must be an easy task. Two other important issues to provide an optimal specification are the cost related to the exchange of patient data, which should be minimal, and the view of the patient demographic information overall system, which must be always updated.

Our approach is different from other efforts in this service [8–9], and is widely known as Patient/Person Master Index (PMI), although it is based on the same standard, PID service of CORBAmed [10]. We propose a new paradigm for the management of IDs in order to have a PMI service. This new service enhances CORBAmed ones with ideas from other standards and other domains like database systems. The federation philosophy forces us to propose solutions to the semantic, functional and instance incompatibilities in our PMI.

1.1. Semantic-Level

The systems do not have the same demographic schema but the concepts in this common semantic domain must be unambiguous. The definition of a common ontology to describe the demographic knowledge is based on CEN, openEHR and PID schemas. We based our work in openEHR because of its philosophy of integrating all the previous efforts. We use OWL as ontology language because it is the standard proposed by the Web 3 Consortium (W3C) and will facilitate the description of the service in OWL-S.

1.2. Functional-Level

The systems are designed independently, hence they have different functionalities. However a unique view of the demographic knowledge about a patient is needed, maintaining the distribution of this information, and allowing each system of the federation to continue working as alone. The standardization of a service to manage this demographic knowledge is needed. Each autonomous system participating in the federation exports its functionality according to the interfaces of the normalized service.

The description of this service should be based on the common ontology developed for semantic integration. Of course the autonomous functionality must be unaltered. We have used the previous work of CORBAmed with the PID service [10] as a starting line. As far as technology is concerned we work with the new architecture of Web Services and the Semantic Web framework, proposed by the W3C. It is a solution strongly coupled with ontology techniques in special if we use OWL-S ontology to describe the services.

1.3. Instance-Level

When data stored in different systems modeling the demographic information about the same patient has to be merged, two new problems appear. Concerning the person identification, object instances from different systems which correspond to the same person must be identified. On the other hand, when the demographic attribute values of the same person in different systems do not match, value conflict resolution arises.

Considering that the systems in the federation continue to support their pre-existing functionality in addition to new federated one, instance incompatibility can be very frequent once the previous problems (semantic and functional) are solved.

2. Using Standards

As previously marked, our work is based on three main standards: OpenEHR [11–13], GPICs (from CEN) [14], and PID Service (from CORBAmed) [10].

To describe the demographic service interface, and solve functional-level incompatibilities, we use PIDS as starting point, but interfaces for federated environments special needs have to be added. The semantic for demographic knowledge provided by the PID service data model is not enough for semantic level integration so it has to be extended.

OpenEHR is an excellent framework for federated EHR, not only for demographic information but for every data (clinical and non clinical) in the EHR. As our approach is based on the philosophy of archetypes, the semantic of demographic knowledge is very open, what forces to describe this with more details using archetypes. For the specification of these archetypes we work with GPIC. This standard gives us a more complex terminology for demographic knowledge.

2.1. OpenEHR Data Model

The aim of openEHR work is the development of an ontology wide enough to accommodate all the previous standardised works about the EHR. This integration philosophy is the main reason for considering this effort an important reference point. The OpenEHR concept of Reference or Information model save the global characteristics of health record entries, how they are aggregated, and the context information required to meet ethical, legal and provenance requirements. The OpenEHR Information models define the set of classes that form the generic building blocks of the federated EHR. It reflects the stable characteristics of an electronic health record, and would be embedded in a federated record server at a programme code level.

One of these information models is the demographic package, showed in Fig. 1 [11]. This is a generalised model of the facts that one might expect to see in a demographic server. The purpose of the model is as a specification of a demographic service, either standalone, or a “wrapper” service for an existing system such as a PMI.

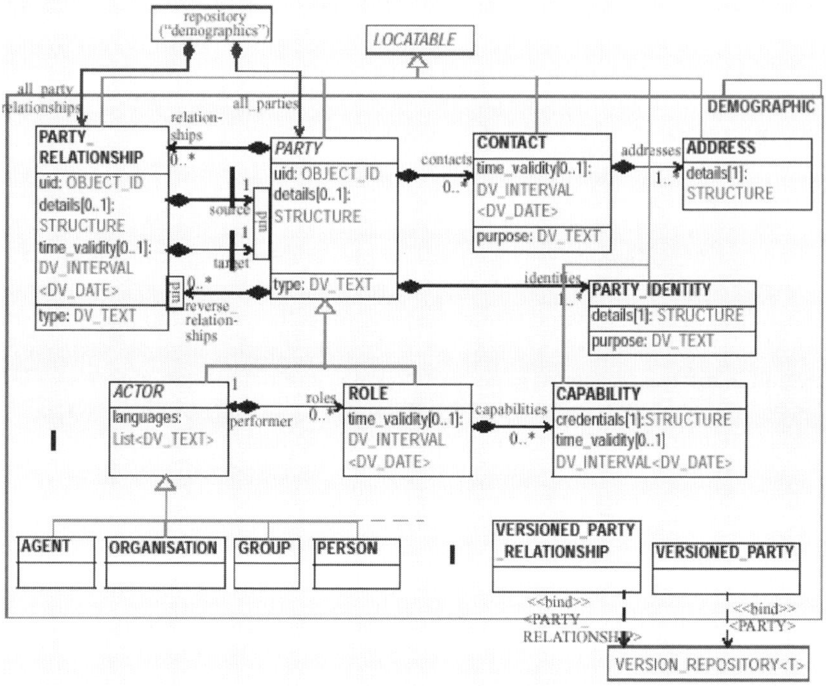

Figure 1. Class diagram for the Demographic Information Model of openEHR.

One of the main design criteria of the model is that it expresses attributes and relationships of demographic entities which exist regardless of particular clinical involvements or participations in particular events. Participations are meaningful only within the context of the health record or other relevant model where they record context-specific relationships between demographic entities and events in the real world.

The identifier concept is very important in a demographic service, common semantic and basic management must be defined for it. In openEHR identifiers are defined in the identification package from the common information model [13]. This package is shown in Fig. 2 and is used by the demographic model for representing person identifiers.

Instances of the classes in the reference model must be serialisable into an EHR Extract in an unambiguous way. The model is designed to be used with archetypes [12], a computable expression of a clinical concept in the form of structured constraint statements, based on this model. The key benefits of archetypes include:

- *Knowledge-enabled systems*: the separation of information and knowledge concerns in software systems, allowing cheap, future-proof software to be built.
- *Knowledge-level interoperability*: the ability of systems to reliably communicate with each other at the level of knowledge concepts
- *Domain empowerment*: to define the informational concepts the specialists work with, and have direct control over their information systems.
- *Intelligent Querying*: to be used at runtime to enable the efficient querying of data based on the structure of archetypes from which the data was created.

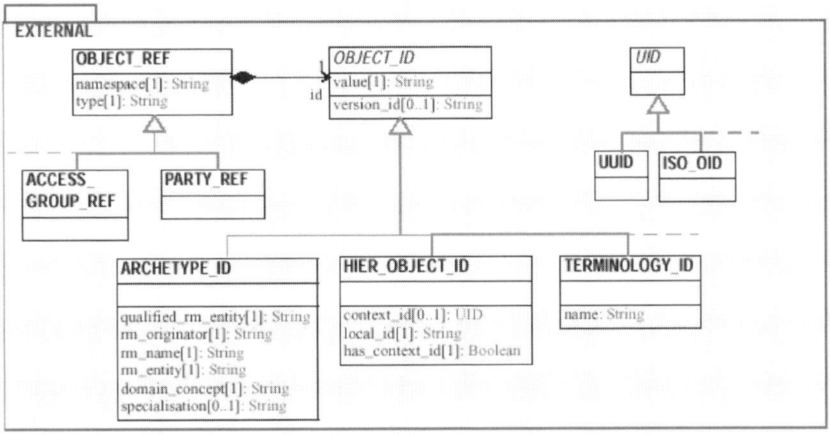

Figure 2. Identification Package in the common Information model. Revision 1.5.

As a result, archetypes can be defined for concepts such as particular kinds of PERSON for actual ROLEs and for party identities and addresses. In our work we are building archetypes with the particular semantic for the demographic knowledge that we manage, based on GPIC standard from CEN.

2.2. CEN GPIC Data Model

In the prEN 14822 the TC251 from CEN defines de General Purpose Information Components (GPIC). This standard addresses the definition and structuring of information relating to entities that are commonly encountered in communications with and between clinical information computer systems. It's a multi-part standard and in part 2, between others are defined components related to subjects of care (including persons and animals), Subject of care related parties and Healthcare agents (including healthcare professionals, organizations and devices). Figure 3 shows a summary of the classes defined for demographic knowledge.

The demographic archetypes needed for an openEHR compliant system can be inspired in GPIC from CEN. This standard gives the specific semantic necessary for this purpose. The effort in standards reconciliation is an important part of our work. The whole EHR is going to be based on openEHR therefore the container of person knowledge must agree with their Demographic Reference Model. The necessary archetypes are going to be based in GPIC non clinical.

2.3. PID Data Model

The Person Identification Service[10], described by CORBAmed group from OMG, defines a data model in IDL that we have summarized in Fig. 4 and Fig. 5 using UML representation.

Some of the main concepts in this model are:

- *Trait*: The characterization of a specific person's attribute is given as a name/value pair and is called "Trait".

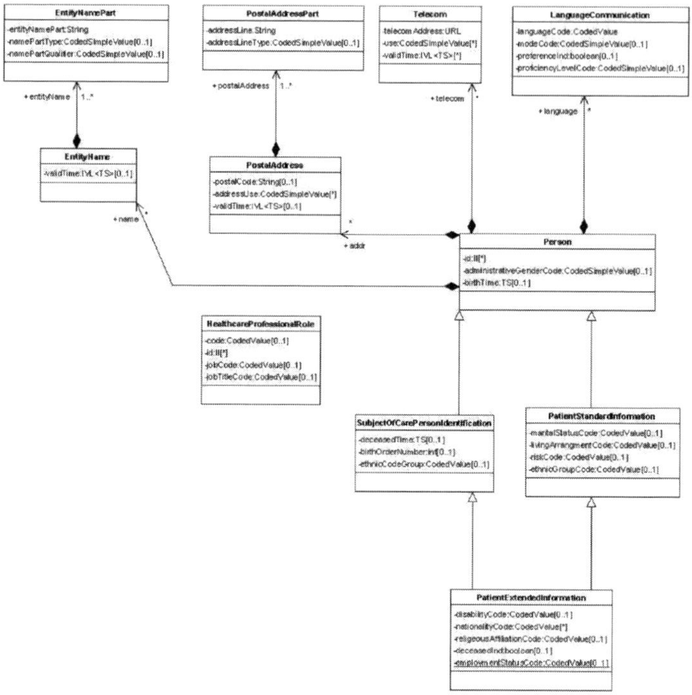

Figure 3. Person in GPIC non clinical.

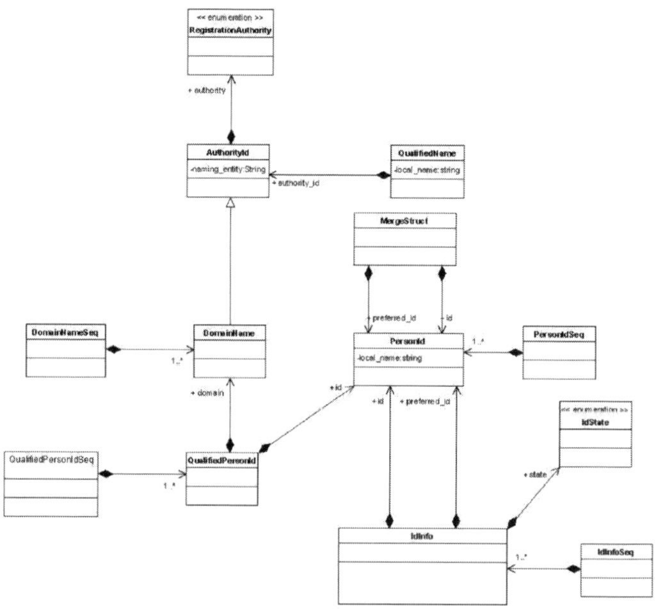

Figure 4. Data model for identifiers in PID service.

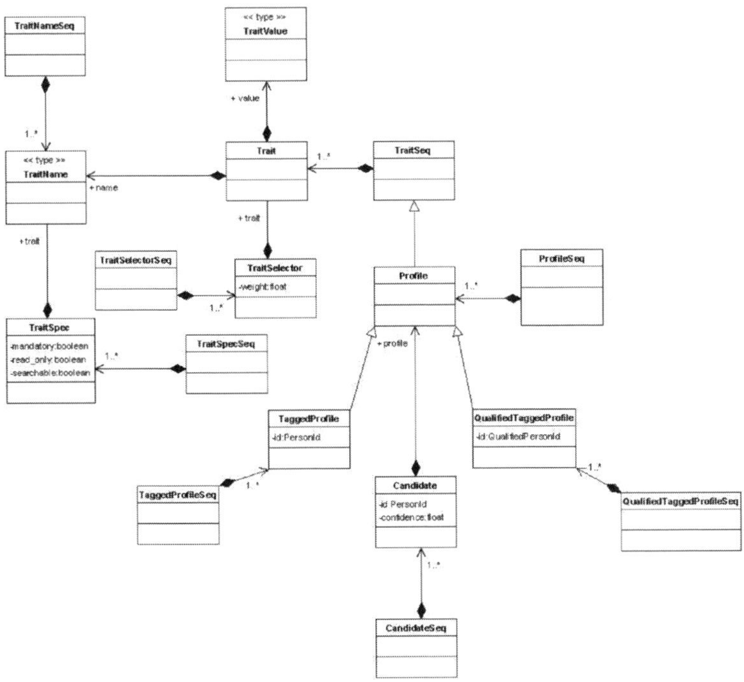

Figure 5. Data model for demographic semantic in PID Service.

- *TraitName*: The name given to the trait of a person as a string. A TraitNameSeq is a sequence of TraitNames and is very useful for specifying the set of traits a client is interested on. PID standard does not specify anything about TraitNames semantic in a particular system.
- *TraitValue*: represents the value of a person's trait. It could be of any type (including multimedia).
- *Profile*: is used when referring to the traits stored by a PIDS and bound to a PersonId. It is also used in the matching process for looking up persons. The term "Profile" is given to these sequences of traits since they are used a lot. This will be a very useful concept in our model and we are going to extend it.
- *Confidence*: is used when a list of candidates is returned after searching for persons. Each candidate contains the ID of the person, a confidence of how well that person's profile matches the profile selector and the set of traits requested in the operation. We are going to use the confidence parameter as support for entity identification and conflicts resolution, the standard says that the use of this parameter is implementation dependent.

2.4. PID Service Model

The PID service organizes person ID management functionality to meet healthcare needs. It is designed to:

- Support both the assignment of Ids within a particular ID Domain and the correlation of Ids among multiple ID Domains.

- Support searching and matching of people in both attended-interactive and message-driven-unattended modes, independent of matching algorithm.
- Support federation of PIDS services in a topology-independent fashion.
- Permit PIDS implementations to protect person confidentiality under the broadest variety of confidentiality policies and security mechanisms.
- Enable plug-and-play PIDS interoperability by means of a "core" set of profile elements, yet still support site-specific and implementation-specific extensions and customisation of profile elements.
- Define the appropriate meaningful compliance levels for several degrees of sophistication, ranging from small, query-only single ID Domains to large federated correlating ID Domains.

PIDS uses the last data model introduced for the specification of several service interfaces. Our interest is centred in correlation and federation tasks and these are supported by the CorrelationMgr interface that includes the methods:

- *load_profiles*: This operation causes the profiles to be loaded into the Correlating ID Domain, from the specified source ID Domains.
- *get_corresponding_ids*: This operation returns the IDs in the destination ID Domains that correspond to the ID passed in.
- *find_or_register_ids*: If this operation is implemented, it causes the profiles to be loaded into the Correlating ID Domain, from the specified source domains. IDs from the Correlating ID domain for each profile are returned.

The system that implements the CorrelationMgr interface acts as SuperID Domain server containing the profiles (set of traits) of every individual in every system of the federation, so demographic information from all participating ID Domains is stored. So correlation is based in centralization of profiles. Our work extends this interface for a more sophisticated correlation method to design a PMI that works over a federation without the centralization of demographic data.

3. Contributions

First we need to extend the PID service, data and functional models, with some useful concepts for correlation of servers. Then we introduce the new PMI server for a federated architecture, compliance with openEHR idea, where semantic and functional conflicts are solved and where value conflicts resolution methods could be easily included.

3.1. Contributions to PID Server

The new paradigm we propose for the federation of demographic services is based on two main concepts of the database domain:

- The *Unique key* is a combination of traits (may be only one) which identifies only one body of information out of several.
- The *Primary key* of a relational table uniquely identifies each record in the table. It can be either a normal attribute that is guaranteed to be unique (such as Social Security Number in a table with no more than one record per person) or it can be generated by the DBMS (such as a globally unique identifier, or GUID, in Microsoft SQL Server). Primary keys may consist of a single attribute or multiple attributes in combination.

In our model the primary key is the Identifier of a person in a system. Normally, not necessarily, it is only an attribute and not a combination of several of them. The concept PersonId, used in CORBAmed PID server, is the equivalent to the primary key in a system or domain. The unique key is any combination of attributes that uniquely identifies any person of the system. This set of attributes must be defined by the system designer. No concept matches exactly with this idea in the PID server defined by CORBAmed. A profile is used when referring to the traits stored by a PIDS and bound to a PersonId. A Trait is the combination of TraitName and TraitValue so a profile is no generic to a system but specific to a person in the system.

We introduce the concept Generic_Profile for referring a set of TraitNames that uniquely identify any person in the system (a unique key). A system can have more than one Generic_Profile.

For correlation task the Server is not going to store demographic information about persons but semantic information about unique and primary key in every system, reducing information duplicity, inconsistency and transaction and augmenting the security and scalability of the system. Once the person is identified his/her demographic knowledge must be quered over the system.

Other new concepts included in server data model are:

- *GenericProfileSeq*: is a sequence of GenericProfiles.
- *QualifiedGenericProfile*: contains a GenericProfile for a domain and the ID Domain.
- *QualifiedGenericProfileSeq*: A sequence of QualifiedGenericProfiles.
- *TraitConfidence*: In order to solve attribute value conflicts we are going to extend the concept of confidence (used only for candidates in the traditional PID) to the trait values for a person. This parameter is a measure of how sure the system is about the validity of that trait value.
- *QualifiedTraitSpec*: TraitSpec is a very useful concept in our PMI model to give specific semantic to Traits, we add some more attributes to Trait Spec to enrich this semantic creating the new type QualifiedTraitSpec.

Some new methods in the server have to be added in the Correlation interface.

- *load_generic_profile*: This operation causes the generic_profiles to be loaded from a source ID Domain into the PMI server.
- *get_generic_profile*: This operation returns from the PMI Server the generic_profiles of the specified source ID Domains.

For semantic conflict resolution the server needs more specific terminology control. As was previously marked PID standard does not specify anything about TraitNames semantic or TraitValues types in a particular system. In our model we are going to add semantic forcing these names corresponds to some concept in a federated ontology and only types from the federated ontology can be used. The demographic server has to inform the client when some TraitName is not agreeing with this federated ontology.

3.2. PMI Server and Federated Architecture

The PMI Server has to interact with the extended PID Servers. We have introduced three new concepts in the service model: Hard-matching, Provisional-Hard-matching and Soft-matching, very close to trait confidence and candidate confidence.

The traits values that are considered with confidence 1 by the PMI Agent are only those introduced by the user. When a search over a domain is made with a profile that includes the traits specified in a GenericProfile for this domain and all the traits have confidence 1 (are directly indicated by user) we refer to HARD_MATCHING (HM). Obviously as the search is made with unique key values the response can only be 0 or 1 candidates and this candidate should have confidence 1. This means that the system is very sure that this is the required person.

When the value of the traits for search has no confidence 1 but the traits corresponds to a GenericProfile we refer to PROVISIONAL_HARD_MATCHING (PHM). 0 or 1 candidate will be returned but as we are not sure about the values of traits the candidate could not have confidence 1. This means that the systems could not be sure about this candidate because he was not sure about some of the traits used for search.

If the search is made with traits that do not correspond to a generic_profile in the domain we refer to SOFT_MATCHING (SM) and the response can be 0, 1 or several candidates. The parameter confidence in these candidates is never going to be 1 and has to be lower that with PHM.

The TraitNames and TraitValues are described in a federated ontology based on GPIC, we have expressed this ontology in OWL language. Only these Traits can be used for communication between PMI server and PIDs and between PMI clients and server.

If the server is going to be included in a EHR architecture compliance to openEHR idea it should be defined in the Service Model [15] manner. The development of this reference model is in a very previous state so our work can be used for this important task. All the data structures used in the PMI server-client interface should be from the openEHR reference model, so archetypes based in the GPIC (our demographic ontology) are specified.

As far as technology is concerned we think that semantic web techniques should be used. We have defined the federated ontology, based on GPIC, in OWL and we are describing the PMI service in OWL-S, this would facilitate the integration in a intelligent agents architecture. For the service description we have written a OWL ontology for the openEHR reference model. About demographic archetypes we are facing the use of OWL instead of ADL, for a more integrated solution.

4. Discussion and Conclusion

Our work is centered in a PMI server that faces the identification of persons and the recovery of their demographic knowledge over heterogeneous clinical information systems. The integration problems for semantic and functional incompatibilities are solved and the value conflict resolution techniques can be deployed in a more easy way.

A great standardization effort is needed for a "universal" EHR because of the difficulties of integration of heterogeneous systems based in different standards. The vision of the problem as the decomposition in normalized services and the merging of different knowledge ontologies is one of the best ways to face this problem.

In our work we make a first discussion in this sense, particularized for the demographic service but with a methodology easily extended to other servers in the EHR. The introduced ideas could be the starting line for the standardization of a PMI service, an important piece in the EHR architecture.

Acknowledgments

This work has been supported by the Spanish Ministry of Science and Technology TIC2003-09300-C04. The authors also wish to acknowledge the contributions of the openEHR members when thoughts and problems about this work have been exposed in their distribution mailing lists. These collaboration efforts are very important for standardization processes.

References

[1] E.P. Lim, J. Srivastava, "Entity Identification in Database Integration: An Evidential Reasoning Approach". Proc. Int'l Conf. Next Generation Database, Fukuoka, Japan, Jan. 1993.

[2] D. Dey, S. Sarkar, "A distance-based approach to entity reconciliation in heterogeneous databases," IEEE Trans. Knowledge and Data Engineering, Vol. 14, No. 3, May/June 2002.

[3] H. Zhao, S. Ram, "Entity identification for heterogeneous database integration — a multiple casifier system approach and empirical evaluation," Information Systems, Vol. 30, pp. 119–132, 2005.

[4] E.P. Lim, J. Srivastava, S. Shekhar, "An evidential reasoning approach to attribute value conflict resolution in database integration," IEEE Trans. Knowledge and Data Enginineering, Vol. 8, No. 5, Oct. 1996.

[5] E.P. Lim, J. Srivastava, "Entity identification in database integration," Proc. IEEE Computer Society Ninth International Conference on Data Engineering, Vienna, Austria, April 19–23, 1993.

[6] E.P. Lim, J. Srivastava, S. Shekhar, "Resolving attribute incompatibility in database integration: an evidential reasoning approach," Proc. IEEE Computer Society Ninth International Conference on Data Engineering, pp. 154–163, 1994.

[7] J. Parsons, Y. Wand, "Attribute-based semantic reconciliation of multiple data sources," Journal on Data Semantics, Vol. 1, LCNS 2800, pp. 21–47, 2003.

[8] D.W. Forslund, R.K. Smith, T.C. Culpepper. "Federation of the Person Identification Service between enterprises," Proc. AMIA Symp. 2000, pp. 240–244, 2000.

[9] S. Facchinetti, D. Berry, S. Pardon, J. Grimson, "Distributed Patient Records require distributed patient ID Management: enter PIDS?" Notes from PICNIC conference.

[10] Person Identification Service (PIDS) Specification. April 2001, Version 1.1. (CORBAmed).

[11] The openEHR Demographic Information Model. Revision 1.4.4. © Copyright openEHR Foundation 2001–2003. All rights reserved. www.openEHR.org.

[12] The archetype object model. Revision: 0.5.1 © Copyright openEHR Foundation 2004. All rights reserved. www.openEHR.org.

[13] The openEHR Common Information Model. Revision: 1.5. © Copyright openEHR Foundation 2001–2003. All rights reserved. www.openEHR.org.

[14] prEN 14822-1:2003 (E)TC 251 WI. Health informatics — General purpose components for messages — Part 2: Non clinical.

[15] The openEHR EHR Service Model. Revision: 0.2. ©2003 The openEHR Foundation. www.openEHR.org.

Medical and Care Compunetics 2
L. Bos et al. (Eds.)
IOS Press, 2005

Telemedicine Training & Treatment Centre "A European Rollout of a Medical Best Practice"

Evert Jan HOIJTINK [a,1] and Ingolf RASCHER [b,2]
[a] *General Manager Portavita BV*
[b] *Director Gesundheitswirtschaft und Krankenhausmanagement, IMO (Institut zur Modernisierung von Wirtschafts- und Beschäftigungsstrukturen)*

Abstract. The project aims at rolling out an already proven eHealth best practice of one of the European countries towards the other European countries. The best practice in this case is the Dutch anti-coagulation approach on treating patients with a high risk of developing coagulation (prevalence of 2%), through specialized "Telemedicine Training/Treatment Centers for Anticoagulation" (TTCA). Specifically the disease management performed by the Dutch anti-coagulation treatment centers results in lower number of complications with patients and a higher customer / patient satisfaction. This is worldwide acknowledged. The TTCA approach has proven itself over the past years to be successful in both medical outcome and patient satisfaction and therefore is ready to be offered to a wider (European) group of patients and medical treatment centers. To prepare this European rollout, all possible medical, organizational, legal and economic issues are investigated in a pragmatic way and measures or action are taken during implementation itself. This project organizes a group of professional organizations in both Germany and The Netherlands. These professionals represent all needed know-how to perform such a new implementation and gather all implementation issues that occur. The investigation is performed in a practical way instead of a theoretical approach. Therefore the project is actually rolled out through a real life pilot with both medical personnel and patients in Germany to gather the real issues by doing. The pilot will be supported by a clinical trial to gather medical and quality of life information.

Introduction

In a TTCA, patients with a high risk to develop coagulation are treated. These patients will get a daily dose of specific medication to thin their blood to a specific degree, called their therapeutic range. If patients stay in their therapeutic range, the risk of complications like a stroke or bleeding will decrease.

This range is monitored on a regular basis in a timeframe between 3 and 28 days, depending on their individual stability.

[1] Oostenburgervoorstraat 83, 1018 MP Amsterdam, The Netherlands; E-mail: evert.jan.hoijtink@portavita.nl.
[2] Dessauer Str. 6, 67663 Kaiserslautern, Germany; E-mail: rascher@imo-institut.de.

The dosing scheme of the medication is adapted depending on the result of a blood analysis (INR) and historical medical data. This blood analysis is performed in one of two possible ways:

- Within a laboratory (for 'regular patients');
- By a self measurement handheld device at home (for 'self measurement patients').

Objective criteria are defined by the FNT[3] to select patients for self-measurement. These patients are trained at the TTCA to teach them the necessary skills. An Internet based e-learning module supports part of this training.

To be able to cost effectively perform this operation of education, blood analysis, calculating and distributing dosing schemes and monitoring patients, a disease management system has been developed.

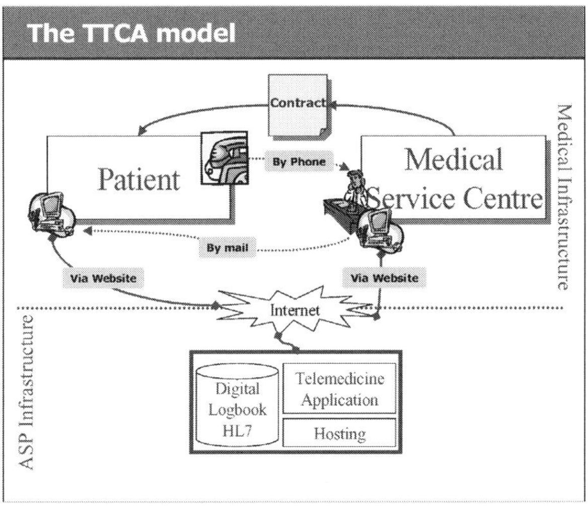

This disease management system is available as an Internet based service (ASP) in the Dutch language. The system is tightly connected to both Laboratory systems (Labosys of Philips Medical Systems) and to self measurement handheld (Coagucheck S of Roche Diagnostics).

Patients have direct access to their medical data in the disease management system through a secure Internet connection. Patients can contact their Medical Service Center by Internet, by phone or visit the center.

This service has been rolled out successfully first in 2003 in the Amersfoort region at the Trombosedienst Eemvallei. The TTCA Eemvallei is a well-established medical organization with internal medics and specialized nurses.

The Netherlands has a worldwide unique infrastructure for accreditation and quality control of anti-coagulation centers. This is done by the FNT, the legal representative of all 62 Dutch anti-coagulation centers.

[3] FNT = The Federatie Nederlandse Trombosediensten is the legal representative of all 62 Dutch Anticoagulation Centers.

The anti-coagulation treatment protocol for regular patients and self measurement patients is approved by the FNT.

Benefits

TTCA is a real life concept with benefits that are proven in several studies. Main benefits are:

Financial

- Use of the disease management system is proven cost effective.

Patient

- Empowerment of the patient to manage his/her own disease;
- More freedom for patient / less patient feeling caused by the use of self measurement devices;
- 7 x 24 hour accessibility of a TTCA decreases insecurity and worries about ability to do things right

Medical quality

- The disease management system forces the medical staff to use approved protocols;
- More responsibility for treatment improves treatment outcome;
- Medical data is always up to date and world wide accessible in case of emergencies.

Technical Architecture

The TTCA Disease Management System is based on leading international standards e.g.:

- Datamodel is based on the latest version of the HL7 Version 3 RIM;
- Workflow engine based on WFMC-specifications;
- Secure internet connection by SSL128 security;
- HTML user interface.

Functional Requirements

For a supporting a Disease Management Clinic with a software solution the following functionality is needed:

- Treatment and Dosing Protocol Conform FNT regulations and using the Dutch Beinema protocol;
- Electronic Health Record based upon the HL7 Version 3 RIM, centrally hosted and accessible by Internet with secure password and personal accounts;
- Roles and functions I.E. Administrations, Help-Desk, Nurse Practitioners, Dosing Doctor
- Workflow Methodology, in which medical personnel works through protocol based tasks.

- Patient Website, with secure account name and password and SSL128 security
- Pricing and Billing model, based upon the Dutch CTG tariffs
- Quality Reporting, based upon the yearly FNT reporting for the quality indices for all Dutch centres.
- INR Measurement infrastructure
    - Connections with Philips Medical Laboratory Infrastructure for regular patients using the Labosys system
    - Connections with Self Management handheld of Roche Diagnostics to read handheld INR values
- eLearning modules, Software to learn how to work with the Coaguchek S handheld through the Internet.

Issues

Main issues that need to be resolved during this project are:

- Medical compliance
- Rescheduling medical roles and functions
- Use of the Internet for modifying medical records (EHR)
- Legal issues / Legislation
- Cost of treatment
- Patient ownership or Patient empowerment
- Transeuropean treatment.

Symposium on Information/Knowledge Management

Medical and Care Compunetics 2
L. Bos et al. (Eds.)
IOS Press, 2005

An Interactive Framework for Developing Simulation Models of Hospital Accident and Emergency Services

Anthony CODRINGTON-VIRTUE [a,b,1], Paul WHITTLESTONE [b], John KELLY [b] and Thierry CHAUSSALET [a]

[a] *Health and Social Care Modelling Group, Cavendish School of Computer Science, University of Westminster, London, UK*
[b] *RKW Healthcare Strategists, London, UK*

Abstract. Discrete-event simulation can be a valuable tool in modelling health care systems. This paper describes an interactive framework to model and simulate a hospital accident and emergency department. An interactive spreadsheet (Excel) facilitated the user-friendly input of data such as patient pathways, arrival times, service times and resources into the discrete event simulation package (SIMUL8). The framework was enhanced further by configuring SIMUL8 to visually show patient flow and activity on a schematic plan of an A&E. The patient flow and activity information included patient icons flowing along A&E corridors and pathways, processes undertaken in A&E work areas and queue activity. One major benefit of visually showing patient flow and activity was that modellers and decision makers could visually gain a dynamic insight into the performance of the overall system and visually see changes over the model run cycle. Another key benefit of the interactive framework was the ability to quickly and easily change model parameters to trial, test and compare different scenarios.

Keywords. Simulation, modelling, accident and emergency

1. Introduction

The Operational Research modelling approach has is useful in helping to understand the internal dynamics of a non-linear hospital structure [1]. The potential of simulation in health care was also observed by Sanchez et al. [2]. In addition, Lowery [3] described simulation as an extremely useful tool for modelling uncertainty which is a major characteristic of illness. As such, Lowery argued, simulation was attractive for modelling health care systems. Despite the potential benefit of modelling and simulation in helping to understand hospital structures, a literature review by Jun et al. [4] showed poor adoption of modelling and simulation in real hospitals. In an effort to help understand the rea-

[1]Corresponding Author: Anthony Codrington-Virtue, RKW Healthcare Strategists, 17, Bentinck Street, London W1U 2SE, UK. Tel.: 020 7486 0434; E-mail: Anthony.Codrington-Virtue@rkw-uk.com; A.Codrington-Virtue@wmin.ac.uk.

Table 1. Model Basic Building (adapted from [5]).

Generic Activities	Generic Processes	Fixed Processes
High abstraction level	Medium abstraction level	Low abstraction level
Flexible enough to model any system and scenario	Flexible enough to model any system which uses similar processes	Can only model and analyse the system it was designed for
Difficult to use; requires knowledge and experience	Simple and intuitive to use after a brief and short introduction	Simple and easy to use after a quick explanation

sons for the poor adoption of modelling with regards to real hospitals, Sinreich and Marmor [5] suggested the reluctance of hospital management to accept change, especially if the suggestions came from a black box. Similarly, Sanchez et al. observed the lack of prevalence of simulation in the health care industry, despite its size and importance, when compared to other industries. Sanchez et al. noted that simulation professionals in health care needed to improve their personal capabilities to: make valid verified models; better understand their customer's business needs; and to provide customers with answers and insights to their business. In addition, Sanchez et al. observed that the simulation and modelling process should help clients understand their process as well as encourage client participation in model development to ensure reliable and valid data. Barnes et al. [6] suggested three key elements to successful simulation in health care: communication and participation; user-friendly simulation software; and using simulation as a decision-making tool.

In the specific context of modelling an emergency department, Sinreich and Marmor recommended that a simulation tool had to be general and flexible enough to model different possible settings, be intuitive and simple to use (so non-professional simulation modellers can easily run the model), and to include default values for all (or most) of the system parameters. This implies that models have a reasonable (medium) level of abstraction (essential for efficiency and flexibility) and simplicity – see Table 1. Generic activities (often the model-building icons or elements of the simulation software package) act as basic building blocks for a model, and often have great flexibility, but a high abstraction level. Consequently, generic activities often require a significant level of knowledge and experience to be utilised effectively. In contrast, fixed processes describe a specific, dedicated model, which tends to be limited but simpler to use. Generic processes offer a pragmatic alternative with medium abstraction levels, yet flexible models to model similar processes.

The view of a reasonable level of abstraction was also supported by Kachitvichyanukul et al. [7], who suggesting that "...the challenge was to build model components that have multiple levels of fidelity that can be changed by the user based on the purpose of the model."

This paper presents a framework for the development of a generic A&E simulation model. In particular, we focus on the front end acting as an interactive framework to input data into the A&E model. This paper will also discuss how the user-friendly front end could effectively manage the level of abstraction towards a generic process whilst remaining flexible enough to model a range of A&E scenarios. As such, the user-friendly front end, could act as a catalyst for communication and participation operating as an intuitive and easy to use tool. This paper will limit itself to the discussion of validation and verification of the interactive framework.

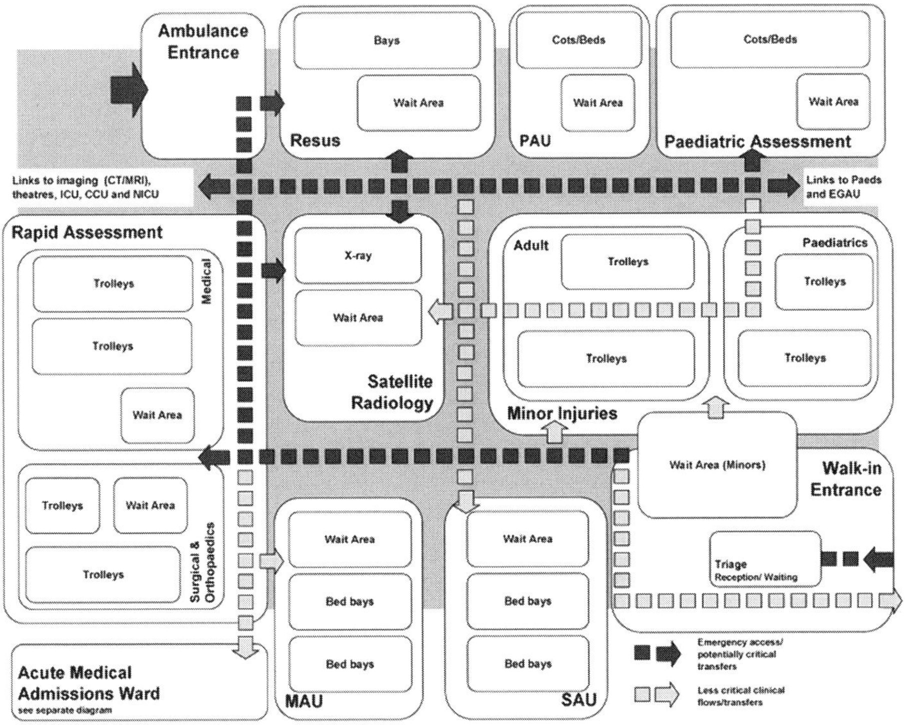

Figure 1. A generic A&E layout. The layout reflects a new service model layout incorporating minor, rapid assessment and resus areas. It shows areas assigned for short-term observation within A&E. These short-term observation areas are shown as assessment units MAU (medical), SAU (surgical) and PAU (paediatric). In this layout, there are separate treatment areas for paediatrics.

2. A "Generic" A&E Department

Although the A&E model aimed to be as generic and re-usable as possible, the layout was based on an A&E department of a proposed hospital build in the UK. The modelled A&E was representative of a modern NHS A&E Department in England drawing on guidance from a number of documents including the New Service Model as defined in Health Building Notes (HBN) 22 [8], Transforming Emergency Care in England [9] and Emergency Assessment Units – A Checklist [10]. The generic A&E layout is shown in Fig. 1.

The A&E model allowed separate entry points through 'Ambulance' and 'Walk In' (Ambulant). Dependent on the assigned route, patients could travel through a number of pathways, but use the same resources independently of the entry point. Clinical areas shown in the A&E model related to injury type, and in order of severity were, minor injuries (adult and paediatrics), rapid assessment (RA) units and resus. Rapid assessment units divided further into medical, surgical and paediatric sub areas. The model also included assessment units that are effectively short-term observation units within A&E. Assessment units were also sub divided into medical (MAU), surgical (SAU) or paediatrics (PAU). A further addition to the model was an X-Ray unit. The model also showed separate treatment areas for adult and paediatrics, reflecting the current desire. Exit points on the A&E model were resus, in-patient, discharge or no-treatment.

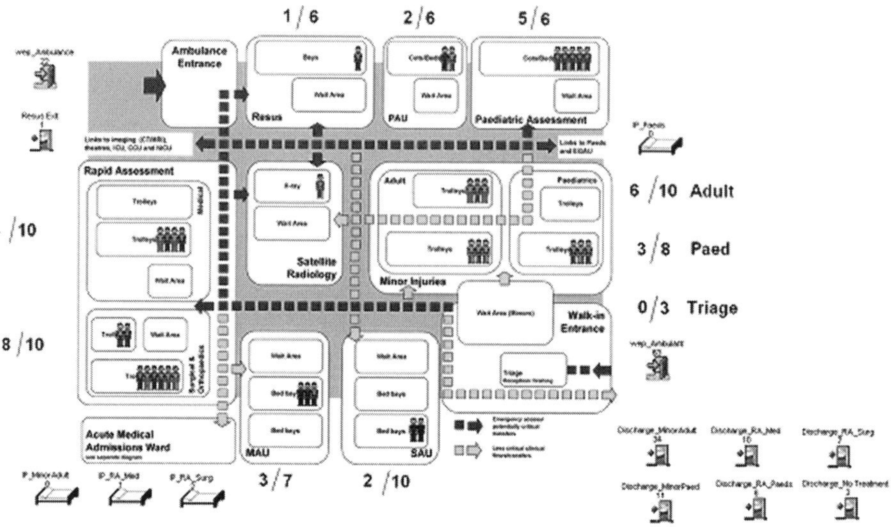

Figure 2. Bitmap generic A&E department. This shows the SIMUL8 A&E model overlaying the generic A&E shown in Fig. 1. A snapshot of patients icons being treated in a number of different areas is shown. During the simulation run patient icons would travel through and exit the A&E according to the their assigned pathway and timings.

3. Model Building

The building process for the A&E model discussed in this paper loosely follows the steps defined by Banks [11] with regards to problem formulation, setting of objectives, model conceptualisation, data collection and model translation. Modelling and simulation was described by Maria [12] as the process of producing a model (modelling) and the operation of a model in a system (simulation).

The software package chosen for the development of the A&E generic model is SIMUL8 [13]. Using Law and Kelton's [14] definitions one might describe SIMUL8 as a stochastic, general-purpose discrete-event simulation package. One of SIMUL8's key features is that it has high visual impact in that the user can see animated items moving on screen in simulation time. To facilitate user acceptance, the simulation model overlays a bitmap file depicting the generic A&E department described previously (see Fig. 2).

In addition, patient icons are colour coded. Therefore, by viewing the A&E model, an A&E clinician or manager can quickly relate to it. As such, during a simulation run, clinicians and managers can see patient flows and activity (i.e. queues building) on a two-dimensional map of an A&E department in simulation time. Furthermore, the structure of the bitmap allows relatively quick modifications in order to depict the actual A&E department of a clinician or manager.

The process of bitmap modification is important as it supports user-friendly connection of the clinician and managers to the model and enhanced dialogue between the model builders and model owners (clinicians and managers). As well as enhanced ownership and dialogue, visual models can provide valuable insight into the modelled process during the simulation run. This leads to further dialogue and allows clinicians and managers to gain further understanding of their processes and interactions, some of which may not be intuitive.

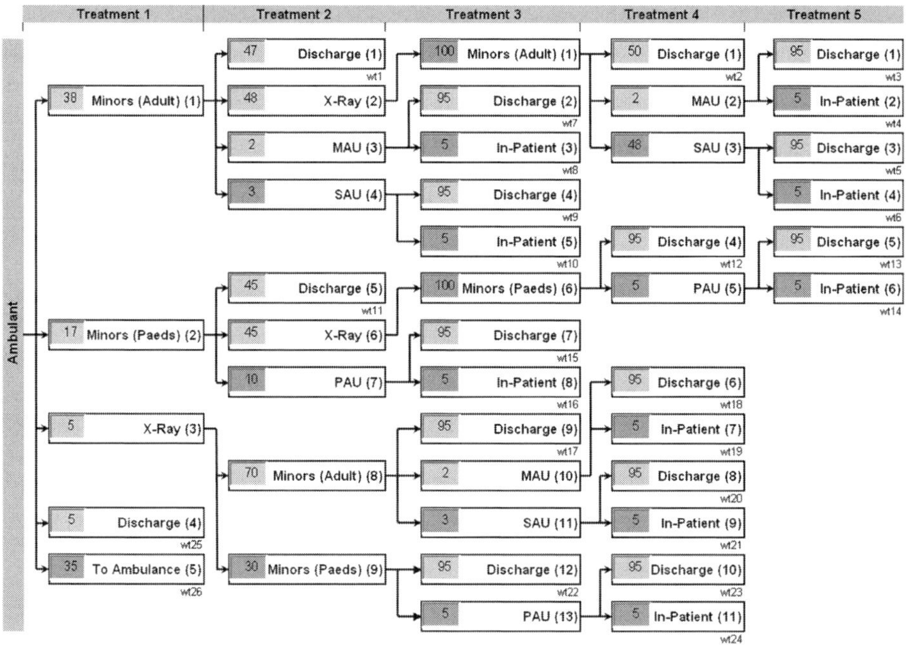

Figure 3. Walk-in (ambulant) pathway. Figure 3 is a screen shot of the user-friendly interface designed to input ambulant pathway routing data. The interface here defines the pathways routings of the ambulant patients and directs the route of travel through the A&E model shown in Fig. 2.

4. Interactive Data Input Interfaces

4.1. Development

To input data into the SIMUL8 A&E model user-friendly interfaces are created using Microsoft Excel enhanced by Visual Basic for Applications (VBA). The user-friendly interfaces facilitate ease and speed of data entry and constrain the parameters for a generic process. They allow patient pathways and corresponding percentages, hourly patient arrivals, patient process times and beds/trolleys/bays allocation to be easily entered. An example of the ambulant pathway routing is shown in Fig. 3.

Therefore, by inputting a percentage value (between 0 and 100) in the pathway boxes, a user can direct flow along predetermined paths. For example, for column Treatment 1, a user can determine the percentage directed to minor (adults), minor (Paeds), X-Ray, discharge or to ambulance (ambulance pathway). An ambulance pathway is also created (not shown in this paper for clarity) and performs in a similar fashion to ambulant pathway described above.

4.2. Validation and Verification

Sargent [15] suggested a number of techniques for validating and verifying models including animation and operational graphics. Animation and operational graphics were the main techniques that were used to validate and verify the interactive interfaces described in this paper. All the patient pathway routings were tested to ensure correct patient flows. Additionally, patient arrivals and departures along routings were tested (in simulation time) to ensure accurate timings. The successful validation and verification of the interactive interfaces shows many potential benefits. Benefits include modellers having the ability to control the level of abstraction leading to user-friendly generic processes. Additionally, the interactive interface described above lends itself well to modification. Therefore, with slight modifications, modellers can quickly generate specific A&E's models if desired. Additionally, the graphical structure of the interfaces works well in harmony with the visual impact of SIMUL8.

5. Conclusion and Future Work

The successful validation and verification of the interactive interfaces showed the potential of how modellers could manage levels of abstraction. Management of abstraction levels by modellers is a vital tool in linking highly abstracted simulation software with generic processes that relate to clinicians and managers. In addition, the interactive framework also supports user-friendly interactions to encourage clinicians and managers to gain a greater understanding and control of their processes and systems.

At the time of writing the authors were in the process of collecting real data from hospitals to validate and verify a full A&E model. The work in this paper was validated and verified with average times generated by SIMUL8. SIMUL8 (and the developed data input interfaces) could process a range of distribution profiles more likely in a real A&E. Analysis of real data might result in a need for greater discrimination of process times within the model. Staff resources and other support activities (e.g. blood testing) were not included in the models above. Inclusion of staff resources and other activities could be considered in future A&E model builds.

Acknowledgements

This work was partly supported by the UK Department of Trade and Industry, Knowledge Transfer Partnership Programme (KTP no 174).

References

[1] P.R. Harper and A.K. Shahani, Modelling for the planning and management of bed capacities in hospitals, *Journal of the Operational Research Society* **53** (2002), 11–18.

[2] S.M. Sanchez, D.M. Ferrin, T. Ogazon, J.A. Sepulreda and T.J. Ward, Emerging issues in healthcare simulation, In *Proceedings of the 2000 Winter Simulation Conference* (2000), 1999–2003.

[3] J.C. Lowery, Getting started in simulation in healthcare, In *Proceedings of the 1998 Winter Simulation Conference* (1998), 31–36.

[4] J.B. Jun, S.H. Jacobson and J.R. Swisher, Application of discrete-event simulation in health care clinics: A survey, *Journal of the Operational Research Society* **50** (1999), 109–123.

[5] D. Sinreich and Y. Marmor, A simple and intuitve simulation tool for analyzing the performance of emergency departments, In *Proceedings of the 2004 Winter Simulation Conference* (2004), 1994–2002.

[6] C.D. Barnes, J.L. Quiason, C. Benson and D. McGuiness, Success stories in simulation in health care, In *Proceedings of the 1997 Winter Simulation Conference* (1997), 1280–1285.

[7] V. Kachitvichyanukul, J.O. Henriksen, C.D. Pegden, R.G. Ingalls and B.W. Schmeiser, Simulation environment for the new millennium (panel), In *Proceedings of the 2001 Winter Simulation Conference* (2001), 541–547.

[8] NHS Estates, *HBN 22 Accident and Emergency Facilities for Adults and Children*, The Stationary Office, London, 2003.
[9] G. Alberti, *Transforming Emergency Care in England* (2004), Department of Health, UK. <http://www.dh.gov.uk/assetRoot/04/09/81/0409781.pdf>, accessed 20 March 2005.
[10] G. Alberti, *Emergency Assessment Units – A Checklist* (2003), Department of Health, UK. <http://www.dh.gov.uk/assetRoot/04/06/08/94/04060894.pdf>, accessed 20 March 2005.
[11] J. Banks, *Discrete-event System Simulation*, 3rd ed., Prentice-Hall International, London, 2001.
[12] A. Maria, Introduction to modeling and simulation, In *Proceedings of the 1997 Winter Simulation Conference* (1997), 7–13.
[13] Simul8 Corporation, *Simul8 Standard R11*, <http://www.simul8.com>.
[14] A.M. Law and W.D. Kelton, *Simulation modeling and analysis*, 3rd ed., McGraw-Hill, New York, 2000.
[15] R.G. Sargent, Validation and verification of simulation models, In *Proceedings of the 2004 Winter Simulation Conference* (2004), 17–28.

Medical and Care Compunetics 2
L. Bos et al. (Eds.)
IOS Press, 2005

A Software Tool to Aid Budget Planning for Long-Term Care at Local Authority Level

Haifeng XIE [a], Thierry CHAUSSALET [a,1], Sam TOFFA [a] and Peter CROWTHER [b]

[a] *Health and Social Care Modelling Group, Centre for Health Informatics Cavendish School of Computer Science, University of Westminster, London, UK*

[b] *Housing and Social Services, London Borough of Merton, London, UK*

Abstract. In this paper, we present a software tool that implements a novel modelling framework developed by the authors to provide useful information to budget planners for long-term care at local authority level. By combining unit costs of care with an underlying survival model for publicly funded residents in long-term care, the software tool is able to provide forecasts on the cost of maintaining the group of elderly who are currently in long-term care (referred to as *known commitments*) for a period of time. User interacts with the tool via a friendly graphical interface that guides them through a set of screens of options in a familiar wizard fashion. This tool was created and tested in collaboration with an English borough. Feedbacks from the care planner and manager show that the tool helps them gain better understanding on the behaviour of length-of-stay of residents under their care, and provides quantitative inputs into their decision making on budget planning for long-term care.

Keywords. Long-term care, budget planning, survival analysis, length of stay analysis, user interface, forecasting, cost

1. Introduction

As people get older, activities of daily living, such as feeding, toileting and self care, can become difficult. In general, long-term care (LTC), which is provided to people who are unable to look after themselves without some degree of support, embraces all form of continuous, social, personal and nursing care, and associated domestic services [1]. In this paper, the term LTC refers to residential care (RC) and nursing care (NC) provided in institutional care homes, eg., residential homes and nursing homes. As the world population is ageing, it is generally believed that LTC will become an even more important issue for an ageing society [2]. Governments around the world have been

[1]Corresponding Author: Thierry Chaussalet, Cavendish School of Computer Science, University of Westminster, 115 New Cavendish Street, London W1W 6UW, UK. Tel.: +44 (0) 20 7911 5000; Fax: +44 (0) 20 7911 5079; E-mail: chausst@wmin.ac.uk.

alerted with the potential difficulties in funding and managing LTC, and are attempting to address the difficulties in their own ways.

Local authorities in England play a major role in running the system of LTC. Under current regulations (ie., the 1990 NHS and Community Care Act and the Care Standard Act 2000), local authorities are responsible for the placement and finance of all publicly funded residents in LTC that conforms to national standards. The ability to discharge elderly patients to LTC is essential in the planning and running of acute hospital care. Under the Community Care (Delayed Discharges, etc.) Act 2003, local authorities have been facing financial penalties since January 2004 for failing to provide vacancies in institutional care homes for hospital discharges [3].

Given limited resources available, local authorities have a keen interest in knowing the behaviour of the LTC system, in particular, how long residents stay in the system, and ultimately, how much the system will cost. From the prospectives of local authorities, the emphasis is placed on the residents who require funding support from the public. A national survey [4] in England showed that 73% of the residents admitted to LTC in 1996 were publicly funded, and most of them were there on a permanent basis, ie., not expected to go back to their own homes.

Extensive studies have been conducted in Britain to develop macro models for projecting the demand and hence the cost of LTC at the national level [5,6]. This type of model, which adopts a "whole system" approach, is useful for strategic planning for a nation. However, at a local level, a methodology that takes into account local characteristics in its forecast will be more suitable. Especially, as far as cost is concerned, local authorities need a method that can help their budget planning and allow evaluation of the potential effects of changes in regulations and financial context on the use of resources and costs. Good budget planning is essential to ensure the successful delivery of LTC that balances demand and provision.

In previous studies [7,8], we developed a modelling framework for predicting the cost of LTC arising from *known commitments* from a local authority perspective. The term known commitments refers to the group of publicly funded residents currently in the LTC system. Knowing the projected cost associated with this group of residents is of particular interest to local authorities as it corresponds to the burden the local authority cannot escape. This information will enable local authorities to identify the fraction of the budget that are already committed due to past admission decisions. Given this information, local authorities will have a fair idea about the resources available for new admissions in a financial year.

In the following section, we briefly describe the modelling framework. In Section 3, we describe a software implementation of the framework that was developed in collaboration with an English borough. Discussion on the usefulness of such a software tool is in Section 4.

2. Modelling Methodology

In England, RC is intended for older people who are frail but still able to manage their activities of daily living; while NC is for older people who are medically stable and have a greater degree of physical and mental disabilities. Residents can be admitted to RC or NC directly. RC residents may be transferred to NC if their conditions deteriorate to such

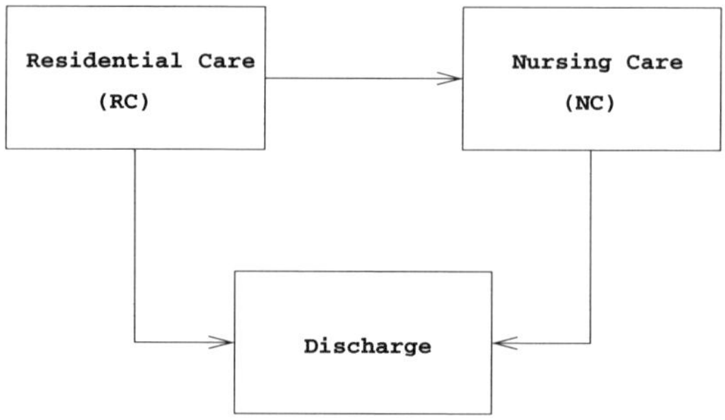

Figure 1. Movements of publicly funded residents in LTC.

an extend that RC is no longer appropriate for their needs. For publicly funded residents, discharges from LTC is predominately by death [9]. The movement of publicly funded residents in LTC is represented in Fig. 1.

2.1. General Modelling Framework

Formally, we seek to forecast the total cost $TC(t)$ of maintaining for t units of time (chosen to be days without loss of generality) a group of publicly funded residents present in LTC at time c. Assuming there are M_R residents in RC and M_N residents in NC at time c this total cost is simply the sum of the cost incurred by each individual in the group, ie.,

$$TC(t) = \sum_{i=1}^{M_R} K(X_i, Y_i) + \sum_{j=1}^{M_N} K(0, Y_j). \tag{1}$$

Where $K(X, Y)$ denotes the cost incurred by a resident during $[c, c + t]$ and can be written as

$$K(X, Y) = K_R(X) + K_N(Y), \tag{2}$$

where $K_R(X)$ and $K_N(Y)$ are the costs for staying in RC for X days and NC for Y days, respectively, during the interval $[c, c + t]$.

From a forecasting perspective, we are interested in the expected total cost. For a more detailed description of the cost framework, see [7]. To produce a good forecast of the total expected cost, the framework needs to take into account future increases in unit prices of care and the pattern of movements of residents in the system. More specifically, the framework needs a model that describes the length-of-stay (or survival) pattern of the residents in RC and NC, and the probability of transfer from RC to NC.

2.2. Survival Model

In a previous study [8], we presented a continuous-time Markov model for the flow of elderly residents within and between RC and NC. Briefly, the model uses a combination of a short-stay state and a long-stay state to capture the flow of residents through each type of care. For instance, a person admitted to RC might stay for a short period

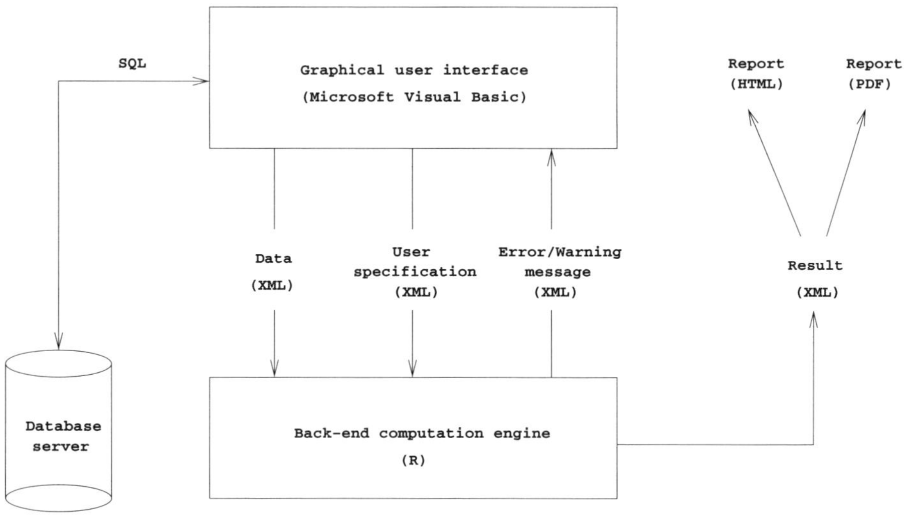

Figure 2. The main components of the software tool and their interactions.

of time, then is either discharged or transferred to NC; or the person might settle down and become a long-stay resident in RC. The state space of the Markov model is aggregated [10] due to the un-observability of the actual short-stay and long-stay states, ie., we observe a person is in RC but do not know whether the person is in short-stay or long-stay state. A procedure for fitting such a model to observational data was developed in [8].

2.3. Data Requirement

The data requirement for this modelling framework is relatively simple. The essential information concerning a resident is: date of admission, type of care, date of discharge (if applicable), destination of discharge (if applicable). An unique identifier for each resident is needed to track movements of a resident in the system. Other information, such as gender and age at admission, might also be useful if more detailed break-down analysis is desired, for example, study male and female residents separately. Such data is already commonly collected by many local authorities for day-to-day administrative purpose. Whilst an increasing number of local authorities are implementing sophisticated information systems to help their management of care services, the required data is becoming more and more widely available.

3. Software Implementation

The cost framework introduced in Section 2 was tested and implemented as a software tool in collaboration with the London Borough of Merton, UK. The aim of the implementation was to develop a decision aid for local authority budget planners and care service managers by providing them with forecast of cost due to known commitments.

The software tool was developed to run on a Microsoft™ WINDOWS™ platform, and consisted of three main components: a graphical user interface (GUI), a back-end computation engine and a component producing final reports (see Fig. 2). The GUI,

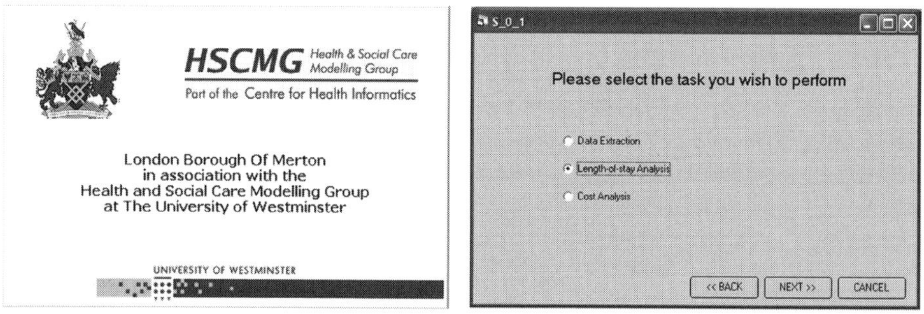

Figure 3. Sample screen shots of the graphical user interface, which guides the user through a set of choices in a familiar wizard fashion.

which is the main point of interaction between the user and the tool, was written using Microsoft™ Visual Basic™. The GUI was designed to guide the user through a set of choices in a friendly and familiar wizard fashion (for sample screen shots see Fig. 3). For example, by clicking on buttons and selecting values from drop-down menus, the user can specify the date range within which data will be extracted for analysis. The sequence of relevant screens presented to the user is determined by the choices made by the user thus far. Once the necessary information and specification is collected, the GUI generates the necessary data by querying (using Structural Query Language (SQL)) a local information system – CAREFIRST. CAREFIRST is a dedicated information system (running ORACLE™ database management system) that contains routinely collected administrative and cost information on residents and their stay in care. This data coupled with other user specified options are fed into a back-end computation engine (written in the open source package – R [11]) that handles the computation and produces forecasted results. These results are further processed to produce final reports in HTML and PDF format. The HTML version of the report is suitable for on-screen browsing and is ready to be published on internal websites; while the PDF version is more suitable for printing and documentation (see Fig. 4).

The software tool was designed with flexibility and extendability in mind. The components of the tool are modular and exchange data with each other via a set of well-defined XML files. The eXtensible Markup Language (XML) is a general and transparent way of exchanging data between programs across different platforms, and has quickly become a communication standard for implementing health care systems [12,13]. The use of XML files in this case increases the interoperability and connectivity among components and allows each component to be implemented using the software tool that is most suitable for its purpose. For example, given the XML file produced by the back-end computation engine, users can produce final reports in different formats with different level of detail by pulling out the relevant information from the XML file, which encapsulates all aspects of the results. Furthermore, additional information can be added to the XML files without breaking existing functionalities as new features are introduced.

During the software development period, regular meetings were held between the developers and the end users. Suggestions and feedbacks were discussed and incorporated into development. The software tool has been demonstrated to potential users at the London Borough of Merton, and a updated version is ready to be released to end users for testing. Early feedbacks suggested that users found the tool was easy to use and the results it produced clear and sensible. However, further forecast are required

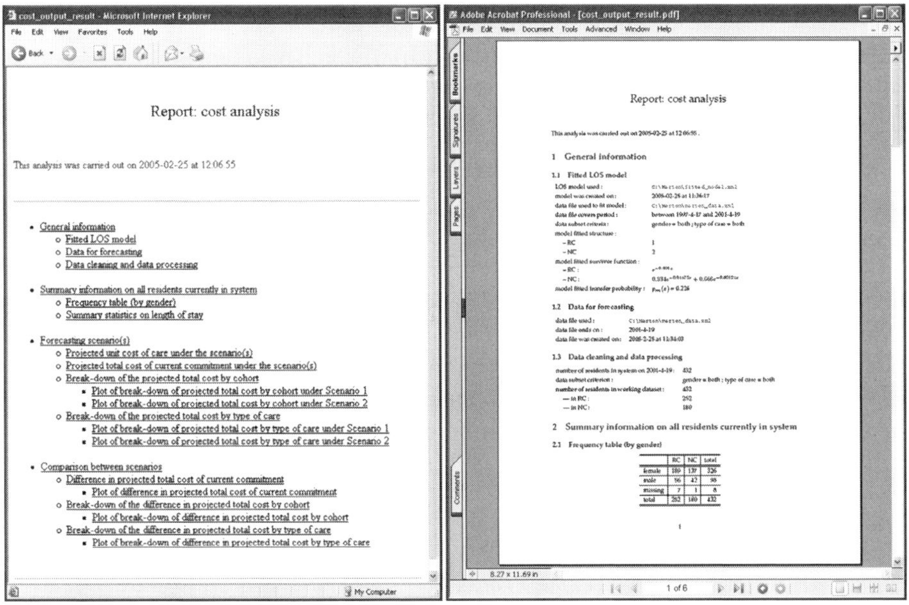

Figure 4. Final reports produced by the software tool. The HTML version (left) is suitable for on-screen browsing. The PDF version (right) is suitable for printing purpose.

to fully validate it use in real-world situations. Our users suggested that the ability of the tool to produce forecast on the cost due to known commitment until the end of the current financial year is the most interesting and useful feature, which allows them to have the most updated assessment of their current position on the budget for LTC in a financial year.

4. Discussion

Local authorities face real challenges when it comes to annual budget planning for funding the system of LTC. Uncertainty about the long-term cost of caring for their current residents in the system, in addition to unknown future admissions, have made the tasks of local authority budget managers very complex and demanding. This software tool quantifies the source of uncertainty related to known and unavoidable commitments and forecasts the resulting financial impact. It also allows the comparison of forecasts under different scenarios, which may reflect possible future pricing or costing policy changes. All these functionalities are of crucial importance to the planning of a successful budget for LTC in a local authority as they enable planners to determine the available budget for new admissions under various scenarios, hence give local authorities a fair idea about their future capacity.

Integrated with the information system of a local authority, this tool allows budget planners to draw on most up-to-date data and produce real time forecasts on demand. In addition to connectivity, interoperability and extendability, another advantage of the chosen implementation of the tool is its cost-effectiveness as it is based on established quality freeware such as R. Cost considerations can be critical in a resource stretched public sector and in non-profit organisations. The development of the software tool presented in this paper serves as an example of fruitful collaboration between academic departments and industry. This tool brings advanced modelling techniques out of research papers into the hands of decision makers in the the public sector and is contributing to improving the delivery of LTC.

Acknowledgements

We thank Mr Roger Simms and Ms Heather Lockwood from the Housing and Social Services Department of the London Borough of Merton, England, UK, for assisting in data extraction and providing feedbacks during software development. This work was partly supported by grants from the UK Engineering and Physical Sciences Research Council (GR/R86430/01) and the London Borough of Merton, UK.

References

[1] W. Laing, *Financing Long-Term Care, the critical debate*, ACE Books, London, 1993.

[2] J. Brodsky, J. Habib and M. Hirschfeld (Eds.), *Key policy issues in long-term care*, World Health Organization (WHO), Geneva, 2003.

[3] D.R. Rowland and A.M. Pollock, Choice and responsiveness for older people in the "patient centred" NHS, *British Medical Journal* **328** (2004) 4–5.

[4] A. Netten, A. Bebbington, R. Darton and J. Forder, *Care Homes for Older People (Volume 1): Facilities, Residents and Costs*, Personal Social Services Research Unit (PSSRU), University of Kent, UK, 2001.

[5] R. Wittenberg, L. Pickard, A. Comas-Herrera, B. Davies and R. Darton, *Demand for long-term care: projections for long-term care finance for elderly people*, Personal Social Services Research Unit (PSSRU), University of Kent, UK, 1998.

[6] R. Wittenberg, L. Pickard, A. Comas-Herrera, B. Davies and R. Darton, Demand for long-term care for older people in England to 2031, *Health Statistics Quarterly* **12** (2001) 5–17.

[7] C. Pelletier, T.J. Chaussalet and H. Xie, A framework for predicting gross institutional long-term care cost arising from known commitments at local authority level, *Journal of the Operational Research Society* **56** (2005), 144–152.

[8] H. Xie, T.J. Chaussalet and P.H. Millard, A continuous-time Markov model for the length of stay of elderly people in institutional long-term care, *Journal of the Royal Statistical Society A* **168** (2005), 51–61.

[9] A. Bebbington, R. Darton and A. Netten, *Care Homes for Older People (Volume 2): Admissions, Needs and Outcomes*, Personal Social Services Research Unit (PSSRU), University of Kent, UK, 2001.

[10] D.R. Fredkin and J.A. Rice, On aggregated Markov processes, *Journal of Applied Probability* **23** (1986), 208–214.

[11] R Development Core Team, *R: A language and Environment for Statistical Computing*, R Foundation for Statistical Computing, Vienna, Austria, 2003.

[12] J. Dudeck, Aspects of implementing and harmonizing healthcare communication standards, *International Journal of Medical Informatics* **48** (1998), 163–171.

[13] R. Schweiger, M. Brumhard, S. Hoelzer and J. Dudeck, Implementing health care systems using XML standards, *International Journal of Medical Informatics* **74** (2005), 267–277.

Medical and Care Compunetics 2
L. Bos et al. (Eds.)
IOS Press, 2005

A Software System for Clinical Monitoring

Jitesh DINESCHANDRA [a,b] and Mike REES [b]
[a] Dendrite Clinical Systems Ltd, Research & Development Department, Ridings House, Raynes Park, UK
[b] Health and Social Care Modelling Group, Centre for Health Informatics, University of Westminster, London, UK

Abstract. Three graphical methods for monitoring clinician performance – the Funnel Plot, the CUSUM and the Variable Life Adjusted Display – are described. In addition the problems associated with incorporating and assessing risk factors into the process are discussed. The software system produced to implement these methodologies is presented; the creation of the user friendly interfaces, the underling algorithms and the structure and connectivity of the database are described. The methodology for piloting and evaluating the system is described. Drawing on developments in experimental usability we propose an experimental procedure aimed at evaluating possible changes in design so as to maximise the use of the system in terms of its accuracy of input and clarity of output.

Keywords. Clinical performance monitoring, funnel plot, variable risk adjusted display, funnel plot, cusum, caché database, usability

Introduction

Current UK Government policy is for the public disclosure of performance statistics for surgeons. However, to date, the results have been patchy. The quality of the data being collected is variable with some hospital trusts putting in little effort. Many hospitals and government departments attempt to profile physicians on the basis of process or outcome measures, or cost, however, each hospital often defines measures differently, consequently there is no universal agreement on the data that should be collected. Furthermore, there has been no agreement on the most appropriate way to risk-adjust the data to allow for the enormous variability between patients [1]. In addition, each hospital includes in their analysis only their own patients, usually a small fraction of a physician's total practice. As a consequence, physicians receive fragmented and confusing feedback on their performance.

Software systems can be developed to carry out these calculations and analyses and implemented in hospital departments. The output from these software systems would give us an indication of the performance level, for example for a particular physician. The main point of interest is to develop software systems where they can be used with ease and output is understood across the board in hospitals and government departments.

In order for the software systems to be implemented in hospitals and to be used by staff at all levels, research needs to be carried out on the usability of such systems, whether 'cosmetic' or technical. Such research would allow us to assess the ease of use of the software and develop software systems that can be used in hospitals across all staff levels. This is essential as software systems are dependent on accurate data entry and knowledgeable use and understanding of both statistical and graphical methods. In order to achieve such goals we need to look at the usability of such software systems and their implementation in the medical environment.

Each hospital trust will produce a database of its results which is the source of information, however they are only of use if they are designed to specification and implemented accordingly to reflect the data stored. A software system for clinical monitoring must be able to draw on all client databases. In this particular case we are not simply interested in where databases are located and how they are linked, but also how they are built and designed. A software system using a well-designed database for acquiring data from clinical processes will be able to take advantage of the database's design and flexibility. By making the software system 'user friendly' the data acquired will be much more accurate, reliable and can be easily retrieved. This data is crucial in the analysis of patient outcome, which will reflect in patient outcome and experience.

1. The Software System

1.1. Software for Monitoring Clinical Performance

It is important that we first establish the software architecture behind the application we are developing. By doing so, we identify available enabling technology required for an effective communication between application process and databases.

There are two main components in the development of the software system: the development environment and the database environment. We first start with the development environment where we establish the visual design of the applications, application processes and logic. At this stage we also setup usability tests. Within the development environment third-party components and dynamic linking libraries may be added to add more functionality and flexibility to the application. These may be graphing components and mathematical functions libraries, which can be accessed from within the development environment. This is illustrated in Fig. 1.

The database is part of the database environment where the data are stored and database administration is performed. The software system under development utilises the Caché database. We are using Visual Basic in our development environment and accessing the database from within the application. The database provides an Object Link Control which is used to access the data in the database from the development environment.

The software system referred to in this paper comprises three tools used in the monitoring of clinical performance: the funnel plot; the variable life adjusted display (VLAD) and the CUSUM chart.

Quality control procedures, and in particular control charts, are widely used in the industrial context where quick detection of problems is essential for efficiency. Monitoring schemes have been introduced in the medical setting where cumulative sums of an outcome measure are plotted as a function of the number of occasions where that outcome could occur [2,3]. However no account is taken of the differences in the risk of occurrence between individuals. In an attempt to account for such risk factors it has

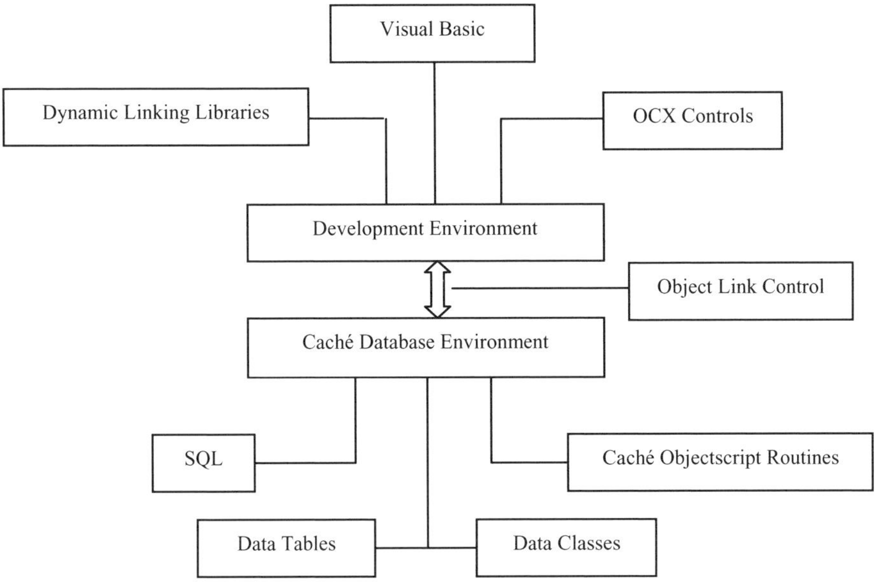

Figure 1. The Software Architecture.

become common practice to plot VLAD values as a function of the number of occasions when the outcome could occur [4].

Funnel Plots are recommended as a graphical aid for institutional comparisons, in which an estimate of an underlying quantity is plotted against an interpretable measure of its precision [5]. Control Limits form a funnel around the target outcome, in a close analogy to standard Shewhart control charts [6].

These tools use the software architecture as described in Fig. 1.

Looking in more detail at the structure we see that data access speeds need to be taken into account. For example, if a hospital's database system contained 5 million records the software tool will be slow in analysing the data. In order to get data speed advantages, most of the data analysis is run within the database environment using SQL, Caché Objectscript routines and Caché classes. This methodology reduces traffic in the link control and only data ready for plotting is channeled through to the development environment.

Figure 2 illustrates how the above tools can be placed in a hospital network.

Ideally there would be a server machine with the Caché Server installed where data are stored through a data gathering system. In addition to the server machine, the clinical monitoring tool would be installed in client machines around the hospital with their Caché server IP address pointing to the IP address of the Caché server machine. Using such setup the client machines are allowed to have a view of the data in the server.

Since the client has a view of the data in the server, it can also fetch the data from the tables. To fetch and analyse this data, for example for a CUSUM plot, objectscript routines are triggered by the clinical monitoring tool through the object link control which provides communication between the database and the tool itself, as illustrated in Fig. 3. A more in-depth analysis would show that all the data analysis is handled between the Caché system in the server machine and the Caché system in the client machine. Once the routines in the server machine have been executed it will pipe the

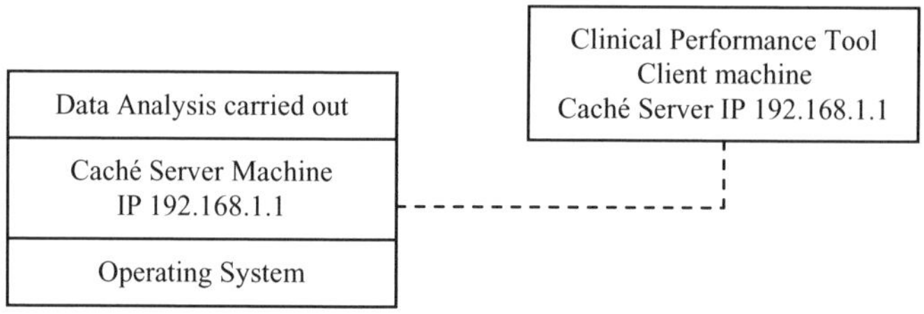

Figure 2. Hospital Network.

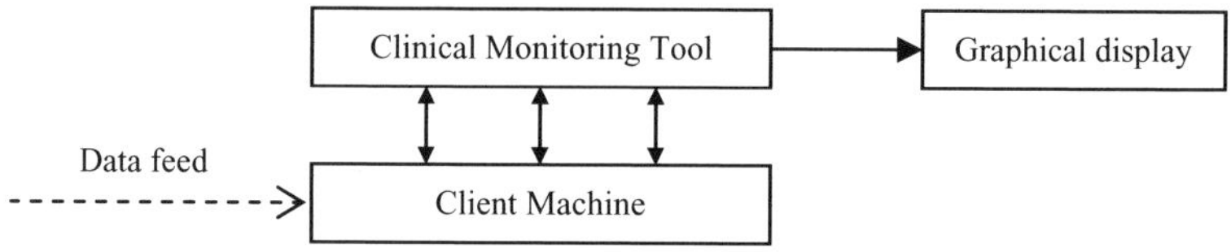

Figure 3. Client side setup.

analysed data through a data feed i.e. link control. By minimizing communication loads betweens the tool and the database we have a faster and more efficient data analysis tool. Once the tool receives the data, it will display the results graphically through a graphical display control.

1.2. Users and their Roles

Once a software system is deployed and implemented, the range of users will be varied. In this particular case, within the healthcare scenario, there are six different types of users across the board:

- Nurses
- Physicians
- Management
- IT Administrators
- Patients
- Societies and User Groups

It is interesting to note that the patient is also a user of the software system in place at hospitals.

Different users have different experiences of the software system. Here, we are interested in maximising their experience through usability so that the information that is displayed can be actioned upon as quickly and as effectively as possible. This will help maximising process effectiveness and hence the whole user experience.

So what roles do each of the user type takes? By looking at each of the users responsibilities within their workplace we can analyse the type of role they take when using the software system. Patients have a 'spectator' role, as they are only able to view information. Nurses have the greatest input in the use of the systems, which carry out most of the data entry. Data entry plays a very important part in software usability, as we will see in the following sections. Physicians carry out some data entry as well as complex data analysis to interpret process efficiency and assess patient outcome. The management will be mostly concerned in analysing data and have no input in terms of data entry and will most often inform on the performance of the medical centre as a whole. IT administrators are mostly involved in the implementation of the software systems and provide technical support such as database connectivity and so forth. Finally, societies and user groups will only use the system to analyse data and make inferences about the data.

Data-entry plays an important part in software usability, as most tasks will involve some kind of data entry or analysis. By facilitating efficient data entry the user will be able to store data more accurately and effectively, minimising errors in the process.

1.3. Data Entry

Data entry tasks can occupy a substantial fraction of the user's time and can be the source of frustrating and potentially dangerous errors [7]. Smith and Mosier [8] offer five high-level objectives as part of their guidelines for data entry:

- *Consistency of data entry transactions.* Similar sequences of actions should be used under all conditions; similar delimiters, abbreviations, and so on should be used.
- *Minimal input by users.* Fewer input actions means greater operator productivity and usually fewer chances for error.
- *Minimal memory load on users.* When doing data entry, users should not be required to remember lengthy lists of codes and complex syntactic command strings.
- *Compatibility of data entry with data display.* The format of data entry information should be linked closely to the format of displayed information.
- *Flexibility for user control of data entry.* Experienced data entry operators may prefer to enter information in a sequence they can control.

We can use the above as a starting point in developing our data entry model with the aim of facilitating data entry and improving user experience. By improving user experience we are improving the software system's usability.

Usability evaluation is the process by which we try to discover just how easy to use a system is, and if it has usability problems, where these lie. There are many usability-testing methods and it is dependent on the context and budget available.

Since the early 1980's there were a shift in attention to user needs and it's a direct indicator of how important usability became as part of the development process. Traditional managers and developers resisted at first but soon witnessed the benefits and demand for usability testing swelled. The remarkable surprise was that usability testing not only sped up projects, but also produced dramatic cost savings [9,10]. Usability increases customer satisfaction and productivity, leads to customer trust and loyalty and inevitably results in tangible costs savings and profitability. Usability returns many benefits (return on investment, or ROI) to products developed for either internal use or sale [11,12].

2. Usability Tests

We now discuss how to set up and run usability tests and look at different kinds of usability tests. The more carefully the set up of usability evaluation is, the more valuable is the data collected is for analysis.

One of the first tasks is to select a group of users 'representative' of the intended user group. Following that we must decide on which indicators to test. This ensures that the test is clearly focused.

Indicators that may be used include:

- How easy it is to learn the application
- Whether a given task can be carried out correctly first time by a new user or a user with one month's experience
- The number of 'breakdowns' (i.e. the user is unable to proceed with the task)
- Time taken to produce a result
- User satisfaction with the ease of use of the product
- A general recording and analysis of a typical working session, to see if there are any usability problems

2.1. Usability Surveys

Written surveys are a familiar, inexpensive, and generally acceptable form for usability tests. Managers and users can easily grasp the notion of surveys and typically large numbers of respondents will produce better data than from potentially biased and highly variable results from small numbers of usability-test participants. Successful surveys have clear set goals and development of focused items that help attain those goals. Experienced surveyors know that care is also needed during administration and data analysis [13].

2.2. Usability Information

Varied information can be extracted from the users in addition to other usability testing mechanisms, which may help in measuring usability of a software system.

Below are some examples:

- Task domain and objects
- Syntax of inputs and design of displays
- Background (age, gender, origins, education, income)
- Experience with computers
- Job responsibilities (which help in identifying user's role)
- Personality style (introvert versus extrovert, risk taking versus risk averse, etc.)
- Familiarity with features (printing, macros, shortcuts)
- Feelings after using an interface (confused versus clear)

2.3. Usability and the Measurement of Clinical Performance

The task of measuring clinical performance can be controversial and it is a complex subject. Many parties are involved such as the Government, medical centres, physicians and patients. Different parties will interpret results differently. On one hand there is the Government, which wants to investigate performance at all levels of medical practice and on the other hand we have the physicians and the patients. A correct interpretation of results is crucial as so there is no misunderstanding of results.

3. Conclusion

Software usability plays an important part in all stages of software development. In clinical software we are not only concerned about the way the software is designed in terms of how it looks but also in terms of its functionally in carrying out a particular task. Problems arising from this are that that the software will not be used correctly or users supposed to use the software will not use it, as they find it difficult. Another problem with software usability, in this case, is the actual understanding of what is being carried out. Clinical systems have a complex design and use a complex statistical methodology. Hence in Clinical Systems, software functionality is closely linked to software usability. By creating an easy to use interface for clinicians, it will have a greater impact on the understanding of the software and the complex statistical methodologies behind it. We will develop the look of the clinical software in terms of its look, design and functionality. On completion of this work a better assessment of clinical assessment tools will be able to be made.

References

[1] B. E. Keogh and R. Kinsman, Fifth *National Adult Cardiac Surgical Database Report 2003*, Dendrite Clinical Systems, 2004.
[2] A. Nix, R. J. Rowlands and K. W. Kemp, Internal quality control in clinical chemistry. *Statistics in Medicine* **6** (1986), 425–440.
[3] G. Gallus, C. Mandelli, M. Marchi and G. Radaelli, On surveillance methods for congenital malformations, *Statistics in Medicine* **5** (1986), 565–571.
[4] J. Lovegrove, O. Valencia, T. Treasure, C. Sherlaw-Johnson and S. Gallivan, Monitoring the results of cardiac surgery by variable life adjusted display, *Lancet* **350** (1997), 1128–1130.
[5] S. Ashley, B. Ridler and R. Kinsman, *National Vascular Database Report 2002,* Dendrite Clinical Systems, 2003.
[6] D. J. Spiegelhalter, Funnel plots for comparing institutional performance, *to appear*, 2005.
[7] B. Shneiderman, C. Plaisant, *Designing the User Interface; Strategies for Effective Human-Computer Interaction*. Addison-Wesley. Fourth ed., 2004.
[8] S. L. Smith and J. N. Mosier, *Guidelines for Designing User Interface Software,* The Mitre Corporation, 1986.
[9] C.-M. Karat, A business case approach to usability. In *Cost-Justifying Usability* (eds R. Bias and D. Mayhew), Academic Press, 1994, 45–70.
[10] J. Dumas and J. Redish, *A Practical Guide to Usability Testing*, Intellect Books, 1999.
[11] R. Bias and D. Mayhew (eds), *Cost-Justifying Usability*, Academic Press, 1994.
[12] A. Marcus, *Return on Investment for usable User-Interface Design: Examples and Statistics*, Aaron Marcus and Associates, 2002.
[13] A. N. Oppenheim, QuestionnaireDesign, Interviewing and Attitude Measurement, Continuum, 2000.

Medical and Care Compunetics 2
L. Bos et al. (Eds.)
IOS Press, 2005

Software Support in Automation of Medicinal Product Evaluations

Radmila JURIC, Reza SHOJANOORI, Lindi SLEVIN and Stephen WILLIAMS
Centre for Health Informatics, Cavendish School of Computer Science
University of Westminster, London, UK

Abstract. Medicinal product evaluation is one of the most important tasks undertaken by government health departments and their regulatory authorities, in every country in the world. The automation and adequate software support are critical tasks that can improve the efficiency and interoperation of regulatory systems across the world. In this paper we propose a software solution that supports the automation of the (i) submission of licensing applications, and (ii) evaluations of submitted licensing applications, according to regulatory authorities' procedures. The novelty of our solution is in allowing licensing applications to be submitted in any country in the world and evaluated according to any evaluation procedure (which can be chosen by either regulatory authorities or pharmaceutical companies). Consequently, submission and evaluation procedures become interoperable and the associated data repositories/databases can be shared between various countries and regulatory authorities.

Keywords. Marketing authorisation procedures, healthcare systems, ICH

Introduction

Medicinal product evaluations, more formally known as marketing authorisation procedures for medicinal product licences, are very important tasks undertaken by government and their regulatory bodies in almost every country in the world. (Please note that the 'marketing authorisation of medicinal product licences' is the procedure out of which a licence may be granted. In our work we refer to this as 'marketing authorisation'). Regulatory systems strictly define marketing authorisation procedures to ensure that all standards on the testing, manufacturing and controlling of medicinal products are achieved. This complex task faces two major challenges today:

(a) Harmonisation of Marketing Authorisation Procedures
Each country has its own marketing authorisation procedures, which differ amongst themselves not only in vocabulary and definitions of medicinal products, but also in the organisational structures and evaluation practices of individual health authorities. This represents a serious drawback for the efficient local and worldwide registration of medicinal products.

(b) Automation of Marketing Authorisation Procedures
Automated software support for marketing authorisation procedures is a critical task that can dramatically improve the efficiency and efficacy of regulatory systems across the world.

In this paper we aim to address both issues by proposing an evaluation framework which consists of regulatory environments, available legislations, databases, healthcare software applications and software solutions that support automated marketing authorisation procedures applicable across local and global regulatory requirements. We believe that by addressing the interoperability of marketing authorisation procedures through software support, we can indirectly enhance current attempts to harmonise them, as initiated within the International Conference on Harmonisation (ICH) procedures (http://www.ich.org).

The paper is organised as follows: Section 1 formulates the problem and discusses the aims of the paper. Section 2 outlines our proposal through the evaluation framework, and through a generic software architectural model. The evaluation framework assists in automation of marketing authorisation procedures, and the generic software architectural model makes marketing authorisation procedures interoperable across various regulatory authorities. Section 3 is centred around the implementation issues for both a database that assists in marketing authorisation procedures, and software application that is built upon it. In Section 5, we conclude and discuss the future works.

1. Problem Formulation and Aims of the Paper

We have examined the procedure for marketing authorisation of medicinal product licensing, as it is defined in the Marketing Authorisation Application (MAA) document (version 5.0) available from the MHRA, Medicines and Healthcare Product Regulatory Agency (available at http://www.mhra.gov.uk), which is a UK regulatory body. In previous works [1–3] we used the New Zealand regulatory document, which is available on Medsafe, and their regulatory authority's web site (http://www.medsafe.gov.nz). In both cases, their practices and legislation overlap with some other regulatory systems, including European Commission Rules Governing Medicinal Products in the European Community (EC), US Food and Drug Administration (FDA, available at http://www.fda.gov/cder /regulatory/ersr/), Australian Therapeutic Goods Administration, Therapeutic Products Program – Health Protection Branch in Canada and World Health Organisation.

However, all these marketing authorisation procedures cannot be exchanged and used instead of each other if we want to save time and efforts when applying for medicinal licenses across the world. Thus the need for rationalisation and harmonisation of regulatory requirements and marketing authorisation procedures is evident. Some conferences and task forces are set up in order to meet the public expectation of reducing the rising cost of health care and ensuring a minimum delay in delivering effective treatment to patients in need. Faster and more efficient marketing authorisation procedures can significantly contribute towards more effective healthcare systems. The ICH works on harmonisation between EC, Japan and American FDA regulatory requirements. The Mutual Recognition Agreement is harmonising regulations among EC members and Australia/New Zealand. The Global Harmonisation Task Force also spans the continents and includes more than 30 countries, various commissions, agencies, agreements, and export/import programs.

In this paper we give a flexible infrastructure, through the evaluation framework, which supports:

1. automatic evaluation of marketing authorisation procedures across various regulatory requirements,

2. interoperability of current and future healthcare systems with databases and software that automates marketing authorisation procedures (with emphasis on systems associated with pharmacological treatments), and
3. compatibility with the procedure of global harmonisation of marketing authorisation.

The first two aims determine the major use of databases, data repositories and software solutions built upon them. However, we must accommodate different levels of automation, which are feasible within marketing authorisation procedures, i.e. a full-scale automation might be neither the most desirable nor a feasible solution [3]. This also means that whichever solution we propose, we need to think in terms of scalability and flexibility of the evaluation framework. We should be able to perform new Marketing Authorisation procedures locally without adding to the cost of incorporating new regulatory requirements or legislation in the system. The automation also influences the third aim and can generate a hierarchy of medicinal product categories and marketing authorisation procedures performed locally and globally [1–3].

2. Our Proposal

We suggest the following goals for our evaluation framework:

(i) We have to automate the submission of licensing applications and semi-automate the evaluation of submitted licensing applications. Hence, marketing authorisation procedures are not fully automated.
(ii) We have to require that each local regulatory authority is responsible for the creation of the *rules* for the licensing application generation and the marketing authorisation procedures performed upon it. These procedures may range from specific local requirements (hybrids with some other regulatory requirements) to global (i.e. *rules* which will result from some harmonisation in the future).
(iii) We have to create databases that store all applications and reports, which have resulted from any marketing authorisation procedures. Such databases/data repositories should be widely available to any regulatory authority and any other healthcare system concerned with pharmaceutical treatments.
(iv) We should assume that basic database functionalities exist for each database involved in the framework. These functionalities include support for database administration functions, the extraction of data for statistical analysis, creation of tools that use our databases for data mining, and availability of various exploratory tools in the healthcare environment.
(v) We leave the design of databases, the applications built upon them, the interfaces, the navigations through various sets of forms, queries and the database reports, outside the scope of this work. We leave readers to refer to our other works to obtain details on our software application design, component deployments, database design and software/database implementations [4–8].

2.1. The Evaluation Framework

The evaluation framework is illustrated in Figs 1 and 2 and described in the next two sections.

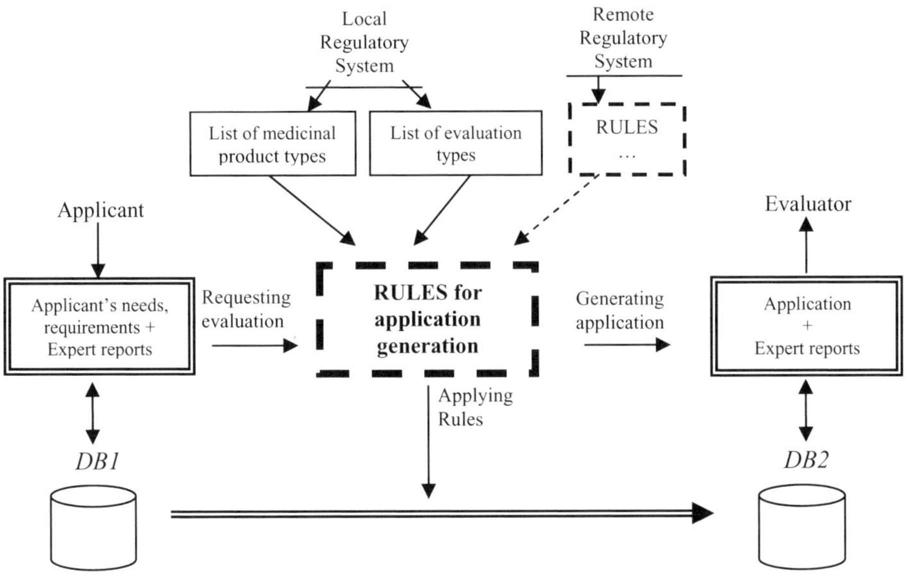

Figure 1. Generating licensing applications within a local regulatory environment.

2.1.1. Workflow for Automated Submission of Licensing Applications

In Fig. 1, we show a dynamic generation and automated submission of licensing applications within a local regulatory authority environment where each applicant formulates the request for evaluation of the medicinal product through their particular requirements. The licensing application is then generated by applying *rules* that determine the type and the format of the application and control the generation of the application. Applying these *rules* can be highly automated and supported by software with minimal (or even without any) evaluator's intervention.

The applicant's data, stored within database DB1, are transformed into the local regulatory authority database, DB2, which stores successfully generated and submitted licensing applications.

All administrative data entry (for example, product information, labelling and packaging, chemical, pharmaceutical and biological documentation) and preliminary checks if the data provided is adequate for a particular applicant's request, should be automated in the *rules*, with various expert's reports – if available – attached to each generated applications. The additional input to the *rules* should also come from the local regulatory system, which lists all types of medicinal products that could be evaluated, and an associated set of marketing authorisation procedures that are locally performed for each medicinal product. This input to the *rules* could be overridden with a similar set of *rules* developed within a remote regulatory system or ICH.

2.1.2. Workflow for Evaluation of Submitted Licensing Applications

In Fig. 2, we show an evaluating procedure and a generation of reports. These reports are stored in database DB3 after applying the evaluation on successfully submitted licensing applications. This is likely to be a semi-automatic process, which cannot be accomplished without a certain degree of evaluator's intervention. However, legislation

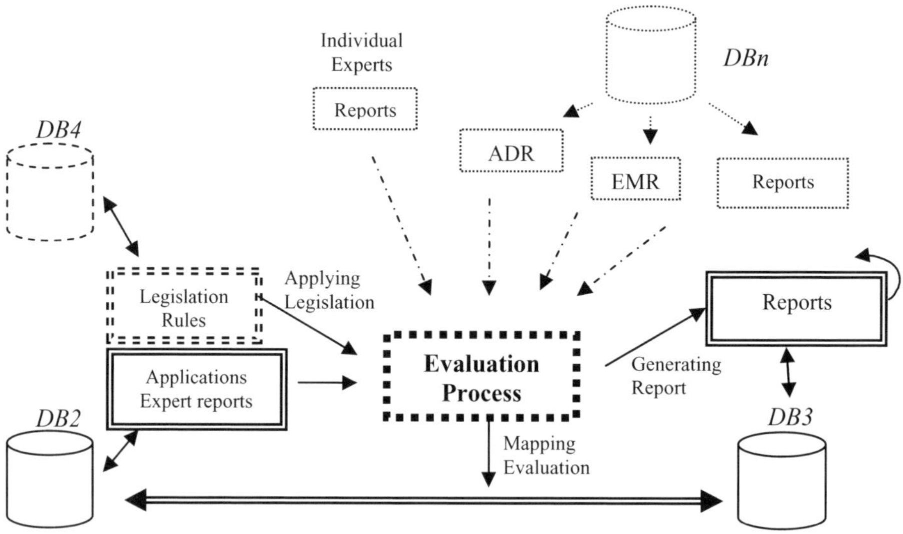

Figure 2. Generating reports through evaluation process.

rules stored within a separate database DB4 may enhance this automation, as well as reports generated by remote regulatory authorities. Opinions/judgements and reports from individual experts, Adverse Drug Reaction (ADR) data from various sources and Electronic Medical Records (EMR) may also contribute to the evaluation and report generation. However, it is unlikely that the use of these (DBn) will be automated and incorporated within a local evaluation procedure without the evaluator's consent. Reports from DB3 should be available for applicants and any remote regulatory authority evaluation procedures.

2.2. Software Architecture for Automation of Marketing Authorisations

In Fig. 3, we show the generic software architectural model that allows automation of marketing authorisations and their applicability across various legislations and regulatory authorities [4].

We use a software architectural level of design because of its important role in achieving security, performance, and modifiability of developing software systems [9]. Software architecture consists of high-level organisation of computational elements named components, interactions between components and the patterns that guide the composition of components into systems [10]. This separation of computation from interaction and the separation of architecture from its implementation are important benefits of software architectures. Components and their interactions participate in various architectural styles, which result from high-level constraints on overall design and should represent the best of all architectural choices for a given problem.

The four-layered architectural model from Fig. 3 uses a component-based technology [11] and its proposed layering is based on how specific/general to our problem requirements each component is. We use a layered architecture as described in [12] where layers are "allowed to use" public facilities of the nearest lower level.

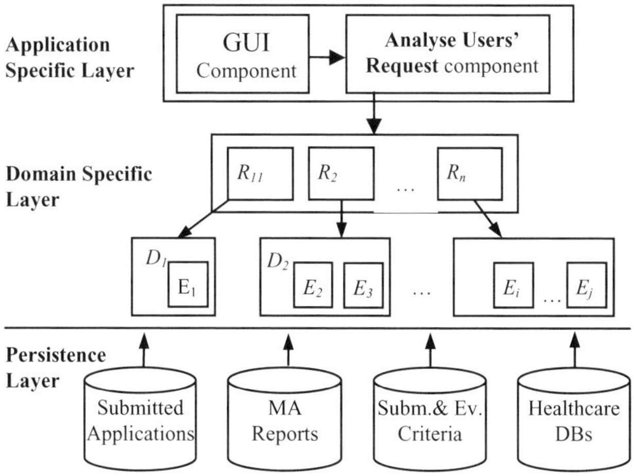

Figure 3. The Generic Software Architecture for Interoperable Marketing Authorisation Procedures.

To illustrate the architecture we use a generic procedure for marketing authorisations, whose functionality is divided into submission and evaluation, as defined in workflows from previous Sections 2.1.1 and 2.1.2:

(i) submission of a licensing application for a marketing authorisation under local regulatory authority rules (***Ri***), and
(ii) evaluation of a submitted licensing application, under evaluation procedure and its rules ***D(Ei)*** available locally/internationally.

The application layer is the most specific layer, whose components are responsible primarily for providing GUI functionality and managing interaction between users and software layers. They also analyse users' requests and route them towards appropriate components of the lower layer(s). This includes the right choice of $\boldsymbol{R_i}$ and $\boldsymbol{D(E_i)}$ components involved in a particular licensing application submission. At this layer we also manage value added services, analyse expert reports, or add users' intervention, which might be essential when automating submissions and evaluations.

The domain layer consists of two families of components. The $\boldsymbol{R_i}$ family of components contains a set of *rules* that are to be followed if we want to have an automated licensing application submission, as in (i) above, within a particular regulatory authority. The $\boldsymbol{R_i}$ family may also include any future set of rules originated within the ICH. The $\boldsymbol{D(E_i)}$ family of components contains all available evaluation procedures and their rules, as in (ii) above, that originate in different regulatory authorities or can be found within future harmonised activities from the ICH.

Components from the domain layer use data repositories and databases stored within components of the persistence layer, where data on submitted licensing applications and reports on their evaluations are kept. Our persistence and domain layers can be seen as a common repository of data and processes, where various applicants (such as pharmaceutical companies, regulatory authorities, and hospitals) can share data and services defined in our component based architecture.

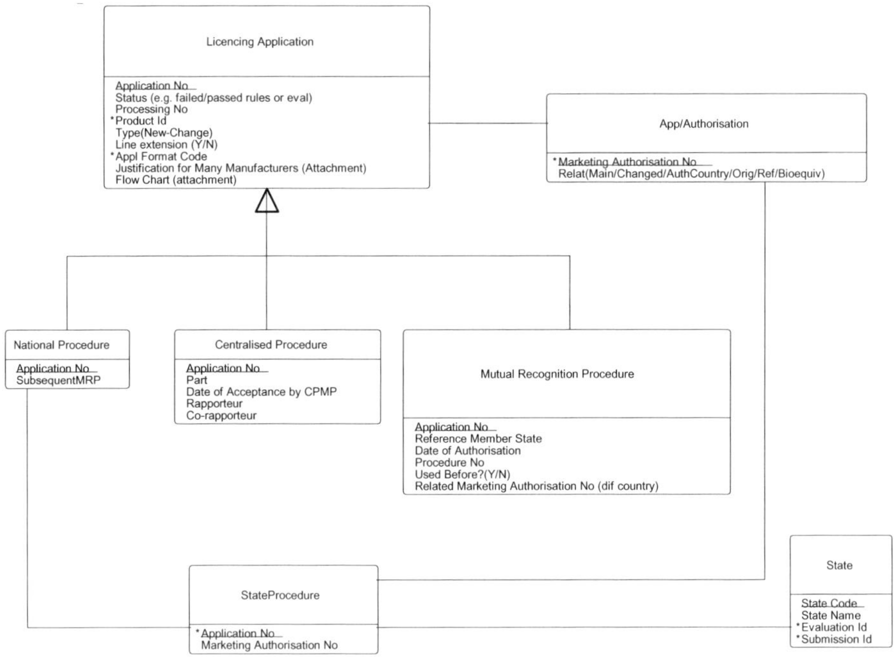

Figure 4. Generalised Licensing Application Entity with its Subtypes.

3. Implementation Issues

A software solution derived from example components in Fig. 3, which assists in the automation of marketing authorisations across the world, is a large-scale distributed data intensive application. It requires sharing of data stored in databases and/or repositories and sharing of processes associated with various marketing authorisation procedures and their prescribed regulations. To ensure (i) transparency of the results of marketing authorisation applications, (ii) sharing of marketing authorisation procedures across regulatory authorities and (iii) interoperation of such procedures with existing healthcare systems, we have implemented the component-based software architecture from Fig. 3 as an EJB application [4]. However, our implementation has had two distinctive pathways.

The first pathway has dealt with databases and data repositories essential for the functioning of such a complex application. When designing and implementing our databases, we had to have in mind that, apart form adhering to the functionality of the software application, they must support the interoperability of marketing authorisations across the world and be reusable across a family of related applications. The former requirement has been addressed by having Mutual Recognition Procedure, National Procedure and Centralised Procedure entities, which are types of marketing authorisation procedures [8]. We have also managed the choice of marketing authorisation procedures by allowing a licensing application to be only of one type (which is done through a specific relationship between database elements). The reusability of our database model was needed in order to judge how generic our solution is and how successfully it can be implemented as a data model across all regulatory authorities. Figure 4 shows an excerpt from our generic database model.

The second pathway has dealt with software application design, choice of a component platform, design of application components, their deployment in a chosen platform and their interconnections with databases and data repositories [4]. We chose the J2EE platform for our implementation, because of our positive experiences of implementing software architecture for interoperable databases as an EJB application [13]. We use design patterns throughout the software application design [6]. Our generic architectural model from Fig. 3 uses the strategy pattern [14] and we deploy our software components following the MVC pattern [15]. We also create patterns that are problem domain specific. Thus such a combination of general and domain specific patterns can be reused in any similar problem domain where workflows, similar to submissions and evaluations from 2.1.1 and 2.1.2, take place. We have also discussed the family of ***Ri*** and ***D(Ei)*** components as being Commercial-Off-The-Shelf (COTS) components [5]. This means that any submission and evaluation procedures that ***Ri*** and ***D(Ei)*** components contain may be developed separately, within any local regulatory authority and plugged into our application whenever needed.

Due to space restrictions, we cannot show all diagrams and models associated with our implementations. We refer our readers to our works referenced in this section.

Conclusions

In this paper we propose a software solution that supports the automation of the submission of licensing applications and their evaluations according to any regulatory authorities' procedures. In Section 2.1 we generate a framework that utilises automation of submissions and evaluations. From the framework we draw the software architecture in Section 2.2 for a distributed and large-scale software application, whose novelty is in allowing licensing applications to be submitted in any country in the world and evaluated according to a chosen evaluation procedure. Thus, submission and evaluation procedures become interoperable and their data repositories/databases can be shared across various countries/regulatory authorities. Our solution has been implemented as an EJB application, using Oracle8i and Sun Studio 7.

At the moment, our prototype implements a certain portion of the functionality depicted in the workflows from Section 2.1. However, our software architectural model addresses many aspects of the problem of automation and harmonisation of marketing authorisation procedures (such as requirements (1)–(3) in Section 1). Our generic architectural model makes authorisation procedures interoperable across the world, because we can choose which procedures we may perform and upon which submitted application (through a choice of ***Ri*** and ***D(Ei)*** software components from Fig. 1). However, it is equally important to note that we have planned for transparency of results of marketing authorisation procedures and for interoperation of such procedures with existing software applications in healthcare systems. Hence, DB2 and DB3 (from Fig. 2) are equivalents for the Submitted Applications and MA Reports databases of our software architecture, in Fig. 3. Healthcare DBs from Fig. 3 can incorporate any repository, which range from the Rules in Fig. 1 to DBn databases in Fig. 2. The technology used for building the software application upon our databases, and the loose coupling between our application and databases that underpin it, make collaborations with any other healthcare software applications feasible.

We are not aware of any other work that addresses the problem of marketing authorisation procedures as we do. There are some attempts to automate such procedures, which are elaborated at [8] and available at the FDA and EMEA websites (http://www.emea.eu.int/htms/human/presub/q24.htm).

Our future works are numerous, and can be extracted from our referenced work. We choose here to comment on two:

1. We will analyse the Health Level Seven (HL7) (available at http://www.hl7.org), which is an ANSI accredited US health industry communication messaging standard. They have extended the protocol for exchange of health-care information towards data repositories that are important for marketing authorisations. We want to see if we can view HL7 as a support in communication between different component layers of our architecture in Fig. 3.
2. We plan to further evaluate our architectural model by testing it in a real life example with more complex submission and evaluation procedures [7]. This will include communicating our solution to the MHRA and pharmaceutical companies in order to address elimination of redundant information that applicants have to provide on different pages of their licensing application.

References

[1] Juric, R. and Juric, J., 1999, "The Application of the UML to the Modelling of Automated Support of Evaluating Medicinal Products across Different Regulatory Requirements", *Proceedings of the 21st Int. Conference on Information Technology Interfaces ITI '99,* pp. 283–291.
[2] Juric R. and Juric, J., 2000, "Applying The UML Modelling Elements in Complex Business Environment", *Proceedings of The Fifth World Conference on Integrated Design and Process Technology*, Society for Design and Process Science Press, ISSN 1090–9389.
[3] Juric R. and Juric, J., 2002, "Applying Component Based Modelling in the Process of Evaluation of Medicinal Products", *Proceedings of the IDPT-2002 conference*, Society for Design and Process Science Press, ISSN 1090–9389.
[4] Juric, R., Williams, S., Slevin, L., Shojanoori R., Courtenage, S., and Milligan, P., 2005, "Component Based Automation of Regulatory Affairs in the Pharmaceutical Industry", to be submitted to the *Journal of Healthcare Informatics*.
[5] Juric, R., and Williams, S., 2005, "Experiences of Generating COTS Components when Automating Medicinal Product Evaluations", submitted to *The Seventeenth International Conference on Software Engineering and Knowledge Engineering, SEKE '05.*
[6] Williams, S., and Juric, R., 2005, "Design Patterns for Distributed Applications in Healthcare Systems", to appear in *Proceedings of the 26th International Conference On Information Technology Interfaces, ITI '05.*
[7] Williams, S., Juric, R., Shojanoori, R., and Slevin, L., 2005, "Submission and Evaluation Rules and Criteria for Marketing Authorisation of Medical Product Licences", *paper in preparation.*
[8] Slevin, L., Shojanoori, R., and Juric, R., 2005, "Developing a Database for Automating Regulatory Affairs in the Pharmaceutical Industry", to appear in Proceedings of the Eighth International Conference on Integrated Design and Process Technology (IDPT).
[9] Bass L., Clements, P., and Kazman, R., 1998, "Software Architecture in Practice", Addison-Wesley.
[10] Shaw, M. and Garland, D., 1996, "Software Architecture, Perspectives on an Emerging Discipline", Prentice Hall.
[11] Szypersky, C., 1998, "Component Software: Beyond Object-Oriented Programming", Addison-Wesley.
[12] Bass, L., and Kazman, R., 1999, "Architecture-Based Development, Technical Report", CMU/sei-99-TR-007, esc-TR-99-007.
[13] Juric, R., and Beus-Dukic, L. J., 2005, "COTS components and DB Interoperability", *Proceedings of the 4th International Conference COTS-Based Software Systems ICCBSS 2005*, pp. 77–89.
[14] Gamma, E., Helm, R., Johnson, R., and Vissides, J., 1995, "Design Patterns", Addison-Wesley.
[15] Alur, D., Crupi, J., and Malks, D., 2003, "Core J2EE Patterns", Prentice Hall.

Medical and Care Compunetics 2
L. Bos et al. (Eds.)
IOS Press, 2005

Crossing Heterogeneous Information Sources for Better Analysis of Health and Social Care Data

N.B. SZIRBIK [a], C. PELLETIER [a,1] and T.J. CHAUSSALET [b]
[a] *Information System Cluster, Faculty of Management and Organisation, Rijksuniversiteit Groningen, NL*
[b] *Health and Social Care Modelling Group, Centre for Health Informatics, Cavendish School of Computer Science, University of Westminster, London, UK*

Abstract. In this paper we describe a methodology that emerged during an implementation of a health-and-social-care-oriented data repository, which consists in grouping information from heterogeneous and distributed information sources. We developed this methodology by first constructing a concrete data repository, containing information about elderly patients flows in the UK's long-term care (LTC) system. In our specific case, the role of the data repository is to allow knowledge extraction about consumption and behavioural tendencies in the elderly people population within the LTC system. These tendencies can be depicted in terms of survival behaviour (modelling), cost evolution, and bed use. Other types of knowledge that can be extracted are typical patient profiles, placement policy in term of rules and criteria effectively applied and, specific features of the business process behind the long-term care provision. A well-constructed data repository can support the discovery (analysis) of hidden aspects about the way patients are placed and accepted in the LTC, and also how the allocated resources are consumed. We argue that the use of this methodology could save time in similar undertakings or in other fields than health and social care.

Keywords. Heterogeneous information sources, decision-making, software project management, health and social care data, modelling

1. Introduction

In this paper we describe a methodology that emerged as a byproduct of an implementation of a health-and-social-care oriented data repository for long-term care (LTC). This repository is grouping information from heterogeneous and distributed information sources, containing information about elderly patients flows in the UK's LTC system. We argue that the use of this methodology could save time in similar undertakings or in other

[1]Corresponding Author: C. Pelletier, Information System Cluster, Faculty of Management and Organisation, Rijksuniversiteit Groningen, Landleven 5, Postbus 800, 9700 AV Groningen, The Netherlands.
Tel.: +31 50 363 7316; Fax: +31 50 363 2275; E-mail:c.m.p.pelletier@rug.nl.

fields than health and social care. We estimate that the possession of knowledge about the best ways to design and implement the data warehouse could have saved significant time and effort to build the repository. This is why we consider important to document and publish our development method. This could help health and social care practitioners, and practitioners from other areas with identical features concerning the data, to speed their data gathering, organization and avoid pitfalls and bad practices.

In 2001, the UK government started a three-year project aiming at improving the quality of health and social care services through better information management [1]. For this purpose, in addition to defining a standard set of data to be collected [2], analysis techniques have to be developed and implemented. These techniques should support better understanding of resource use and population needs, particularly the health and social care services for the elderly. In such contexts, the knowledge of tested methods and established frameworks is very useful to improve data gathering about the flows of the patients through the entire system and also studying what are the different tendencies in the provision of patient cares, and especially of the patient trajectories within the care system.

The paper is organized as follows: Section 2 deals with the general description of our specific project, Section 3 presents the methodological framework we have build and propose for further use, Section 4 elaborates on two of the most interesting lines of research that have been open by our work, and finally Section 5 discusses the limitations of frameworks and their applicability, and draws the main conclusions.

2. Problem

In the context of the studies of the long-term care for elderly people, the role of the data repository is to allow knowledge extraction about consumption and behavioural tendencies in the elderly people population within the LTC system [3]. These tendencies can be depicted in terms of survival behaviour (modelling) [4], cost evolution [5], and bed use. Other types of knowledge that can be extracted are typical patient profiles, placement policy in term of rules and criteria effectively applied [6] and, specific features of the business process behind the long-term care provision. A well-constructed data repository can support the discovery (analysis) of hidden aspects about the way the patients are placed and accepted in the LTC, and also how the allocated resources are consumed (see [7]).

In many complex social organisations, like health and social services, the decision making process is distributed. There are a number of different stakeholders, with rather different goals, who have access to different, and disconnected sources of data. This leads to local 'views', usually narrow and biased. Local decisions can be supported by their views. Nevertheless, the impact of these decisions on a larger scale cannot be estimated. For global decisions (e.g. a consolidated budget) the stakeholders have to meet and negotiate. Due to the fact they hold views that have been grown from partial and sometimes conflicting perspectives, the decision taken can be just biased in the favour of the strongest negotiator.

A data repository that gathers information from the different areas of the social and health care stakeholders leads to the possibility to have a holistic perspective of the investigated social and health care system. Also, this centralisation allows various analysis, data flow and process mining that search for global estimations and global understanding of otherwise hidden phenomena. A global-view data analysis tool of crossed historical data about LTC patients is the main instrument to achieve better coordination between stakeholders. Such a tool should allow to analyse the use of the resources for LTC in the past, to identify possibilities for improvement, to discover the path patterns (trajectories) of the patients in the system (eventual bottlenecks), and to establish patient's profiles based on their experience in the system.

The results of the analysis will enable tactical and strategic managers to have a better understanding of the system and leads to a better utilization of the existing and planned resources. Our approach is to allow a continuous re-grouping (with a rate of update of 3–6 months) of the historical data concerning the LTC patient, across the various organizations that own and use these data.

3. The Methodology

The proposed methodology consists of six steps or phases. Compared with the software and database developments models known in software engineering, this methodology is close to the well-known waterfall model [8]. This model has been criticised for its lack of flexibility via iterative development, but in our case, the iterative style of development can be anyway applied over the steps of the proposed methodology. This can be done by viewing the steps as milestone-ending phases, containing many short term iterations that can implement small parts of functionality and data schema of the overall project. In this view, one can see the methodology as an extension of the UP (the Unified Process), or any other iterative development methodology as Agile Development or XP (extreme programming), where short iterations that are strongly time-boxed (i.e. these has to start and end at a very precise time) and are part of more "elastic" phases. These phases are defined by methodological constraints (and not project dates), and the end of these can be seen as conceptual milestones for the project manager – opposed to time/budget milestones.

The first step (phase) ends when the development team has identified and solved the most critical requirement for the building of the data warehouse. Also, the developers should be able to convince the stakeholders that they have a sound solution for this critical requirement. For example, in a typical warehouse that collects weather data, the elimination of "noise" (unwanted data) is crucial. For a warehouse that stores data about potential terrorist communication, fast search for certain text patterns is the most important. In genome research, structuring algorithms have to be discovered before the warehouse is built. Every application tends to have its own core set of critical requirement.

The strongest requirement about the data in an LTC warehouse (at borough, county or national level) is that the data should be anonymous according to the UK Data Protection Act and Health and Social Care Act. Our methodology considers that in the implementation of such a repository, the first step is to establish clear ways to ensure that the privacy requirement (via anonymity of the records in the repository) is achievable. Our point is that this requirement should be identified from the start and tackled first. The implementers should show the data owners and the stakeholders that there is a way to align to this requirement. This can be done using mapping files, owned by the owners of the data sources. In a mapping file, the unique identity of the patient (given by his social services number) is associated with a unique identifier generated by our system. To disclose the identity of the patient, access to this mapping file is necessary, and the access is limited only to the updating sessions of the central repositories.

All data contributed by stakeholders to the central (academically kept) repository where they are kept and used for model testing and validation must be anonymous. By developing a "cookie-based" stakeholder owned key-mapping mechanism, that allows the cyclic update of the central repository without using the names, social services numbers or other non-anonymous information from the local records, we are able to start our project. For project management, reaching this milestone (i.e. the solving of the critical aspect(s)), can be viewed as the "go/no-go" decision point in the project.

The second step, which we refer to as "scope and granularity" analysis, is to identify the quality and scope of each data source and also the rate of updating (depending on the dynamics of the entities to which the data refer). This step also concerns the complementarities of the data sources, usually raising all kinds of potential inconsistencies. For example, after crossing two sources, we have found patients who were still in the system as alive after their registered death or appeared with a different gender in different states. Most of these situations are due to data input mistakes and should be eliminated or fixed. These aspects are critical to any data integration effort and various software filters and inconsistency detectors should be developed before other software applications that are necessary for the repository. Sometimes, for data gathering projects where the data volumes are low, but the structure of the data is very complex (e.g. the data contain a lot of unstructured or semi-structured text), some filtering and consistency procedures should be designed to be done by hand by human operators. These procedures have to be established and validated early in the project. We apply here the same development principle as in the UP (unified process – see [8]) that states that the critical aspects of a project should be tackled in its early stages. One good final advice in this phase is to validate the collection of data by running one (small-scope) collection exercise.

The third step is to match the potentially collectible data with the results that are desired by the stakeholders and the decision makers. This will reduce the scope of the data gathered and will simplify the schemas of the data repository. In our case, the scope reduction is also a consequence of the analysis tools that have been already developed. However, such an intention of the scope should be made with care, and the implementers should consider that it is possible that new tools and models can be added to the analysis methods and certain data that are currently not used can be valuable in the future. Another aspect in this phase is to determine what are the factors that can increase the speed of the analysis. The speed factor is dependent on the availability of data – or search time. In any data repository, there are data that are used very often and buffered in small "cache"s, or the navigability of the database schemas is designed in a way that shortens the path to those records that are queried often. Data that are considered immediately useful for the analysis tools, should be easily reachable, and data that are not, could be placed "at distance" from the main query starting points. If necessary, the new queries can be written for new tools, or the old queries can be rewritten. In extreme cases, the whole schema of the database could be changed, and simple porting software can be used to migrate the whole information in the repository towards a database with a different operational structure (but containing the same information).

The fourth step consists in building an ontology that maps the relevant terms in the scoped universe of discourse. This is necessary because in distributed environments, the denominators for data attributes and values can be different (depending on local technical jargon and/or background of the local data collectors). The central data repository schema and architecture should be based on this common ontology, which can be also shared via mapping the terms and concepts to the local database schemas. What we have observed in our work is that different people, from different environments and with different backgrounds use local specialised languages that are incomprehensible to outsiders. This makes enormously difficult the task to group stakeholders to discuss together their local decisions. A very important byproduct of the development of the data integration is that the stakeholders that are also decision makers learn to communicate better and subsequently to understand better the problems of others, enabling in this way the possibility to achieve win-win decisions through collaborative negotiation. We observed that the ontology makers are also perceived as third-trusted parties (not only the developers of the integrated repository). Looking retrospectively, we consider now that the achievement of this milestone could be the most important outcome of such a project.

The next two phases can be grouped under the name maintenance. However, the scope and goals of the two are different. The fifth step is to establish the update policy for each local source and estimate the costs involved. Besides the speed and intensity of local change, granularity is an important aspect, because different databases can store the same kind of information with a different temporal or spatial scope. For example, costs can be recorded as per week, per month or per year; or in a hospital, per clinic, department or bed (or individual case). This leads to the transformation into a unique (adapted for analysis) granularity. This can involve the writing of software that adjust granularity to the desired level, but can also involve manual procedures where the granularity conversion cannot be achieved by simple routines. At this level, a manager can consider that the project is terminated. However, we include as a last step the post-validation and training phase. Validation should happen at each iteration (functionality and data models created at that iteration are thoroughly tested) and this eliminates the need for an explicit testing as in the waterfall model of development. Therefore, we consider the first operational use of the system (first effective collection of data) as a last maintenance and bug-fixing stage.

Hence, the sixth step is the first real-life gathering of the data, and by this testing if the filtering software deposits correctly the right information into the repository. The sources should be analyzed with the simplest methods and after the data collected should be analyzed immediately with the same methods to detect anomalies that are induced by the data gathering process. In our case, we discovered in this phase that it is necessary to enact some methods to "clean" automatically the gathered data from noise. The development of this "combing" software is tedious and the implementers should plan their project in a way that allows slack in this step. However, if a few records generate the noise it is better to handcraft ad-hoc some simple queries that eliminate these. In other projects – with different nature of information gathered, we believe that other problems can appear in this phase. Our advice for this stage is to include some slack iterations (two, but this depends on the scale of the project), to iron out the discovered problems without the pressure to launch the repository for decision making analysis. This does not imply that the users should not work already with the system, offering them a good opportunity to obtain final training for system use.

Throughout the whole project, the stakeholders should be heavily involved. Each iteration (we recommend 3–4 weeks for an iteration, with 2–4 iterations per methodology step) should end with a presentation of the existing functionality to the stakeholders.

These should provide feedback and approve the course of action. Changes of the functional requirements should lead to the changes in the operational plans (number of iterations and their content), plus the time/buget re-arrangements that arise from this desired changes.

4. Future Work

We consider there are two very important aspects yet to be investigated. Our proposed methodology for development is actually a "methodological framework" that shows "what" has to be done and in which order these issues have to be solved. But it has no clear mapping onto a project management structure. We have made a link with iterations, but we have not offered yet clear guidelines of how to plan the project, how to link the plan to a team and how to link these to a budget and control mechanism. The other interesting avenue for future research is related to ontological engineering.

The methodology suggest the use of the waterfall model. This model in software development is still used today because of the desire for predictability. Project managers and strategy planners cannot work by not having a clear idea of how much it will cost to integrate data and how long it will take to make it usable. Predictive approaches in project management look to do work early in the project in order to yield a greater understanding of what has to be done later. This way, stakeholders can reach a point where the latter part of the project can be estimated with a reasonable degree of accuracy. With predictive planning, a project has two stages. The first stage (usually up to the "go/no-go" decision) comes up with plans as a final product and is difficult to predict, but the second stage is much more predictable because the plans are in place.

However, there is a debate about whether software projects can be really predictable [9]. The core of this problem is requirements elicitation. The main sources of complexity in software or database centric projects is the difficulty in understanding the requirements of the stakeholders. These tend to change even later in the development process. The requirement changes are usually making a predictive plan impossible. Freezing the requirements early on and not permitting changes is possible, but this leads typically in the outcome of delivering a system that does not fulfill the real requirements of its users.

Requirements change is clearly unavoidable, and it is impossible to stabilize requirements sufficiently in order to use a predictive plan. This leads to the need to advocate adaptive/iterative planning. The difference between a predictive project and an adaptive project is that planning is done at the beginning rather than continuously. Changing requirements will just change the iteration structure and content. Of course, this will lead to changes in the initial contract. With a predictive plan, one can develop a fixed-price/fixed-scope contract. Such a contract says exactly what should be built, how much it will cost, and when it will be delivered. Such fixing is not possible with an adaptive plan. However, it is possible to fix from the start a budget and a time for delivery, but this will not fix exactly what functionality will be delivered. An adaptive contract assumes that the users will collaborate with the development team to regularly reassess what functionality needs to be built and in extreme situations will cancel the project if progress ends up being too slow.

For stakeholders, the adaptive approach is less desirable, as they would prefer greater predictability in the project. However, predictability depends on a precise, accurate, and stable set of requirements. If the development team can demonstrate to the stakeholders that they cannot stabilize their requirements early, a flexible, iterative project planning and management should be forced upon them. However, we have not yet developed a clear framework for project planning and control and how this is mapped on the methodological steps proposed in the previous section. This is subject for further research and will need input from other cases of software development involving database integration. Also, we should extend the framework by including team organisation tips, and also a mapping to a model that includes the time/budget constraints of the project.

Another line of research we consider valuable to continue is the development of the activities in step 4 (ontology construction). For environments where the interaction of the stakeholders is not really important, this step can be even ignored. However, in our case, as mentioned, the building of the ontology triggered a conscious effort of the stakeholders to better the understanding of each other. We would like to investigate if this has happened in other projects and also to extend the ontology building process from a mere step in the framework to a full process that takes place in parallel with the development process (and supporting it), from the beginning. Also, it is very interesting to study the novel technologies offered by the ontology building research in the field of the Semantic Web (especially those investigations in the Genome Ontology Project – involving huge data gathering, see [10]). These can bring new insights in how the parallel process of ontological construction in the project can be supported, automated and integrated with the development process and stakeholder feedbacks.

5. Discussion and Conclusions

One of the biggest problems with any framework (for software development or other domains) is that it covers partial aspects and there are always too many gaps, at conceptual and also at implementation levels. Though, by trying to fill these gaps, the understandability of the framework is always reduced and the potential user is lost in too many details. The content of this paper reflects the incomplete state of our knowledge and also the gaps that need to be filled and extensions to be developed. Anyway, all of the above proposed ideas are in fact based on the idea that it is a bad thing to start a data integration project without a methodological framework. We have discovered a pattern for a specific approach and we consider that the pattern is generic enough to be applicable in other contexts. What was not a goal of this paper is to demonstrate the applicability of the methodological framework in other domains with similarities with our project. Nevertheless, this lack of proof is not a negation of the applicability either, on the opposite, our intuition is that the methodology could be very useful, especially for environments with lots of heterogeneity (in terms of domains, people's skills and backgrounds, goals, and especially information systems).

In conclusion, we claim that a lot of effort can be saved in a data integration undertaking if the development team identifies the correct methodological pattern. Our methodological framework can at least play the role of a guideline or of an inspiration point. We have presented the outlines of our project and the derived framework steps:

1. identification and solving of the most critical issue(s)
2. identification of the scope and granularity of the data sources, including the data overlapping identification

3. identification of the most needed data in the repository
4. ontological alignment of the data and also of the people
5. identification of the update policies
6. validation and fine-tuning via the first real data-gathering

We also claim that this (smallest) framework can be used for practical implementations. It has been argued in the paper that the development team (by realizing step 4) is playing the role of third trusted party that teaches the stakeholders a common shared language, enhancing mutual understanding. The main conclusion here is that in distributed decision making the process core boils down to mere negotiations. Insight into the problems faced by other (by understanding its language, data, and the analysis results of this data), can lead negotiators to win-win situations. This should be the social result of any project that collects data for better decision making leading to enhanced global outcomes.

Acknowledgements

We thank Teresa Temple and Peter Crowther from the London Borough of Merton Social Services Department for data provision, and Peter Millard, visiting professor at the University of Westminster, for his expert advice. This work was partly supported by the Engineering and Physical Sciences Research Council (GR/R86430/01).

References

[1] *DOH, Making it happen – The key areas for action*, <www.publications.doh.gov.uk/ipus/socialcare/happen/>, accessed 27 November 2004.
[2] *NHS, Single Assessment Process (SAP) Dataset*, <www.nhsia.nhs.uk/datasets/pages/ds_older.asp>, accessed 27 November 2004.
[3] C. Pelletier, T.J. Chaussalet, N. Szirbik and C. Vasilakis, Integration of Data on Long-Term Care from Heterogeneous Sources for Research Purposes, In *Proceedings of MEDICON 2004*, Ischia, Italy, 31 July – 5 August 2004.
[4] H. Xie, T.J. Chaussalet and P. Millard, Continuous-time Markov models for the flow of elderly people in institutional long-term care, *Journal of the Royal Statistical Society, Series A* **168** (2005), 51–61.
[5] C. Pelletier, T.J. Chaussalet and H. Xie, A framework for predicting gross institutional long-term care cost arising from known commitments at local authority level, *Journal of the Operational Research Society* **56** (2005), 144–152.
[6] H. Xie, T. Chaussalet, W. Thompson and P. Millard, Modelling Decisions of a Multidisciplinary Panel for Admission to Long-term Care, *Health Care Management Science* **5** (2002), 291–295.
[7] H. Xie, *Modelling issues in institutional long-term care: placement, survival and costs*, Department of Computer Science, University of Westminster, London, 2004.
[8] P. Kruchten, *The Rational Unified Process, An Introduction*, 3rd. Edition, Addison Wesley, Object Technology, 2004.
[9] M. Fowler, *The New Methodology*, <www.martinfowler.com/articles/newMethodology.html>, accessed 19 March 2004.
[10] Gene Ontology Consortium, *An Introduction to the Gene Ontology*, <www.geneontology.org/GO.doc.shtml>, accessed 19 March 2004.

Medical and Care Compunetics 2
L. Bos et al. (Eds.)
IOS Press, 2005

Clinical Knowledge Management: An Overview of Current Understanding

Rajeev K. BALI[a] and Ashish DWIVEDI[b]
[a] *Knowledge Management for Healthcare (KMH) research subgroup, Biomedical Computing Research Group (BIOCORE), Coventry University, United Kingdom*
[b] *Hull University Business School, The University of Hull, United Kingdom*

Abstract. This chapter outlines contributions to a workshop for ICMCC 2005. We details some of the central issues surrounding the incorporation of the Knowledge Management (KM) paradigm for the healthcare and clinical sectors. The complex nature of KM is discussed, together with some essential theories and some contemporary applications of the tools and techniques are presented.

Keywords. Clinical knowledge management, healthcare knowledge management, healthcare informatics, clinical informatics

Introduction

This workshop will examine some of the key issues surrounding the incorporation of the Knowledge Management (KM) paradigm for clinical and healthcare environments. What is KM? Whom does it benefit? How is it carried out? Questions such as these will be addressed as well as discussions as to whether it would be beneficial for healthcare stakeholders to adopt the KM paradigm so as to facilitate effective decision-making and integration in the context of healthcare delivery. The key to the success of KM in the clinical and healthcare sectors is to achieve an effective integration of technology with human-based clinical decision-making processes. By doing so, healthcare institutions are free to disseminate acquired knowledge in a manner which ensures its availability to other healthcare stakeholders. This is of paramount importance as clinical and healthcare management continues its growth as a global priority area.

1. Clinical Knowledge Management

Advances in Information and Communication Technologies have made it possible for healthcare institutions to transform large amounts of medical data into relevant clinical information but an average physician still spends about 25 percent of his/her time managing information and has to learn 2 million clinical specifics [1]. Biomedical literature is doubling every 19 years, a fact which further compounds the problem of information overload [2]. The notion of incorporating KM in Healthcare has been put forth as a possible solution to this problem [3–5].

Healthcare managers are being forced to examine costs associated with healthcare and are under increasing pressure to discover approaches that would help carry out activities better, faster and cheaper [6,7]. Workflow and associated Internet technologies are being seen as an instrument to cut administrative expenses. Specifically designed IT implementations such as workflow tools are being used to automate the electronic paper flow in a managed care operation, thereby cutting administrative expenses [7].

One of the most challenging issues in healthcare relates to the transformation of raw clinical data into contextually relevant information. Advances in IT and telecommunications have made it possible for healthcare institutions to face the challenge of transforming large amounts of medical data into relevant clinical information [8]. This can be achieved by integrating information using workflow, context management and collaboration tools, giving healthcare a mechanism for effectively transferring the acquired knowledge, as and when required [9].

2. Workshop Outline

The workshop presented and discussed various case studies which allow us to understand better the multifarious nature of KM in the clinical and healthcare sectors.

2.1. Merging Knowledge Management and Information Technology in Healthcare

In the last 10 years, the Information and Communication Technologies (ICTs) revolution has redefined the structure of the 21st century healthcare organization. It is clear that the 21st century healthcare organization will bring about new healthcare services and that traditional management and technological concepts would not be the appropriate conduit for disseminating these new healthcare services. A Knowledge Management (KM) solution would allow healthcare institutions to give clinical data context, so as to allow knowledge derivation for more effective clinical diagnosis. It would also provide a mechanism for effective transfer of the acquired knowledge in order to aid healthcare workers as and when required. Using data inputs from a collaborating organization, we argue that healthcare institutions that integrate KM and ICT into their main organizational processes are more likely to survive and prosper. These organizations would have a profound understanding of how to use clinical information for creating value in tangible and intangible terms.

2.2. Object Orientation Technologies for Collaborative Applications

Advances in information and communication technologies (ICT), together with the search for effective and efficient ways to deliver healthcare, have resulted in the emergence of new heath delivery systems such as Community Health Information Networks (CHIN) and Telemedicine applications. We explore the feasibility of combining OO technologies with healthcare-based workflow management systems (WFMS). We introduce the concept of workflow technologies and discuss the main advantages and limitations of WFMS. We detail the circumstances in which the use of WFMS could be considered and the technological factors necessary for its successful implementation.

2.3. A Conceptual Model for Healthcare Knowledge Management

We present the notion that changes caused by the information technology revolution have been so widespread that, theoretically speaking, the healthcare sector can use the same technology to innovate. As a consequence, all the adopters of a similar technology would have matching technological advantages that are easily duplicatable, thereby denying anyone a unique competitive advantage. However, the lack of an explicit and generic KM framework for adopting KM hinders its rapid acceptance. We present a novel theoretical KM framework that could help organisations to navigate this difficult change process.

2.4. KM as an Enabling Paradigm for Healthcare Stakeholders

Contemporary thinking amongst different healthcare stakeholders (HSs) indicates tremendous interest in new paradigms, concepts and frameworks like Clinical Governance (CG), Evidence Based Medicine (EBM), Community Health Information Networks (CHIN), Knowledge Management (KM) and Integrated Care concepts like Integrated Health Care Delivery Systems (IHCDS), Integrated Quality Development, Integrated Patient Pathways (IPP). We explore the rationale behind these frameworks and analyse them based on their support for people, processes and technology.

2.5. Implications for Clinical Knowledge Management and Practice

The objective of this section is to determine the future for Knowledge Management (KM) applications that focus on healthcare processes. This is achieved by tracing the evolution of KM by examining how different sectors have formulated industry-specific KM applications, then discussing the key constraints that these sectors have faced whilst formulating industry specific KM applications. We detail how these constraints can impede the coming of age of KM applications for healthcare. The results of several case studies on the future of healthcare KM applications are presented.

Conclusions

This chapter has presented the concept of knowledge management (KM) and its efficacy for the clinical and healthcare environments. We have discussed the nature of KM and have introduced the complex relationships and obstacles that exist and presented some novel solutions which can go towards overcoming these obstacles.

References

[1] A. Dwivedi, R.K. Bali, A.E. James and R.N.G. Naguib. The Efficacy of using Object Oriented Technologies to build Collaborative Applications in Healthcare and Medical Information Systems, *Proc.of the 2002 IEEE CCECE Conf. Canada*. 2002.

[2] J.C. Wyatt, "7. Intranets," *Jnl. of The Royal Soc of Med*, **(93):10**, pp. 530–534, 2000.

[3] AN Dwivedi, RK Bali & RNG Naguib (2003) "Organization Current Knowledge Design (OCKD): A Knowledge Management Framework for Healthcare Institutions", *Proc of the IEEE-EMBC 25th Ann Int Conf of the IEEE Eng in Med and Biol Soc (EMBS)*, 17–21 September 2003, Cancun, Mexico, 1236–1239.

[4] SM Malone, Knowledge Management: White knight or white elephant? *Topics in Health Information Management*. Frederick: Feb 2001. **(21):3**; 33.

[5] S Lutz, D Chin. "Charting the landscape of healthcare in the next decade", *Managed Healthcare*. Cleveland: Nov 1999. **(9):11**; 29.

[6] M. Davis and J. Klein, Net holds breakthrough solutions. *Modern Healthcare*, Supplement: Eye on Info. Feb 7, pp. 14–15, 2000.

[7] G.B. Latamore "Workflow tools cut costs for high quality care", *Health Management Technology*, Atlanta, 20 (4), 32–33, 1999.

[8] A. Dwivedi, R.K. Bali, A.E. James and R.N.G. Naguib. 2001, "Workflow Management Systems: the Healthcare Technology of the Future?," *Proc of the IEEE EMBC-2001 23rd Annual International Conference of the IEEE Engineering in Medicine and Biology Society (EMBS)*, Istanbul, Turkey, 2001, pp. 3887–3890.

[9] A. Dwivedi, R.K. Bali, A.E. James and R.N.G. Naguib, "The Efficacy of Using Object Oriented Technologies to build Collaborative Applications in Healthcare and Medical Information Systems," *Proc of the IEEE Canadian Conference on Electrical and Computer Engineering (CCECE) 2002.* Winnipeg, Canada, **2,** 2002, pp. 1188–1193.

Symposium on Patient Empowerment

Medical and Care Compunetics 2
L. Bos et al. (Eds.)
IOS Press, 2005

Health Informatics: A Roadmap for Autism Knowledge Sharing

Ron OBERLEITNER[a], Rebecca WURTZ[b] M.D., Michael L. POPOVICH[b], Reno FIEDLER[b], Tim MONCHER[b], Swamy LAXMINARAYAN[c], and Uwe REISCHL[d] M.D.

[a] *e-Merge Medical Technologies (Boise, ID)*
[b] *Scientific Technologies Corporation, Tucson Arizona*
[c] *Institute of Rural Health and Biomedical Research Institute, Idaho State University*
[d] *Center of Health Policy, Boise State University*

Abstract. With the prevalence of diagnosed autism on the rise, increased efforts are needed to support surveillance, research, and case management. Challenges to collect, analyze and share typical and unique patient information and observations are magnified by expanding provider caseloads, delays in treatment and patient office visits, and lack of sharable data. This paper outlines recommended principles and approaches for utilizing state-of-the-art information systems technology and population-based registries to facilitate collection, analysis, and reporting of autism patient data. Such a platform will increase treatment options and registry information to facilitate diagnosis, treatment and research of this disorder.

Background

Autism spectrum disorder (autism) is characterized by a range of neurological anomalies that typically include varying degrees of communication deficits and repetitive negative social behaviors. A tenfold increase in the incidence of autism over the past 15 years has been documented and is regarded as a significant public health concern. Despite the documented increase in the incidence of autism, the cause(s) of this disorder and appropriate treatment remain mysterious. The NIH road map emphasizes the need for developing phenotypic signatures based on available evidence including documentation of behavioral, clinical and genetic traits, as well as contributions by the basic sciences and applied bioengineering such as medical imaging outcomes, auditory phenomenology, neuroscience, and brain modeling studies.

Current population-based databases include a number of cross sectional studies sponsored by the CDC (Autism and Developmental Disabilities Monitoring Network [ADDM Net] and NIMH). These involve partnerships between a variety of governmental agencies, universities, and leading nonprofit organizations. Database initiatives that have been spearheaded include the Autism Genetic Resource Exchange, Autism Treatment Network, and Autism Tissue Program. Each of these offer contributions to the understanding of autism, but have significant limitations in terms of ease of use, costs to build and maintain, and interoperability with other database projects.

In the National Institute of Mental Health's April 2004 *Congressional Appropriations Committee Report on the State of Autism Research*, the authors list the following obstacles, among others, to understanding the causes of and treatments for autism:

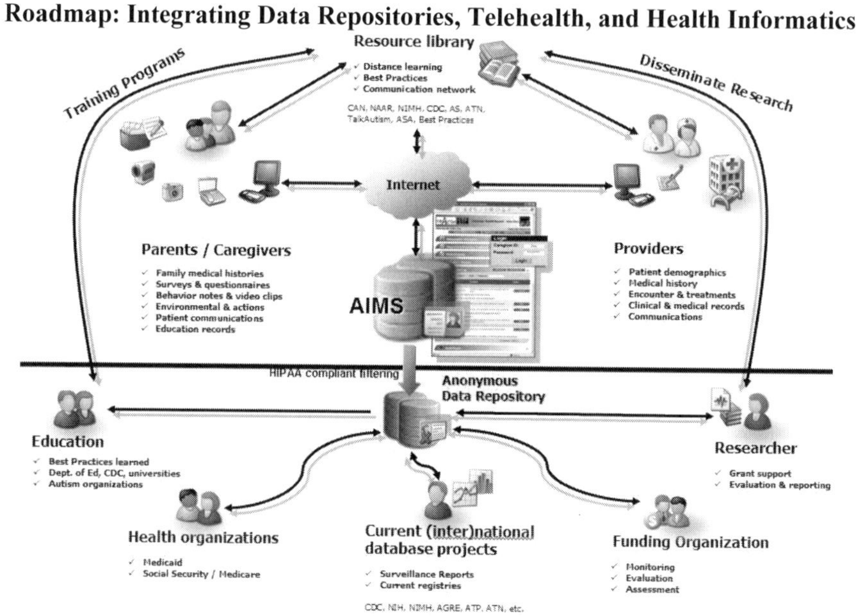

Figure 1. Illustration of AIMS™ to Service Patients, Parents, and Healthcare Providers, while Supporting Researchers, Health Organizations, and Funding Agencies in Understanding More about Autism Spectrum Disorders.

- Lack of a national autism twin registry that would allow researchers to access a large sample of well-defined twins where at least one twin is affected by autism.
- Lack of multi-site, high-risk population studies (i.e. pregnancies and infant siblings of individuals with autism) that would allow for increased knowledge about risk factors, early development of autism, and enhanced characterization of the disorder.
- Need for enhanced mechanisms to involve voluntary organizations, industries and potential donors in all stages of research design and implementation.

The shortcomings related to a lack of information resources can be overcome by the design and implementation of a longitudinal, person-based autism registry that would leverage the benefits provided by telehealth and the benefits offered by an interoperability infrastructure which integrates and builds on information already generated by the above referenced initiatives. This paper outlines a vision for such a registry.

Complementary to necessary in-person examinations, the value of telemedicine and information technology to support the evaluation, diagnosis, and treatment of autism by the community of parents, health care providers, educators, and researchers has been outlined. (Oberleitner 2004). To date, the ability to create a sharable information resource to support the diverse community of stakeholders is limited. The following illustration provides the concept for a new Autism Information Management System (AIMS). This system is designed, in part, to create a complementing patient registry that will be interoperable in relation to the current database initiatives, while providing a platform of sharable information to support the mission and goals of the various stakeholders.

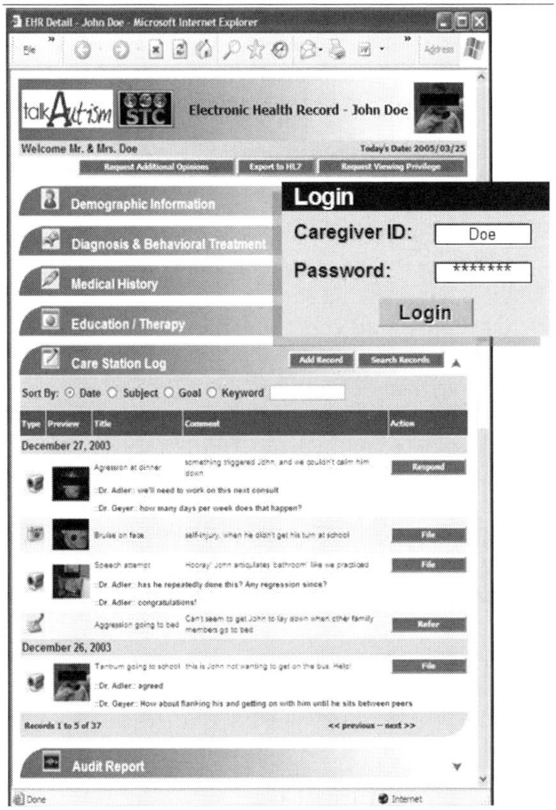

Figure 2. Sample view of an autism EHR as developed by e-Merge/TalkAutism (Boise, ID) and STC (Tucson, AZ) →.

Caregivers and Providers: The primary concept for the AIMS is a "Parent/Provider driven Person-Centric Information Environment" enabled by a web-based electronic health record (EHR), designed and maintained to enhance treatment options for caregivers. Caregivers would own the data and would have final jurisdiction in matters of access by providers. Providers (clinics, health professionals, therapists, specialized educators etc.) and caregivers (parents, other family members, paraprofessionals, respite workers, therapists, etc.) could complement in-person visits by communicating directly via a telehealth platform.

To help foster optimal use of this EHR, the system should incorporate an always-updating online portal resource library tailored to the caregivers and providers. Such a library will increase access to distance learning, updatable resource directories, and online communication forums involving other caregivers and health professionals is optimal to provide support and incentive to update the EHR.

An EHR can be used to capture and transmit patient behavior in a natural environment via input into text, and data capture devices like stethoscopes, or even cell phones and videophones. For example, images and video clips from a digital camera can send date linked to the treatment activities, milestones, or concerning behaviors. This can facilitate patient case management by providing visibility and insights into episodes that occur in their natural environment, and will allow a provider to remotely evaluate situations occurring at the moment of concern, and without delays or distractions found in a typical office environment. This type of system minimizes the impact on the individual with autism while maximizing the utilization of the provider. The system also offers the opportunity of the parent/guardian to record accurate information in a timely fashion, which is of utmost concern to most.

By providing such support and communication benefits, the platform is also a convenient medium for researchers to request voluntary information to facilitate research via surveys, questionnaires or with unique data capturing technology. And as seen in other applications of telemedicine, there is savings realized by reduced travel for both professionals and families, comparable satisfaction to inperson visits, and advantages of accurate case documentation – all contributing to justify the technology hosting fee for this platform.

'Patient Case' to 'Anonymous Data' Repository: The design of the AIMS targets the need for researchers, health professionals, and educators to collect information about populations of individuals with autism. The vision is to allow anonymous data sets to be built based upon individual patient cases propagated in an individual's EHR, that can be integrated and coexisting with other database projects. De-identified information will be combined to create an extended knowledgebase to support applied research as well as information sharing of "best practices." Funding organizations would also be provided the ability to use the information to monitor and evaluate the impact of their service support.

Technical characteristics of this system would follow recent public health information development standards (CDC PHIN, 2002) and would build upon the lessons learned in developing population based registries such as immunization information tracking systems (Scientific Technologies Corp, 2002). Specifically, the system would exhibit the following features:

- Would utilize a secure web-based technology to support data collection and information retrieval in an easy to use format.
- The information database would be relational and person-centric to support individual case management, individual encounters, and would include treatment based tracking.
- The system would include appropriate tools needed to capture and link video clips, family observations, and health histories related to time and space (i.e. environmental conditions).
- The system would include the necessary tools to support documentation, research, and reporting.

In order to achieve these goals, the AIMS must have the capability to electronically transfer information in a secure environment. The use of a Master Patient Index (MPI) to uniquely identify patients and to protect confidentiality will be essential. The underlying patient / provider database would contain defining data fields and code sets to support patient management including the following:

- Patient identification and demographics
- Family history
- Longitudinal medical history
- Epidemiologic questionnaires: i.e. exposures.
- Time stamped behavior characteristics with attached video clips
- Treatment plans and parent progress reports
- Clinical and medical records

In addition to the core components, the system would allow attachment of added code sets such as:

- Co-morbidity (eg. ADHD, sleep disorders, etc.)
- School records and reports.
- Online Treatment survey data
- Family observations of treatment efficacy

One of the essential design criteria will be to guard against information overload. In addition to the controls embedded in the data collection tools, it is recommended that "rule based" algorithms be employed to search for specific criteria, automating alerts for rapid provider notification and assessment.

Rationale

The typical health information system is one that is driven by patient encounters and maintained by providers or payers. These types of information systems currently do not support patient nor parent / guardian needs. They do not support research and reporting requirements. As such, additional information systems must be developed for clinical trials, patient registries, and statistical reporting. Resources are duplicated, additional costs incurred, and the ability to share lessons learned is curtailed or non-existent.

AIMS will be designed to collect information from diverse sources, store and share person-based case data and video, and monitor and report all value added benefits. For example, there could be a module that can integrate school data in parallel. The ability to protect the privacy and confidentiality of individuals, providers, and research initiatives will require that information resources be limited to registered users and managed and controlled in compliance with HIPAA security standards.

The autism caregiver community should be especially motivated to adopt and propagate an accessible electronic health record that is easy to update and offers enhanced treatment for the affected individual(s) in their care. Many families maintain meticulous health history information because they typically visit multiple health providers and must therefore coordinate multiple stakeholders' understanding of their child's medical history. In schools, current best practices frequently require data collection and analysis to determine treatment effectiveness. Various technology options are appearing on the market to support families and educators in this regard.

There are a number of reasons why a patient-centric autism community telehealth platform is feasible at this time. National objectives have been established through current federal initiatives to facilitate the implementation of electronic health records (EHR). These initiatives require that health care information technology providers work with the community to establish standards for communication and data transfer. The relatively recent use of standard "case" definitions and data elements encourages the development of population-based data bases for information sharing about population health indicators. This can directly lead to a better understanding of autism.

The national push towards more extensive use of electronic health records will encourage technology vendors to develop improved next-generation online health records systems. As more health data is created and stored electronically, there will be increasing opportunities to share information and more incentives to establish resources capable of recording longitudinal data on individuals. The impact of HIPAA to support patient confidentiality has also forced the information technology community to focus more on security and thus establish improved methodologies for protecting and sharing data.

In addition to national trends and standard implementation, there are recent examples of registries that have succeeded. Chronic disease and medical registry models including population-based immunization registries are being implemented and maintained by public health departments. These systems acquire data through the participation of both private and public health care providers. There are now technology, business practice and policy solutions available that capture patient demographics and health information electronically. These systems are also available through easy-to-use Web-based applications and protect patient and provider confidently. These systems can be used as models for the implementation of autism based registries.

Conclusion

A strong partnership between parents, providers, and teachers will be necessary to address the challenges of early diagnosis, treatment, and care of the children with autism. New telehealth technologies and electronic medical records storage and retrieval systems offer new opportunities for parents, providers and researchers to communicate their observations and findings to each other. We recommend the development of a new Autism Information Management System (AIMS) that will create a complementing patient registry that is interoperable in relation to current database initiatives while providing a platform of sharable information to support the mission and goals of parents, health care providers, teachers, and researchers involved with the autism spectrum disorder.

References

[1] Oberleitner, R, Laxminarayan, S (2004); Information technology and behavioral medicine: impact on autism treatment & research, In: Studies in Healthcare Technology and Informatics;103:215–22.

[2] Oberleitner, R (2004), Talking to the autism community [interviewed by Semahat S Demir], IEEE Eng Med Biol Mag. 2005 Jan-Feb;24(1):14–5, 19.

[3] Oberleitner, R.; Laxminarayan, S.; Suri, J.; Harrington, J.; Bradstreet, J. (2004), The Potential of a Store and Forward Tele-Behavioral Platform for Effective Treatment and Research of Autism, In: IEEE Eng Med Biol Soc, EMBC 2004. Conference Proceedings. Volume 2, 3294–3296.

[4] Congressional Appropriations Committee Report on the State of Autism Research, April 2004. http://www.nimh.nih.gov/autismiacc/CongApprCommRep.pdf.

[5] CDC Publication, Public Health Information Network Functions and Specifications, December 2002. http://www.cdc.gov/phin.

[6] Scientific Technologies Corporation, Immunization Information Systems, A Resource Guide, 2002, a collection of white papers.

Author Index